HOLLYWOOD FILM HISTORY

A CUSTOM EDITION

KEVIN SANDLER, EDITOR
FILM AND MEDIA STUDIES
ARIZONA STATE UNIVERSITY

Custom Publishing

New York   Boston   San Francisco
London   Toronto   Sydney   Tokyo   Singapore   Madrid
Mexico City   Munich   Paris   Cape Town   Hong Kong   Montreal

Cover photograph courtesy of the John Kobal Foundation/Getty Images.

Copyright © 2009 by Pearson Custom Publishing
All rights reserved.

This copyright covers material written expressly for this volume by the editor/s as well as the compilation itself. It does not cover the individual selections herein that first appeared elsewhere. Permission to reprint these has been obtained by Pearson Custom Publishing for this edition only. Further reproduction by any means, electronic or mechanical, including photocopying and recording, or by any information storage or retrieval system, must be arranged with the individual copyright holders noted.

All trademarks, service marks, registered trademarks, and registered service marks are the property of their respective owners and are used herein for identification purposes only.

Printed in the United States of America

2007420627

LR/JW

Pearson Custom Publishing is a division of

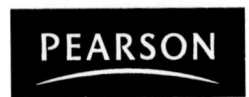

www.pearsonhighered.com

ISBN 10: 0-558-06508-2
ISBN 13: 978-0-558-06508-9

Acknowledgments

Grateful acknowledgment is made to the following sources for permission to reprint material copyrighted or controlled by them:

"The Cinema of Attractions," by Tom Gunning, reprinted from *Early Cinema: Space, Frame, Narrative* (2008), first published in *Wide Angle Magazine*, 1986.

"Founding Father: Louis Lumière in Conversation with Georges Sadoul," by Georges Sadoul, reprinted from *Projections 4: Film-makers on Film-making* (1995), Farrar, Straus & Giroux.

"The Birth of a Nation," by Daniel Bernardi, reprinted from *Film Analysis: A Norton Reader* (2005), W.W. Norton & Company.

"The Birth of a Nation: Reconsidering Its Reception," by Janet Staiger, reprinted from *Interpreting Films: Studies in the Historical Reception of Cinema* (1992), by permission of Princeton University Press. Copyright © 1992 by Princeton University Press.

"Reply to the New York Globe," by D.W. Griffith, reprinted from *The Birth of a Nation* (1994).

"How I Made the Birth of a Nation" and "The Rise and Fall of Free Speech in America," by D.W. Griffith, reprinted from *Focus on D.W. Griffith* (1971), Prentice-Hall, Inc., a Pearson Education Company.

"Fourteen," by Charlie Chaplin, reprinted from *Charlie Chaplin: My Autobiography* (1992), published by Bodley Head, by permission of The Random House Group Ltd.

"Pie and Chase," by Donald Crafton, reprinted from *Classical Hollywood Comedy* (1995), Routledge Publishing, a division of Taylor & Francis Group LLC.

"Response to 'Pie and Chase'," by Tom Gunning, reprinted from *Classical Hollywood Comedy* (1995), Routledge Publishing, a division of Taylor & Francis Group LLC.

"Interview with Marion Mack," by Raymond Rohauer, reprinted from Buster Keaton's *The General* (1975), by permission of Rizzoli Publications.

"The Fallen Woman Film and the Impetus for Censorship," by Lea Jacobs, reprinted from *The Wages of Sin: Censorship and the Fallen Woman Film* (1991), by permission of The University of California Press.

"Columbia Pictures," by Tino Balio, reprinted from *Post-Theory* by David Bordwell (1996). Copyright © 1996 by the Board of Regents of the University of Wisconsin System. Reprinted by permission of The University of Wisconsin Press.

"Authorship and Genre," by Jim Kitses, reprinted from *The Western Reader* (1969), Amadeus Press.

"The White Man's Indian," by John O'Connor, reprinted from *Hollywood's Indian: The Portrayal of the Native American in Film* (2003), University Press of Kentucky.

"John Ford Talks to Philip Jenkinson," by Philip Jenkinson, reprinted from *John Ford: Interviews* (2001), first published in *The Listener*.

"Introduction," by Richard Dyer, reprinted from *Heavenly Bodies: Film Stars and Society* (1987), Palgrave Publishers Ltd.

"Ingrid from Lorraine to Stromboli," by James Damico, reprinted from *Journal of Popular Film* 4, no. 1 (1975), Heldref Publications.

"Are Stars Necessary?" and "The Enjoyment of Fear," by Alfred Hitchcock, reprinted from *Hitchcock on Hitchcock: Selected Writings and Interviews* (1995), by permission of The University of California Press.

"HUAC, the Blacklist, and the Decline of Social Cinema," by Brian Neve, reprinted from *The Fifties: Transforming the Screen, 1950-59* (2003), by permission of The University of California Press.

Acknowledgments

"Making the Film: Contemporary Accounts," by Jarrico et. al., reprinted from *Salt of the Earth* (1978), by permission of The Feminist Press.

"Introduction: Hollywood in the Home," by Christopher Anderson, reprinted from *Hollywood TV: The Studio System in the Fifties* (1994), by permission of The University of Texas Press. Copyright © 1994 by Christopher Anderson.

"A Face in the Crowd," by Jeff Young, reprinted from *Kazan: The Master Director Discusses His Films* (1991), Newmarket Press.

"From Roadshowing to Saturation Release," by Justin Wyatt, reprinted from *The New American Cinema*, edited by Jon Lewis (1999), by permission of Duke University Press. Copyright © 1999 by Duke University Press.

"Goldfinger," by Albert Broccoli, reprinted from *When the Snow Melts: The Autobiography of Cubby Broccoli* (1999), by permission of Pan MacMillan, London. Copyright © 1999 by Cubby Broccoli.

Excerpts from "CARA and the Emergence of Responsible Entertainment," by Kevin S. Sandler, reprinted from *The Naked Truth: Why Hollywood Doesn't Make X-Rated Movies* (2007), by permission of Rutgers University Press. Copyright © 2007 by Kevin S. Sandler

"The Last Good Time We Ever Had," by Noel King, reprinted from *The Last Great American Picture Show* (2004), University of Amsterdam Press.

"Taxi Driver," by Ian Christie and David Thompson, reprinted from *Scorsese on Scorsese* (2004), Farrar, Straus & Giroux.

"The New Hollywood," by Thomas Schatz, reprinted from *Film Theory Goes to the Movies* (1993), Routledge Publishing, a division of Taylor & Francis Group LLC.

"Batman," by Mark Salisbury, reprinted from *Burton on Burton* (2006), Farrar, Straus & Giroux.

"sex, lies, and marketing: Miramax and the Development of the Quality Indie Blockbuster," by Alisa Perren, reprinted from *Film Quarterly* 55, no. 2 (2001), by permission of the University of California Press.

"Blockbusters and Independents: 1975 to the Present," by Jesse Algeron Rhines, reprinted from *Black Film/White Money* (1996), reprinted by permission of Rutgers University Press. Copyright © 1996 by Jesse Algeron Rhines.

"Spike Lee's Bed-Stuy BBQ," by Marlaine Glicksman, reprinted from *Spike Lee: Interviews* (1989), Film Society of Lincoln Center.

"Just Another Girl Outside the Neo-Indie," by Christina Lane, reprinted from *Contemporary American Independent Film: From the Margins to the Mainstream* (2005), Routledge UK, a division of Cengage Learning.

Contents

Introduction — 1

Screening Film History — 3
"Hollywood Film History: An Introduction," Kevin Sandler — 5

The Rise of Hollywood and the Coming of Sound — 11

1. The Birth of Cinema — 13
"The Cinema of Attractions: Early Film, Its Spectator and the Avant-Garde," Tom Gunning — 15
"Founding Father: Louis Lumière in Conversation with Georges Sadoul," edited and translated by Pierre Hodgson — 21

2. Narrative Integration — 27
"*The Birth of a Nation* (1915): Integrating Race into the Narrator System," Daniel Bernardi — 29
"*The Birth of a Nation*: Reconsidering Its Reception," Janet Staiger — 37
"Reply to the *New York Globe*," D. W. Griffith — 52
"How I Made The Birth of a Nation," D. W. Griffith — 54
"The Rise and Fall of Free Speech In America," D.W. Griffith — 57

3. Slapstick and the Silent Period — 59
"Pie and Chase: Gag, Spectacle and Narrative in Slapstick Comedy," Donald Crafton — 61
"Response to 'Pie and Chase'," Tom Gunning — 72
"Interview with Marion Mack," Raymond Rohauer — 74
"Fourteen," Charlie Chaplin — 80

The Studio Era — 85

4. The Production Code — 87
"The Fallen Woman Film and the Impetus for Censorship," Lea Jacobs — 89

5. The Studios — 107
"Columbia Pictures: The Making of a Motion Picture Major, 1930–1943," Tino Balio — 109

6. Genres — 121

"Authorship and Genre: Notes on the Western," Jim Kitses — 123
"The White Man's Indian: An Institutional Approach," John E. O'Connor — 130
"John Ford Talks to Philip Jenkinson about Not Being Interested in Movies," Philip Jenkinson — 136

7. Stars — 139

"Introduction to *Heavenly Bodies*," Richard Dyer — 141
"Ingrid From Lorraine to Stromboli: Analyzing the Public's Perception of a Film Star," James Damico — 152
"Are Stars Necessary?," Alfred Hitchcock — 161
"The Enjoyment of Fear," Alfred Hitchcock — 163

The Television Broadcasting Age — 167

8. Anti-Communism and Hollywood — 169

"HUAC, the Blacklist, and the Decline of Social Cinema," Brian Neve — 171
"Making the Film: Contemporary Accounts on *Salt of the Earth*" — 189

9. Television's Impact on Hollywood — 197

"Introduction: Hollywood in the Home," Christopher Anderson — 199
"*A Face in the Crowd*: An Interview with Kazan," Jeff Young — 212

10. The Birth of the Blockbuster — 223

"From Roadshowing to Saturation Release: Majors, Independents, and Marketing/Distribution Innovations," Justin Wyatt — 225
"*Goldfinger*," Albert R. Broccoli — 239

11. The Rating System — 247

"CARA and the Emergence of Responsible Entertainment," Kevin S. Sandler — 249

12. Auteur Renaissance — 265

"'The Last Good Time We Ever Had': Remembering the New Hollywood Cinema," Noel King — 267
"*Taxi Driver*," Ian Christie and David Thompson interviewing Martin Scorsese — 279

The Conglomerate Era — 283

13. The Contemporary Hollywood Blockbuster — 285

"The New Hollywood," Thomas Schatz — 287
"*Batman*," Mark Salisbury Interviewing Tim Burton — 307

14. Independents: Miramax and Black Film — 313

"sex, lies and marketing: Miramax and the Development of the Quality Indie Blockbuster," Alisa Perren — 315

"Blockbusters and Independents: 1975 to the Present," Jesse Algeron Rhines — 325

"Spike Lee's Bed-Stuy BBQ," Marlaine Glicksman — 340

15. Women Directors and Hollywood — 347

"Just Another Girl Outside the Neo-indie," Christina Lane — 349

Introduction

Screening Film History

Hollywood Film History: An Introduction

By Kevin Sandler

The motion picture is a mighty art form. Whether we are among hundreds of strangers in a theater, at home in front of the television with a few friends, or alone in front of a computer screen or iPod, movies appeal to our dreams, aspirations, and fears. Who could forget the exhilarating spectacle of Indiana Jones running from a giant rolling boulder in *Raiders of the Lost Ark* (1981)? The climatic moment of *Jerry McGuire* (1996) when Tom Cruise says to Renée Zellweger, "You complete me." Or the irresistible self-confidence of "McLovin" in *Superbad* (2007)? These movies, like most others in Hollywood film history, repeatedly engage us on an emotional and visceral level unmatched by any medium.

However, Hollywood filmmaking is also a commercial enterprise. Since the 1920s, a small handful of corporations—now multinational media conglomerates—have controlled the production, distribution, and exhibition of the vast majority of American movies. The typical two-hour Hollywood story—one in which a sympathetic character overcomes a series of obstacles to achieve his or her desire—is less an art form to these companies than a commodity, a narrative experience sold to audiences around the world. Just the shear commercial scale and worldwide consumption of Hollywood films demands that we consider them as a business designed to make money.

Richard Maltby confronts these contradictions by providing us with a model for understanding Hollywood cinema as both an art and a business. He argues that a Hollywood movie, in the first instance, must be approached as a commercial commodity in a capitalistic marketplace before its existence as a creative work, political commentary, or social document. For Maltby, Hollywood's essential business approach—beyond any technological, stylistic, or institutional shifts the industry experienced—has remained the same for most of the twentieth century: "entertaining its audiences, producing the maximum pleasure for the maximum number for the maximum profit."[1] He refers to this continuity of economic purpose as Hollywood's "commercial aesthetic," positioning film style in service to the larger commercial ambitions of the industry itself. As a result, Hollywood's business strategies can never be fully separated from their aesthetic practices because the industry's products are also formally organized in a way "to turn pleasure into a product we can buy."[2] This affirmative cultural function, what we commonly call "Hollywood entertainment," nonetheless has powerful ideological effects and social and cultural resonance for audiences. They do not call it a "dream factory" for nothing and that is what makes Hollywood films ripe for examination.

To study Hollywood as an industrial and formal system, *Hollywood Film History* embraces a method offered by Douglas Gomery and pursues the key question that guides his periodization: "How did a collection of major studio corporations (Hollywood) come to dominate the production, distribution, and exhibition of movies and continue to maintain its control through the coming of sound, the innovation of colour and widescreen images, and the diffusion of television and home video?"[3]

---

[1] Richard Maltby, *Hollywood Cinema*, 2nd Ed. (Malden, MA: Blackwell, 2003), 15.
[2] Maltby, 52.
[3] Douglas Gomery, "Hollywood as Industry," in *American Cinema and Hollywood: Critical Approaches*, John Hill and Pamela Church Gibson. ed. (Oxford: Oxford University Press, 2000), 20.

Introduction

Part I: The Rise of Hollywood to the Coming of Sound explores the evolution of movie viewing in the United States, from novelties of showmen in the final years of the nineteenth century to the consolidation of the feature film industry by the late 1920s. Part II: The Studio Era examines the domination of the production, distribution and exhibition of films throughout the 1930s and 1940s by an oligopoly of eight studios. Part III: The Television Broadcasting Age explores Hollywood struggling and adjusting to a new economic model brought on by the Paramount antitrust decrees, suburbanization and the baby boom, and competition from television between the late 1940s and the early 1970s. Part IV: The Conglomerate Era examines Hollywood rebuilding itself into various subsidiaries of highly diversified media conglomerates from the mid-1970s onward. The essays that comprise each section are based on canonical readings from major film scholars as well as articles and interviews from film practitioners—including directors, executives, and stars. Together, these readings reveal the workings of Hollywood as a delicate balance between industry and art, between entertainment and commercial enterprise, between "show" and business.

Lesson One: The Birth of Cinema begins this historical journey by examining Hollywood's evolution as a storytelling medium between 1907 and 1913—the "narrativization" of the cinema as Tom Gunning describes it. Prior to this time, he argues, early cinema was dominated by a "cinema of attractions"—the exhibition of spectacles for viewers to admire and be astonished by rather than one of psychologically motivated characters. It was a cinema of showing rather than telling, composed of close-ups, visual tricks, gags, and incidents that were interesting in and of themselves. Louis Lumière, who along with his brother Auguste, was one of the founding fathers of cinema, provides a first-hand account of the "cinema of attractions" in France. He describes building the *cinématographe*—a film projector more portable and practical than Thomas Edison's Kinetograph—as well as the first paid screening of projected motion pictures at the Grand Café in Paris in March 1895.

Lesson Two: Narrative Integration focuses on the lasting impact of D. W. Griffith's 1915 epic, *The Birth of a Nation*. Griffith is widely considered to have created the modern cinematic grammar that we associate with the Classic Hollywood style, conventions designed to enhance narrative clarity and coherence. Despite its artistic achievements, notes Daniel Bernardi, *The Birth of a Nation* perpetuates a story of white racism, reinforcing a romantic representation of the Old South, miscegenation, and social segregation. According to Bernardi, "How can we simultaneously acknowledge the film's contribution to storytelling technique while challenging its systematic embrace of racism? Can racism in film be at once ugly and painful and at the same time artistic and romantic?" The outrage that *The Birth of Nation* prompted in viewers fuels Janet Staiger's investigation of the film. She historicizes the reception of the film from its initial screening to the series of debates and responses that greeted the film decades later. For Staiger, the racism in *The Birth of a Nation* operates not only as propaganda but intersects with ongoing debates regarding media effects, film scholarship, and leftist politics. Griffith himself vehemently denied any such racism in the film, defending his storytelling techniques and historical accuracies in a series of editorials and interviews at the time of its release. Interestingly, as his pamphlet on motion picture censorship makes clear, Griffith was a staunch defender of free speech, a right that would not be extended to the cinema in the United States until 1952.

Lesson Three: Slapstick and the Silent Period explores the work of Charles Chaplin, Buster Keaton, and Charlie Chase whose silent film comedies rivaled the Griffithesque historical fictions as the dominant forms of cinema expression in the 1920s. Donald Crafton opposes these two strands of Hollywood cinema, arguing that "the disruptive gags of slapstick can be regarded as an anachronistic manifestation of the cinema of attractions." Slapstick embraces the spectacle of nonnarrative intrusions and disruptions while Classical Hollywood cinema prioritizes story linearity and clarity, what Crafton metaphorically calls the "pie" and "chase." Ultimately, he suggests, feature-length comedies such as Keaton's *The General* and Chaplin's *The Gold Rush* subsumed slapstick into their cause-effect narrative structures. The chapter's first-person accounts of slapstick comedy include Marion Mack, Keaton's love interest in *The General*, who details the timing and precision of the stuntwork as well as Chaplin who discusses the great deal of invention that went into his gags. However, "If a gag interfered with the logic of events," he stated in his autobiography, "no matter how funny it was, I would not use it."

Lesson Four: The Production Code examines the self-regulatory operations of the Motion Picture Producers and Distributors of America (MPPDA), the trade organization formed by the major studios in 1922 after the notorious star scandals of Fatty Arbuckle and William Desmond Taylor prompted calls for reform in Hollywood. The industry hired former U. S. Postmaster General Will Hays to run the MPPDA and establish a set of production guidelines—what would ultimately become the 1930 Motion Picture Production Code—to deal with cuts by state censors boards and threats of economic boycotts from Catholics. Of great concern to reformers (and by extension the industry) was what Lea Jacobs calls the "fallen woman film"—a genre that emphasized female independence, sexuality, and social mobility over normative definitions of female chastity, domesticity, and fidelity. Jacobs demonstrates that the MPPDA failed to adequately eliminate enough controversial material from fallen woman films between 1930 and 1934 to satisfy the industry's detractors. Amidst this growing public relations problem, the MPPDA created the Production Code Administration (PCA) to oversee the "Code," with Joseph I. Breen at its helm to ensure studio compliance. For over twenty years, Hollywood films "arranged" under the PCA were as much a product of Breen's Catholic sensibility as they were the product of a studio executive, a studio house style, or a star's image.

Lesson Five: The Studios is the first of three lessons looking closely at the Hollywood studio system, a vertically integrated oligopoly dominated by five major companies (Loew's—parent company to MGM, Paramount, RKO, Twentieth Century-Fox, and Warner Bros) and three minor ones (Columbia, Universal, and United Artists). Due to the high cost of making, promoting, and distributing movies, the "Big Five" and the "Little Three" each worked to structure their business so they would be less vulnerable to risk. Production supervisors and studio chiefs like Irving Thalberg (MGM) and Daryl Zanuck (Warner Bros. and then Fox) standardized their products, developing "house" styles for their companies based around a star-genre formula. Tino Balio examines Columbia's role in the studio system, from its beginnings on Poverty Row to a producer-distributor specializing in "B" pictures that played on the bottom half of double bills in independent theaters. The studio did not have a house style, per se, though it specialized in screwball comedies in the second half of the 1930s. In its quest for profits, Columbia largely produced economy models of "A" pictures and developed a few "A" pictures of their own with stars loaned out by the Big Five. Frank Capra was responsible for most of these pictures as Columbia's most important contract director. Despite Clark Gable's and Claudette Colbert's prima donna behavior during the filming of *It Happened One Night* (1934), Capra's film swept all five major Academy Awards that year.

Lesson Six: Genres explores the genre systems of the Studio Era. These formulas consisted of a fixed body of characters and story types, settings and situations, themes and iconography, whose conventions were shared by other films of its kind. Genres compensated for the risk inherent in filmmaking; since each new picture was an unproven commodity, Hollywood needed to produce proven formula pictures with slight variations to "guarantee" a certain return at the box office. Major movie genres of this time include musicals, melodramas, science-fiction, horror films, comedies, and war films. This lesson focuses on the Western, the genre composing almost one-quarter of all Hollywood pictures produced between 1926 and 1967. Jim Kitses discusses the Western's versatility and enduring mythology through a series of antinomies arranged around "Wilderness vs. Civilization" that reveal the basic contradictions at the heart of America: imperialism, rugged individualism, and manifest destiny. John E. O'Connor demonstrates how Native American stereotypes served this mythology. In discussing the various dramatic, commercial, and political considerations that influenced, shaped and transformed the artistic representations of Native Americans in Hollywood films, he reveals the industry's carelessness in portraying historical events and presenting the complexity of Native American cultures. In one of his rare interviews, John Ford, the director most associated with the Western, reflects on the genre's mythology and his role (or lack thereof) in contributing to some of its more egregious ideologies.

Lesson Seven: Stars examines another form of standardization in classical Hollywood that continues to this day: the star system. Like genres, the movie star provided the studios with a tangible commodity, an image that could be created, marketed, and advertised for profit. The right star's name in the opening credits or on the marquee could draw huge audiences to a film. Richard Dyer argues that a star's image lies not only in his or her films, but also in studio promotion (pin ups, interviews, press coverage), writings about the star (film criticism, fan magazines), and the way he or she is used in other contexts (songs, advertisements, novels). The whole intertextual, multimedia construction and audience absorption of the star, he says, is grounded in the notion of the "real": "What is the star really like?" James Damico analyzes the 1949 controversy surrounding Ingrid Bergman and her extramarital affair with director Roberto Rossellini through this critical lens. Audiences were unable to reconcile her offscreen behavior with her onscreen persona, an image characterized by beauty, spirituality, and saintliness despite the sexual nature of many of her roles, particularly in *Notorious* (1946). Alfred Hitchcock directed Bergman in this film and two others (*Spellbound*, 1945, and *Under Capricorn*, 1949), and the "master of suspense" clearly understands the psychology behind star imagery. His essays, "Are Stars Necessary?" and "The Enjoyment of Fear" reveal a filmmaker closely attuned to the artistic and business dimensions of Hollywood moviemaking.

Lesson Eight: Anti-Communism in Hollywood explores the beginning of the post-WWII period in which dramatic economic, cultural, and social changes transformed Hollywood and the films it made. In the 1950s, the film industry witnessed an end to its stability and affluence. The 1948 *Paramount* decree forced the major studios to divest themselves of their theater holdings. In 1952, the U.S. Supreme Court also awarded First Amendment protection to films, forever changing the nature of Hollywood's products. At the same time, the massive post-war shift in American leisure time, the baby boom, and the mass movement to the suburbs led to an irreversible decline in motion picture attendance. By 1952, ticket sales had fallen almost 50% from their most profitable level in 1946. Also of great consequence were the House Committee on Un-American Activities (HUAC) hearings during the late 1940s and early 1950s, a period in which Brian Neve makes clear when Hollywood adapted its policies and practices for a new era of American Cold War leadership. Hollywood blacklisted more than 200 suspected communists and produced films that offered affirmative images of an America of economic abundance and class consensus. *Salt of the Earth* (1952) was a remarkable attempt by blacklisted artists to fight back against the Hollywood establishment through its efforts to depict the social reality of women, organized labor, and racial minorities. Producer Paul Jarrico, director Herbert J. Biberman, actress Rosaura Reveultas, and crew member Jules Schwerin share their stories here.

Lesson Nine: Television's Impact on Hollywood examines the motion picture industry's redefinition of itself in the 1950s as it competed for leisure time with spectator sports, hi-fi sets, bowling, and of course, television. During the war years, almost 25% of all U. S. expenditures for recreation were paid in movie admissions; by 1962 that percentage plummeted to 4.5%. Hollywood responded to this sudden loss of the mass audience by phasing out "B" pictures, dropping contracts with creative personnel, and offering sights and sounds television could not duplicate. The studios produced fewer but more expensive films, exhibited pictures with stereophonic sound, and developed widescreen formats. However, Hollywood also embraced the new medium of television, emerging as the primary suppliers of television programming in the 1950s. Chris Anderson identifies the significance of this period as one in which movies studios became subsidiaries of transnational media and leisure conglomerates. The shift to television production in Hollywood, he says, also signaled a growing trend toward the integration of the media industries, a consolidation of capital and diversification of products through corporate mergers. Director Elia Kazan, a "friendly" witness at the HUAC hearing who "named names" of Communist Party members in the film community, was one of several filmmakers who made feature films critical of television and television personalities. The hypnotic power and disdain he feels for the small screen comes through in his interview for *A Face in the Crowd* (1957), a political satire about a country singer turned television demagogue.

Lesson Ten: The Birth of the Blockbuster examines Hollywood in the first half of the 1960s adapting to the technological, economic, and social changes that took place during the 1950s. With the collapse of the studio system, film companies now primarily acted as distributors for independent producers who made the pictures themselves. Hollywood rented out production space and facilities to these independents, financed their production wholly or in part, and distributed and marketed their pictures. Yet, the independents did not stray far from the aesthetic practices of the majors that preceded them. They still submitted films to a now antiquated Production Code Administration and largely relied on popular novels, musicals, and plays as source material to attract mass audiences. As foreign films and their freedom of content increasingly became more popular with college students and the cultural elite, Hollywood returned to the most visually enticing spectacles and genres from earlier eras to attract dwindling audiences: biblical epics, westerns, and musicals. Justin Wyatt demonstrates how the aesthetics of these big-budget films—what later would be commonly referred to as blockbusters—substantially transformed the distribution practices of Hollywood. From roadshow experiments in the 1960s to saturation releases in the 1970s and beyond, the majors finally found the formula for filmmaking in the post-studio era: high concept projects (stars, genre, an exploitable premise) that could be marketed visually to different audience segments. Also at this time, production and distribution increasingly became internationalized, the result of the financial savings of co-productions, access to diverse casts and locations, and the growing importance of foreign markets to the bottom line. *Goldfinger* (1964) was one of these films. It was distributed by United Artists and independently co-produced by Albert "Cubby" Broccoli, whose autobiographical accounts illuminates these very changes.

Lesson Eleven: The Rating System explores the creation of the Code (later Classification) and Rating Administration (CARA), which replaced the Production Code Administration (PCA) in 1968. Shifting cultural mores, cinematic free expression, declining attendance, and independent film and foreign film competition had undermined the credibility of the single-seal-for-all films approach of the PCA for more than a decade. To adapt, much belatedly, to this changing marketplace, the Motion Picture Association of America (MPAA, changed from MPPDA in 1945), under the presidency of Jack Valenti and with the cooperation of the National Association of Theatre Owners (NATO), abandoned the moral absolutism of the Production Code for a rating system, dividing movies into four age categories: G (suitable for general audiences); M (allowing unrestricted admission but with caution to parents with children); R (restricting attendance to those over 16 to be accompanied by an adult); and X (restricting attendance to those over 16).[4] Kevin Sandler demonstrates how classification enabled Hollywood to update its business practices (a rating system permitting free expression) without changing its business model (entertainment for all ages). The MPAA and NATO member companies accomplished this feat by completely and collusively abandoning the use of the X rating by the early 1970s. In doing so, the industry could once again ensure the quality of Hollywood products to both its audience and detractors. This new model of entertainment, what Sandler identifies as "responsible" entertainment, along with a series of obscenity rulings handed down in 1973, he believes, played a large role in the box office recovery of Hollywood.

Lesson Twelve: Auteur Renaissance examines a brief moment of aesthetic adventure in U.S. cinema from the late-1960s to the mid-1970s commonly referred to as the Auteur Renaissance or New American Cinema. Like the film industries of Europe and Japan, the industry at this time was more of a director's cinema, providing a higher measure of authorial control than ever had been granted in the Studio Era. Against a backdrop of political and social unrest (Vietnam, Watergate, and the civil rights movement), an increasingly younger cinemagoing audience, a generation of film school graduates, and the unprecedented freedom of the rating system, Hollywood directors explored sex and violence in vivid detail, critically examined aspects of American culture, and wildly experimented with cinematic narrative and form. It was a period, as Noel King suggests, that linked the "traditions of classical Hollywood genre filmmaking with the stylistic innovations of European art cinema"; it was a time before the predominance of mall and multiplexes, synergies and franchises. As a result, the Auteur Renaissance became a benchmark against which future developments in contemporary American filmmaking would be measured, and as King makes clear, have failed to live up to. Martin Scorsese is considered one of those exceptions. He continues to produce work of philosophical depth and aesthetic innovation. Scorsese discusses one of his most celebrated works, *Taxi Driver* (1976), and ironically, one the critics commonly associated with the end of the Auteur Renaissance.

Lesson Thirteen: The Contemporary Hollywood Blockbuster examines the beginnings of the diversification and expansion of the American film industry into new media conglomerates that would

---

[4]In 1970, the M category became GP (when the age restriction was raised to 17); in 1972, the GP became PG (for Parental Guidance); in 1984, the PG-13 was added for additional caution to parents and children; and in 1991, the X was changed to NC-17 for (no children 17 and under admitted).

shape Hollywood's attitudes toward moviemaking for the remainder of the century. Deregulation during the Reagan administration enabled giant multinational companies such as Coca-Cola (who bought Columbia in 1982) and News Corporation (who purchased Twentieth Century-Fox in 1985) to control the entertainment marketplace more completely than the studios ever did in the Studio Era. At the core of Hollywood's production strategies in "New Hollywood," states Thomas Schatz, were blockbusters, "multi-purpose entertainment machines that breed music videos and soundtrack albums, TV series and videocassettes, video games and theme park rides, novelizations and comic books." In 1975 and 1977, *Jaws* and *Star Wars* recalibrated the potential profit of a Hollywood hit, and their directors, Steven Spielberg and George Lucas, established the importance of sequels and franchises to the business of contemporary Hollywood. Yet, it was *Batman* (1989), the product of the recently merged and then largest media company in the world, Time Warner, which ushered in the synergies of the modern "event" picture. Tim Burton, the film's director, discusses the complications involved in adapting an iconic character in the wake of the merger and tremendous fan hype.

Lesson Fourteen: Independents: Miramax and Black Film explores the independent movie scene of the 1980s and 1990s, a production gap left over by the MPAA studios' abandonment of the auteur picture and commitment to the blockbuster film. Unlike Hollywood's economic model of reaching international mass audiences with high-concept pictures, independent companies target a more select, narrow demographic with low-budget exploitation or art-house films. After several not-so-fortunate independent distributors went bankrupt by the end of the 1980s, Miramax thrived by replicating event pictures on a smaller scale through exploitation marketing, ushering in the era of what Alisa Perren calls the "indie blockbuster." Miramax's release of *sex, lies and videotape* (1989), she argues, set the standard for success for low-budget, niche distribution as well as laid the groundwork for the creation of the major-independents: specialty art-house divisions like Paramount Classics and Fox Searchlight purchased or created by the MPAA distributors and their conglomerates. This period also saw the rise of Black independent cinema, films by and about African Americans whose culture and stories were all but ignored by Hollywood. Jesse Algeron Rhines examines the Black Filmmakers Foundation, Island Pictures, and New Line Cinema, independent companies that distributed features by black filmmakers who later joined the Hollywood establishment to make movies with crossover potential. One of these directors, Spike Lee, has gone from one Hollywood major to another, sometimes more successfully than others, in depicting black life while often returning a profit to the distributor. He speaks about the challenges facing African Americans in the industry in regard to his most celebrated film, *Do the Right Thing* (1989).

Lesson Fifteen: Women Directors and Hollywood Cinema examines the talents and challenges facing female directors in the 1990s working in independent films and Hollywood. Despite the numerous success stories of certain male directors like Quentin Tarantino and Joel and Ethan Coen, the economic phenomenon of the indie blockbuster and the establishment of the major-independents did not greatly benefit women filmmakers and tales about women. Christina Lane explores the production-distribution context that affected the decreased visibility and opportunities for women in contemporary Hollywood, contributing to what she sees as the "homogenization of new indie cinema." Two factors, she states, have placed women at a disadvantage: first, the Sundance Film Festival, originally a grassroots venue fostering independent cinema and now an acquisition site and publicity event for Hollywood; and second, the major-independents and independent distributors themselves, companies more concerned with making profits than with making statements now that independent films were fixtures in multiplexes. As a result, women filmmakers and "female" genres have become "less marketable and less marketed." Male-oriented gangster films, thriller genres, and quirky "loser" films are considered more "auteurist" and promotable (i.e. commercial) while female-oriented films are considered didactic and feminist (i.e. non-commercial).

The study of the U. S. film industry and American cinema is a fascinating and complex one. This reader examines only a small part of this rich history between executives and directors, stars and regulators, politicians and distributors. Together, these accounts reveal the tenuous relationship between art and business in Hollywood, one that directly and indirectly shapes American identity, culture, and ideology.

The Rise of Hollywood and the Coming of Sound

LESSON ONE

The Birth of Cinema

The Cinema of Attractions
Early Film, Its Spectator and the Avant-Garde

Tom Gunning

Writing in 1922, flushed with the excitement of seeing Abel Gance's *La Roue*, Fernand Léger tried to define something of the radical possibilities of the cinema. The potential of the new art did not lie in 'imitating the movements of nature' or in 'the mistaken path' of its resemblance to theatre. Its unique power was a 'matter of *making images* seen'.[1] It is precisely this harnessing of visibility, this act of showing and exhibition, which I feel cinema before 1906 displays most intensely. Its inspiration for the avant-garde of the early decades of this century needs to be re-explored.

Writings by the early modernists (Futurists, Dadaists and Surrealists) on the cinema follow a pattern similar to Léger: enthusiasm for this new medium and its possibilities; and disappointment at the way it has already developed, its enslavement to traditional art forms, particularly theatre and literature. This fascination with the *potential* of a medium (and the accompanying fantasy of rescuing the cinema from its enslavement to alien and passé forms) can be understood from a number of viewpoints. I want to use it to illuminate a topic I have also approached before, the strangely heterogeneous relation that film before 1906 (or so) bears to the films that follow, and the way a taking account of this heterogeneity signals a new conception of film history and film form. My work in this area has been pursued in collaboration with André Gaudreault.[2]

The history of early cinema, like the history of cinema generally, has been written and theorized under the hegemony of narrative films. Early filmmakers like Smith, Méliès and Porter have been studied primarily from the viewpoint of their contribution to film as a storytelling medium, particularly the evolution of narrative editing. Although such approaches are not totally misguided, they are one-sided and potentially distort both the work of these filmmakers and the actual forces shaping cinema before 1906. A few observations will indicate the way that early cinema was not dominated by the narrative impulse that later asserted its sway over the medium. First there is the extremely important role that actuality film plays in early film production. Investigation of the films copyrighted in the US shows that actuality films outnumbered fictional films until 1906.[3] The Lumière tradition of 'placing the world within one's reach' through travel films and topicals did not disappear with the exit of the Cinématographe from film production. But even within non-actuality filming—what has sometimes been referred to as the 'Méliès tradition'—the role narrative plays is quite different from in traditional narrative film. Méliès himself declared in discussing his working method:

> As for the scenario, the 'fable,' or 'tale,' I only consider it at the end. I can state that the scenario constructed in this manner has no importance, *since I use it merely as a pretext for the 'stage effects,' the 'tricks,' or for a nicely arranged tableau.*[4]

Whatever differences one might find between Lumière and Méliès, they should not represent the opposition between narrative and non-narrative film-making, at least as it is understood today. Rather, one can unite them in a conception that sees cinema less as a way of telling stories than as a way of presenting a series of views to an audience, fascinating because of their illusory power (whether the realistic illusion of motion offered to the first audiences by Lumière, or the magical illusion concocted by Méliès), and exoticism. In other words, I believe that the relation to the spectator set up by the films of both Lumière and Méliès (and many other film-makers before 1906) had a common basis, and one that differs from the primary spectator relations set up by narrative film after 1906. I will call this earlier conception of cinema, 'the cinema of attractions'. I believe that this conception dominates cinema until about 1906–7. Although different from the fascination in storytelling exploited by the cinema from the time of Griffith, it is not necessarily opposed to it. In fact the cinema of attractions does not disappear with the dominance of narrative, but rather goes underground, both into certain avant-garde practices and as a component of narrative films, more evident in some genres (e.g. the musical) than in others.

What precisely is the cinema of attractions? First, it is a cinema that bases itself on the quality that Léger celebrated: its ability to *show* something. Contrasted to the voyeuristic aspect of narrative cinema analysed by Christian Metz,[5] this is an exhibitionist cinema. An aspect of early cinema which I have written about in other articles is emblematic of this different relationship the cinema of attractions constructs with its spectator: the recurring look at the camera by actors. This action, which is later perceived as spoiling the realistic illusion of the cinema, is here undertaken with brio, establishing contact with the audience. From comedians smirking at the camera, to the constant bowing and gesturing of the conjurors in magic films, this is a cinema that displays its visibility, willing to rupture a self-enclosed fictional world for a chance to solicit the attention of the spectator.

Exhibitionism becomes literal in the series of erotic films which play an important role in early film production (the same Pathé catalogue would advertise the Passion Play along with 'scènes grivoises d'un caractère piquant', erotic films often including full nudity), also driven underground in later years. As Noël Burch has shown in his film *Correction Please: How We Got into Pictures* (1979), a film like *The Bride Retires* (France, 1902) reveals a fundamental conflict between this exhibitionistic tendency of early film and the creation of a fictional diegesis. A woman undresses for bed while her new husband peers at her from behind a screen. However, it is to the camera and the audience that the bride addresses her erotic striptease, winking at us as she faces us, smiling in erotic display.

As the quote from Méliès points out, the trick film, perhaps the dominant non-actuality film genre before 1906, is itself a series of displays, of magical attractions, rather than a primitive sketch of narrative continuity. Many trick films are, in effect, plotless, a series of transformations strung together with little connection and certainly no characterization. But to approach even the plotted trick films, such as *Voyage dans la lune* (1902), simply as precursors of later narrative structures is to miss the point. The story simply provides a frame upon which to string a demonstration of the magical possibilities of the cinema.

Modes of exhibition in early cinema also reflect this lack of concern with creating a self-sufficient narrative world upon the screen. As Charles Musser has shown,[6] the early showmen exhibitors exerted a great deal of control over the shows they presented, actually re-editing the films they had purchased and supplying a series of offscreen supplements, such as sound effects and spoken commentary. Perhaps most extreme is the Hale's Tours, the largest chain of theatres exclusively showing films before 1906. Not only did the films consist of non-narrative sequences taken from moving vehicles (usually trains), but the theatre itself was arranged as a train car with a conductor who took tickets, and sound effects simulating the click-clack of wheels and hiss of air brakes.[7] Such viewing experiences relate more to the attractions of the fairground than to the traditions of the legitimate theatre. The relation between films and the emergence of the great amusement parks, such as Coney Island, at the turn of the century provides rich ground for rethinking the roots of early cinema.

Nor should we ever forget that in the earliest years of exhibition the cinema itself was an attraction. Early audiences went to exhibitions to see machines demonstrated (the newest technological wonder, following in the wake of such widely exhibited machines and marvels as X-rays or, earlier, the phonograph), rather than to view films. It was the Cinématographe, the Biograph or the Vitascope that were advertised on the variety bills in which they premièred, not *Le Déjeuner de bébé* or

The Black Diamond Express. After the initial novelty period, this display of the possibilities of cinema continues, and not only in magic films. Many of the close-ups in early film differ from later uses of the technique precisely because they do not use enlargement for narrative punctuation, but as an attraction in its own right. The close-up cut into Porter's *The Gay Shoe Clerk* (1903) may anticipate later continuity techniques, but its principal motive is again pure exhibitionism, as the lady lifts her skirt hem, exposing her ankle for all to see. Biograph films such as *Photographing a Female Crook (1904)* and *Hooligan in Jail* (1903) consist of a single shot in which the camera is brought close to the main character, until they are in mid-shot. The enlargement is not a device expressive of narrative tension; it is in itself an attraction and the point of the film.[8]

To summarise, the cinema of attractions directly solicits spectator attention, inciting visual curiosity, and supplying pleasure through an exciting spectacle—a unique event, whether fictional or documentary, that is of interest in itself. The attraction to be displayed may also be of a cinematic nature, such as the early close-ups just described, or trick films in which a cinematic manipulation (slow motion, reverse motion, substitution, multiple exposure) provides the film's novelty. Fictional situations tend to be restricted to gags, vaudeville numbers or recreations of shocking or curious incidents (executions, current events). It is the direct address of the audience, in which an attraction is offered to the spectator by a cinema showman, that defines this approach to film making. Theatrical display dominates over narrative absorption, emphasizing the direct stimulation of shock or surprise at the expense of unfolding a story or creating a diegetic universe. The cinema of attractions expends little energy creating characters with psychological motivations or individual personality. Making use of both fictional and non-fictional attractions, its energy moves outward towards an acknowledged spectator rather than inward towards the character-based situations essential to classical narrative.

The term 'attractions' comes, of course, from the young Sergei Mikhailovich Eisenstein and his attempt to find a new model and mode of analysis for the theatre. In his search for the 'unit of impression' of theatrical art, the foundation of an analysis which would undermine realistic representational theatre, Eisenstein hit upon the term 'attraction'.[9] An attraction aggressively subjected the spectator to 'sensual or psychological impact'. According to Eisenstein, theatre should consist of a montage of such attractions, creating a relation to the spectator entirely different from his absorption in 'illusory depictions'.[10] I pick up this term partly to underscore the relation to the spectator that this later avant-garde practice shares with early cinema: that of exhibitionist confrontation rather than diegetic absorption. Of course the 'experimentally regulated and mathematically calculated' montage of attractions demanded by Eisenstein differs enormously from these early films (as any conscious and oppositional mode of practice will from a popular one).[11] However, it is important to realize the context from which Eisenstein selected the term. Then, as now, the 'attraction' was a term of the fairground, and for Eisenstein and his friend Yutkevich it primarily represented their favourite fairground attraction, the roller coaster, or as it was known then in Russia, the American Mountains.[12]

The source is significant. The enthusiasm of the early avant-garde for film was at least partly an enthusiasm for a mass culture that was emerging at the beginning of the century, offering a new sort of stimulus for an audience not acculturated to the traditional arts. It is important to take this enthusiasm for popular art as something more than a simple gesture to *épater les bourgeois*. The enormous development of the entertainment industry since the 1910s and its growing acceptance by middle-class culture (and the accommodation that made this acceptance possible) have made it difficult to understand the liberation popular entertainment offered at the beginning of the century. I believe that it was precisely the exhibitionist quality of turn-of-the-century popular art that made it attractive to the avant-garde—its freedom from the creation of a diegesis, its accent on direct stimulation.

Writing of the variety theatre, Marinetti not only praised its aesthetics of astonishment and stimulation, but particularly its creation of a new spectator who contrasts with the 'static', 'stupid voyeur' of traditional theatre. The spectator at the variety theatre feels directly addressed by the spectacle and joins in, singing along, heckling the comedians.[13] Dealing with early cinema within the context of archive and academy, we risk missing its vital relation to vaudeville, its primary place of exhibition until around 1905. Film appeared as one attraction on the vaudeville programme, surrounded by a mass of unrelated acts in a non-narrative and even nearly illogical succession of performances. Even when presented in the nickelodeons that were emerging at the end of this period, these short films always appeared in a variety format, trick films sandwiched in with farces, actualities, 'illustrated songs', and, quite frequently, cheap vaudeville acts. It was precisely this non-narrative variety that placed this form of entertainment under attack by reform groups in the early 1910s. The Russell Sage Survey of popular entertainments found vaudeville 'depends upon an artificial rather than a natural human and developing interest, these acts having no necessary and as a rule, no actual connection'.[14] In other words, no narrative. A night at the variety theatre was like a ride on a streetcar or an active day in a crowded city, according to this middle-class reform group, stimulating an unhealthy nervousness. It was precisely such artificial stimulus that Marinetti and Eisenstein wished to borrow from the popular arts and inject into the theatre, organizing popular energy for radical purpose.

What happened to the cinema of attractions? The period from 1907 to about 1913 represents the true *narrativization* of the cinema, culminating in the appearance of feature films which radically revised the variety format. Film clearly took the legitimate theatre as its model, producing famous players in famous plays. The transformation of filmic discourse that D. W. Griffith typifies bound cinematic signifiers to the narration of stories and the creation of a self-enclosed diegetic universe. The look at the camera becomes taboo and the devices of cinema are transformed from playful 'tricks'—cinematic attractions (Méliès gesturing at us to watch the lady vanish)—to elements of dramatic expression, entries into the psychology of character and the world of fiction.

However, it would be too easy to see this as a Cain and Abel story, with narrative strangling the nascent possibilities of a young iconoclastic form of entertainment. Just as the variety format in some sense survived in the movie palaces of the 20s (with newsreel, cartoon, sing-along, orchestra performance and sometimes vaudeville acts subordinated to, but still coexisting with, the narrative *feature* of the evening), the system of attraction remains an essential part of popular film-making.

The chase film shows how, towards the end of this period (basically from 1903 to 1906), a synthesis of attractions and narrative was already underway. The chase had been the original truly narrative genre of the cinema, providing a model for causality and linearity as well as a basic editing continuity. A film like Biograph's *Personal* (1904, the model for the chase film in many ways) shows the creation of a narrative linearity, as the French nobleman runs for his life from the fiancées his personal column ad has unleashed. However, at the same time, as the group of young women pursue their prey towards the camera in each shot, they encounter some slight obstacle (a fence, a steep slope, a stream) that slows them down for the spectator, providing a mini-spectacle pause in the unfolding of narrative. The Edison Company seemed particularly aware of this, since they offered their plagiarized version of this Biograph film (*How a French Nobleman Got a Wife Through the New York Herald 'Personal' Columns*) in two forms, as a complete film or as separate shots, so that any one image of the ladies chasing the man could be bought without the inciting incident or narrative closure.[15]

As Laura Mulvey has shown in a very different context, the dialectic between spectacle and narrative has fuelled much of the classical cinema.[16] Donald Crafton in his study of slapstick comedy, 'The pie and the chase', has shown the way slapstick did a balancing act between the pure spectacle of gag and the development of narrative.[17] Likewise, the traditional spectacle film proved true to its name by highlighting moments of pure visual stimulation along with narrative. The 1924 version of *Ben Hur* was in fact shown at a Boston theatre with a timetable announcing the moment of its prime attractions:

    8.35 *The Star of Bethlehem*
    8.40 *Jerusalem Restored*
    8.59 *Fall of the House of Hur*
    10.29 *The Last Supper*
    10.50 *Reunion*[18]

The Hollywood advertising policy of enumerating the features of a film, each emblazoned with the command, 'See!' shows this primal power of the attraction running beneath the armature of narrative regulation.

We seem far from the avant-garde premises with which this discussion of early cinema began. But it is important for the radical heterogeneity which I find in early cinema not to be conceived as a truly oppositional programme, one irreconcilable with the growth of narrative cinema. This view is too sentimental and too ahistorical. A film like *The Great Train Robbery* (1903) does point in both directions, towards a direct assault on the spectator (the spectacularly enlarged outlaw unloading his pistol in our faces), and towards a linear narrative continuity. This is early film's ambiguous heritage. Clearly in some sense recent spectacle cinema has reaffirmed its roots in stimulus and carnival rides, in what might be called the Spielberg-Lucas-Coppola cinema of effects.

But effects are tamed attractions. Marinetti and Eisenstein understood that they were tapping into a source of energy that would need focusing and intensification to fulfil its revolutionary possibilities. Both Eisenstein and Marinetti planned to exaggerate the impact on the spectators, Marinetti proposing to literally glue them to their seats (ruined garments paid for after the performance) and Eisenstein setting firecrackers off beneath them. Every change in film history implies a change in its address to the spectator, and each period constructs its spectator in a new way. Now in a period of American avant-garde cinema in which the tradition of contemplative subjectivity has perhaps run its (often glorious) course, it is possible that this earlier carnival of the cinema, and the methods of popular entertainment, still provide an unexhausted resource—a Coney Island of the avant-garde, whose never dominant but always sensed current can be traced from Méliès through Keaton, through *Un Chien andalou* (1928), and Jack Smith.

Notes

First published in *Wide Angle* vol. 8 no. 3/4, Fall 1986.

1. Fernand Léger, 'A critical essay on the plastic qualities of Abel Gance's film *The Wheel*', in Edward Fry (ed.), *Functions of Painting*, trans. Alexandra Anderson (New York: Viking Press, 1973), p. 21.
2. See my articles 'The non-continuous style of early film', in Roger Holman (ed.), *Cinema 1900–1906* (Brussels: FIAF, 1982), and 'An unseen energy swallows space: the space in early film and its relation to American avant garde film' in John L. Fell (ed.), *Film Before Griffith* (Berkeley: University of California Press, 1983), pp. 355–66, and our collaborative paper delivered by A. Gaudreault at the conference at Cerisy on Film History (August 1985) 'Le cinéma des premiers temps: un défi à l'histoire du cinéma?'. I would also like to note the importance of my discussions with Adam Simon and our hope to investigate further the history and archaeology of the film spectator.
3. Robert C. Allen, *Vaudeville and Film:* 1895–1915, *A Study in Media Interaction* (New York: Arno Press, 1980), pp. 159, 212–13.
4. Méliès, 'Importance du scénario', in Georges Sadoul, *Georges Méliès* (Paris: Seghers, 1961), p. 118 (my translation).
5. Metz, *The Imaginary Signifier: Psychoanalysis and the Cinema,* trans. Celia Britton, Annwyl Williams, Ben Brewster and Alfred Guzzetti (Bloomington: Indiana University Press, 1982), particularly pp. 58–80, 91–7.
6. Musser, 'American Vitagraph 1897–1901', *Cinema Journal,* vol. 22 no. 3, Spring 1983, p.10.
7. Raymond Fielding, 'Hale's tours: Ultrarealism in the pre-1910 motion picture', in Fell, *Film Before Griffith,* pp. 116–30.
8. I wish to thank Ben Brewster for his comments after the original delivery of this paper which pointed out the importance of including this aspect of the cinema of attractions here.

9. Eisenstein, 'How I became a film director', in *Notes of a Film Director* (Moscow: Foreign Language Publishing House, n.d.), p. 16.
10. 'The montage of attractions', in S. M. Eisenstein, *Writings* 1922–1934, edited by Richard Taylor (London: BFI, 1988), p. 35.
11. Ibid.
12. Yon Barna, *Eisenstein* (Bloomington: Indiana University Press, 1973), p. 59.
13. 'The variety theater 1913' in Umbra Apollonio (ed.), *Futurist Manifestos* (New York: Viking Press, 1973), p. 127.
14. Michael Davis, *The Exploitation of Pleasure* (New York: Russell Sage Foundation, Dept. of Child Hygiene, Pamphlet, 1911).
15. David Levy, 'Edison sales policy and the continuous action film 1904–1906', in Fell, *Film Before Griffith,* pp. 207–22.
16. 'Visual pleasure and narrative cinema', in Laura Mulvey, *Visual and Other Pleasures* (London: Macmillan, 1989).
17. Paper delivered at the FIAF Conference on Slapstick, May 1985, New York City.
18. Nicholas Vardac, *From Stage to Screen: Theatrical Method from Garrick to Griffith* (New York: Benjamin Blom, 1968), p. 232.

Founding Father

Louis Lumière in conversation with Georges Sadoul, edited and translated by Pierre Hodgson

Introduction

Spring 1994. I have a new job, helping out in a French government agency set up to promote the centenary of film, *L'Association Premier Siècle du Cinéma*. France being France, this is a big deal. I am not quite sure what I have been hired to do. Somewhat unenthusiastically, I start rummaging through the shelves, familiarizing myself with all the videotapes people have sent in. I slot another VHS into the machine. There is no label to say what it is. Only the name of the distributor, 'Lobster Films, Paris', a firm which specializes in clearing out attics in search of old films.

An image appears on the screen. The sound is not quite in sync, the picture flickering black and white. The first words emerge: *'Monsieur Louis Lumière, dans quelles circonstances avez-vous commencé à vous intéresser aux photographies animées?*' ('Mr Louis Lumière, in what circumstances did your interest in animated photography arise?') And I realize what this is. This is the only extant television interview with the man who invented cinema, recorded on 6 January 1948.

The interview—a transcript of which is translated here in honour of the centenary—was published in France in the 1960s in book form. The original television and radio versions have almost never been seen or heard.

Many men, apart from Louis Lumière, have a claim on the title of founding father of cinema. Thomas Edison in America, for instance, or Max Skladanowski in Germany. But it was Lumière who designed, built and marketed the first all-round film machine, which worked as a camera, a projector and printer all at once. It was he who called it the 'cinematograph', the word by which in most countries the film business, or some aspect of it, is known today. And it was he who started the first continuous, fee-paying public screenings at the Grand Café in Paris just one hundred years ago.

Louis Lumière never expected cinema to be more than a passing fad (though, as he says in this interview, he was experimenting with 3-D films in 1935, forty years after the original invention). But because his camera doubled as a projector, it laid the foundations of an industry. Within months of the first fee-paying public screening, on 28 December 1895, Lumière had sent projectionists all over the world—to Mexico and St. Petersburg and Saigon—where they showed footage of France to pay for the cost of shooting pictures to send home. The new fad spread like wild fire.

Most of the 1,500 or so Lumière films which have survived (average length 40–50 seconds) are documentaries of exotic places, state visits, army training courses, of comic scenes from everyday life. The subject matter is rarely of much interest. But Louis Lumière was an accomplished photographer* and he used this skill to develop cinematography of great modern beauty. The first fifty or so films in the catalogue were shot by him personally, and the rest by a handful of cameramen whom he trained. In this interview, Lumière denies he was ever a film director, but if he was not that, we can safely say he was the first *auteur*.

*The original Lumière family business was manufacturing high quality photographic plates (the firm was eventually taken over by Ilford).

After the First World War, the Lumière film business declined, and the brothers' interest moved off in different directions, but the historical connection remained. When it was decided to hold a film festival in Cannes, it was thought that the president of the jury ought to be the man who, forty-five years earlier, had laid the foundations for the industry—Louis Lumière.

That was in early September 1939, quite possibly the worst timing there has ever been. War broke out, and the festival was postponed until 1946, by which time Lumière was too old to be president. Nevertheless, he attended the first Cannes Film Festival as a member of the public and there he met the historian of early cinema, Georges Sadoul. A few weeks later, Sadoul received a huge envelope through the post containing an alarming number of corrections to the definitive work he had just published.

Not long before these events, General de Gaulle had set up an organization called RTF designed to emulate or perhaps to rival the BBC. As it happened, Sadoul was on the staff of this organization, employed, partly at least, to experiment with a new form called television.

When he received Lumière's package, Sadoul did two things. He set about producing a revised edition of his book, and he decided to interview Louis Lumière for television. Perhaps the irony of it appealed to him. Here was the founding father of film, now almost on his death bed, just present at the birth of the next mass medium.

The old man had long refused to give any interviews, but on this occasion he agreed. He invited Sadoul and his wife to come and visit him at his house at Bandol, on the coast between Marseilles and Cannes, and said the television crew could come in after lunch. After a few technical mishaps, the interview was recorded and Louis Lumière died very shortly afterwards.

The interview itself is strange, not at all what we think of as television. There is no attempt at naturalism. Louis Lumière reads from a prepared typescript, rather like a cautious lawyer giving a press statement after a difficult trial. He wears a suit and a medal of high rank in the Légion d'honneur, the French equivalent of a knighthood. It seems as though the occasional cutaways to the interviewer were added later, with spurious questions designed to dress up a formal statement as a conversation. Lumière's great age and frailty are obvious. The typescript shakes in his hand. His voice is cracked. But his determination to set the record straight is impressive. Here is a man who, in his lifetime, has seen the toy he invented become by far the most popular form of entertainment in the world, wanting to tell people how it all happened; the man who invented cinema, in at the start of television.

GEORGES SADOUL: *Mr Louis Lumière, in what circumstances did your interest in animated photography arise?*
LOUIS LUMIÈRE: My brother Auguste and I started work in the summer of 1894. At this time, Marey, Edison and Demeny had conducted useful research, but no one had yet projected images on to a screen. No one had found a way of driving film through a camera. My brother Auguste experimented with a serrated cylinder, similar to that used by Léon Boully in some other invention, but this system was too violent. It could not work and it never did.
GS: *Did Mr Auguste Lumière then suggest any other solutions to the problem?*
LL: No. My brother lost interest in the technical side of cinematography as soon as I had discovered a workable method of driving film through a camera. The patent was taken out by us jointly because we always took joint credit for research and patents, regardless of whether or not each of us had made a contribution. The fact is that I am the sole author of cinematography, just as my brother was sole author of other inventions patented jointly by us.
GS: *What was your solution to the problem?*
LL: One night, sick in bed and unable to sleep, I had a brainwave. The answer was to adapt, for use in cinematography, a device similar to the presser foot which shifts cloth through a sewing-machine. I tried a circular eccentric gear, then soon replaced it with a similar, but triangular mechanism.
GS: *And so you built a prototype along these lines?*
LL: The first machine was built by Mr Moisson, chief engineer in our factories, according to a series of sketches which I gave him. There was no celluloid in France at that time, so our first experiments

were conducted using strips of photographic paper manufactured in our factories. I cut the strips and perforated them myself. The first results were excellent, as you can see.

GS: *Quite. There is something very moving about that long strip of paper which you have donated to the Cinémathèque française. The images are perfectly sharp.*

LL: Those strips were for experimental purposes only. You could not project images from such negatives because paper is too opaque. But in the laboratory I was able to imagine the effect of animation by holding paper images up to a strong light. The results were very good.

GS: *Was it long before celluloid came in?*

LL: I would have used celluloid from the beginning if I had been able to obtain sufficiently supple and transparent supplies in France. But it was available neither in France nor in England. In the end I sent one of our heads of department to America, to the New York Celluloid Company, where he found sheets of plain celluloid which we were able to coat, cut into strips and perforate in Lyons. It was Mr Moisson who devised a perforating-machine, according to the same principles as a sewing-machine.

GS: *The emulsion you produced was of a much higher quality than that made by Kodak for Edison's films. That is obvious, now we can compare the two. Photographically speaking, the earliest American films are of an indifferent quality, whereas yours are as good as today's. When did you make your first film on celluloid?*

LL: I made my first film towards the end of the summer of 1894. It is *La Sortie des usines Lumière* (Workers Leaving the Lumière Factories). You've probably noticed that the men are in straw boaters and the women in summer dresses. At that stage, I needed a great deal of sunlight to shoot such a sequence because I had only a poor quality lens. I could not have shot that sequence in autumn or winter. *La Sortie des usines Lumière* was shown for the first time in Paris, rue de Rennes, at the Society for the Encouragement of National Industry on 22 March 1895. At the end of the screening, I was invited by Mascart, an eminent physicist and member of the Académie française, to give a lecture. I also projected on to a screen a picture of a photographic image undergoing development. This presented certain difficulties I won't go into here.

GS: *Was your invention already called cinematography?*

LL: I don't think so. Our first patent, taken out on 13 February 1895, had no particular name. We called it 'a machine designed to take and show chronophotographic prints'. The word 'cinematography' came a few weeks later.

GS: *We're all so familiar with the word 'cinema' nowadays, but at the time people thought it barbarous and unpronounceable. Did you never think of calling it anything else?*

LL: My father, Antoine Lumière, couldn't bear the word 'cinematograph'. His friend Lechère, who was a sales representative for Moët et Chandon champagne, persuaded him to call the thing 'domitor'.

GS: *What did that mean?*

LL: I'm not sure. I think Lechère thought it up. The root concept is probably something to do with domination. Neither my brother nor I ever accepted this word. We never used it.

GS: *But if you had accepted it, instead of talking about going to the cinema, we'd say going to the domitor, and instead of cinematography we'd say domitory, because it was the success of the machine which you called 'cinematograph' that laid the foundations of a new art form and a new kind of entertainment. Were there any particular technical problems associated with the perfection of the domitor, I mean cinematograph?*

LL: One thing that bothered me was: how strong is celluloid? At the time, this was an unknown quantity. We did not know what the properties of celluloid were. So I devised a series of experiments which involved piercing strips of film with needles of different diameters and suspending various weights on the needles. In this way, I discovered that the perforations could, without inconvenience, be larger than the diameter of the sprocket over which they passed. This caused no loss of strength compared to a perforation exactly the same diameter as its sprocket.

GS: *Was the cinematograph built in your factories?*

LL: No, we weren't equipped to do such work. After a lecture I gave in Paris in 1895, an engineer named Jules Carpentier asked if he could manufacture our cameras in his works, which had just started production of a first-class stills camera. Carpentier and I became close friends, and remained close friends until he died. I accepted his proposition, but he was not able to complete cameras for delivery until early in 1896, so until then I had to make do with the prototype we had built in Lyons.

GS: *Since, in 1895, you only had one instrument, which doubled up both as a camera and as a projector, you must have been personally responsible for shooting every film made that year.*

LL: That is right. All the films shown in 1895, either at the Photographic Conference in Lyons in June, or at the *Revue Générale des Sciences* in Paris in July, or in the basement of the Grand Café from 28 December on, all these films were shot by me, with one single exception: *Les Brûleuses d'herbe* (The Girls who Burn Grass), which my brother Auguste shot while on holiday at our house at La Ciotat. I should add that, not only did I shoot these films, but the first films shown at the Grand Café were developed by me in enamel hospital pails containing developer, water and fixative, and it was I who made the prints, using a white, sun-drenched wall as a light source.

GS: *For half a century now these films have been world famous. They mark the dawn of cinematography. They are:* Boat Leaving Harbour, Game of Cards, Arrival of a Train in the Station at La Ciotat, Demolishing a Wall, Lunch for Baby *and* The Gardener Takes a Shower. *Can you tell us something about* Game of Cards, *for instance.*

LL: The players are my father, Antoine Lumière, who is the one lighting a cigar; and opposite him, his friend, Trewey, dealing. Trewey was our agent in London and he organized the cinematograph screenings there. He appears in several of my films, *Assiettes tournantes* (Turning Plates) for instance. The third player, the one pouring out beer, is my father-in-law, Winkler, the brewer from Lyons. The footman was an employee. He was from Gonfaron. A true-blooded, silver-tongued southerner. He had an answer to everything and always made us laugh with his pranks.

GS: *What about* Arrival of a Train?

LL: I shot that in La Ciotat in 1895. On the platform, there is a little girl hopping. She is holding her mother's hand on one side and her nanny's on the other. That is my eldest daughter, Madame Trarieux, now four times a grandmother. My mother, Madame Antoine Lumière, is in the picture too wearing a Scottish shawl.

GS: *The arrival of the train was your big hit at the Grand Café. When the locomotive appeared on the screen, spectators shrank back terrified. They thought they were going to be run over. What about* Demolishing a Wall?

LL: It was shot by me in our factory in Monplaisir (Lyons) while the builders were in. The man in shirt sleeves is my brother Auguste, telling the men what to do.

GS: *At the Grand Café, from January 1896 onwards, the film was shown backwards, which made it look as though a wall was building itself. A kind of special effect—the first ever. What about* Lunch for Baby?

LL: It was shot in the garden of our house in Lyons. The man is my brother Auguste, the woman is his wife and the baby is their daughter.

GS: *The first ever close-up. People were amazed not just by the expression on the baby's face, but also by the way the bushes moved in the sun. Now tell us about* The Gardener Takes a Shower.

LL: I am not 100 percent certain, but I think the idea for the script came from a prank of my younger brother Edward. Unfortunately, he was killed as a pilot in the 1914–18 war. He was too young to play the part of the boy with his foot on the hose, so I found an apprentice in the works instead. His name was Duval and he was our chief packer for nearly forty-two years. The gardener is played by our gardener, Monsieur Clerc. He worked in the factory for forty years too, and is still alive today. He retired to somewhere near Valence.

GS: *Did you shoot any other films during 1895, apart from these eight famous ones?*

LL: I must have shot about fifty, though I can't be certain. Each film was seventeen metres in length and the screening lasted for about one minute. Seventeen metres may seem an odd sort of length, but it was governed by the capacity of the magazine containing the negative.

GS: *Can you recall the names of any other films you shot during 1895?*

LL: We produced a few comedies featuring relatives, friends and employees. One such was *Le Photographie* (The Photographer) starring my brother Auguste and Maurice, the photographer, who was to hold the franchise of our cinematograph at the Grand Café. We also made a film called

Charcuterie américaine (American Pork Butcher), starring a sausage-making machine. The pig went in one end and sausages came out the other, and vice versa. My brother and I had great fun building the machine at our house in La Ciotat. On the side, we inscribed the words *Crack, charcutier à Marseille* (Crack of Marseilles, Pork Butcher). Perhaps I should mention *Debarquement des congressistes à Neuville-sur-Saône* (Arrival of Conference Members at Neuville-sur-Saône), which is really the first newsreel footage. I shot it during the conference in June 1895 and projected it the very next day.

GS: *Did you make any further films after 1895?*

LL: Very few. I left that to the cameramen I trained: Promio, Mesguisch, Doublier, Perrigot and others. Within a few years, they filled our catalogue with more than 1,200 films shot across five continents.

GS: *When did you abandon your cinematographic activities?*

LL: My last work was done in 1935, when I invented a form of three dimensional cinema. I showed the results in Paris, Lyons, Marseilles and Nice. I have always been a technician and a researcher. I have never been what is called a director. I can't see myself in a modern studio. As a matter of fact, I am unable to move now. I can scarcely leave Bandol.

LESSON TWO

Narrative Integration

The Birth of a Nation (1915)
Integrating Race into the Narrator System

Daniel Bernardi

Context

Set during the American Civil War and Reconstruction, *The Birth of a Nation* (1915) is a powerful story about the plight of two upper-class families: the Stonemans of the North and the Camerons of the South. A historic epic, this classic film offers its audience a tender portrait of two families' struggle for unity in the dense fog of war. Yet it is committed also to a romantic vision of the "Southern Legend" in its depiction of the Reconstruction era. Beset by revengeful black brutes, self-righteous white politicians, plundering carpetbaggers, manipulative mulatto mistresses, plotting mulatto politicians, and the graphic death of a Confederate daughter, the Stonemans and the Camerons endure this turbulent period of American history, eventually coming together in a marriage that symbolizes a reunited nation.

Produced and directed by David Wark Griffith (1875–1948), *The Birth of a Nation* is widely considered to be the most important American film in history. Since its initial screening, critics and scholars have proclaimed it the first feature-length film to offer audiences a powerful melodrama told with artistic subtlety. Indeed, this classic work led American cinema into the era of the Hollywood style, a system of narrative filmmaking that marshals cinematic technique—from cinematography to editing—in the service of character psychology, causal, plot development, and moral endings. Although refined and even challenged over time, this style of filmmaking is still dominant today. And for this reason, Griffith is widely considered to be the father of American cinema—"the Shakespeare of the screen."

The Birth of a Nation is based on two of Reverend Thomas Dixon Jr.'s novels, *The Clansman: An Historical Romance of the Ku Klux Klan* (1905) and *The Leopard's Spots* (1902). Not surprisingly, it is known also for perpetuating some of the most repulsive stereotypes of African Americans in history. Borrowing from the Dixon novels, Griffith offers us a binary caricature of former slaves: either "faithful souls" loyal to the belief in white superiority or overly sexualized "brutes" out for revenge. Yet with few exceptions, European American actors play African American characters in blackface, making the film more about the way in which whiteness imagines blackness than it is about blackness itself. Griffith, it is widely reported, went so far as to segregate the cast, refusing to allow black actors to touch white actresses. For the famous director, whites must remain united in their quest for racial purity and national dominance. As one of the last intertitles of the film explains: "The former enemies of North and South are united in common defense of the Aryan birthright." Using the techniques of filmmaking to support the story of white supremacy, Griffith casts the Ku Klux Klan as heroes—romantic men in white hoods who ride with apparent honor and virtue in defense of white women, white families, and, via didactic metaphor, a white nation.

The importance of this complex film lies not simply in either its contribution to the art of cinematic storytelling or its overt racism, but in the relationship between these forces in the context of film history. Segregating Griffith's contribution to the craft of narrative filmmaking from his racist imagery undermines the impact that *The Birth of a Nation* had—and continues to have—on cinematic storytelling. In many ways, Griffith developed his style of filmmaking to tell unambiguous stories of an American color line. In *The Birth of a Nation*, this color line marks a clear hierarchy of races reinforced by a romantic representation of the Old South, social segregation, antimiscegenation laws, disenfranchisement, and the natural—divine—right of white rule into the future.

Analysis

Despite the trend among critics and scholars to either ignore or excuse the articulation of white supremacy in *The Birth of a Nation* in favor of focusing on the film's artistic achievements, and despite the criticism, on the other side, that this work is nothing more than racist propaganda, Griffith's epic reveals an important moment in film history, when cinematic storytelling developed as popular art in the service of racism. In what ways does *The Birth of a Nation* reflect history? How are the techniques of cinema employed in the film to facilitate and refract the story of white supremacy? More broadly, how can we simultaneously acknowledge the film's contribution to storytelling technique while challenging its systematic embrace of racism? Can racism in film be at once ugly and painful and at the same time artistic and romantic?

Reflecting History

It is difficult and perhaps unproductive to view *The Birth of a Nation* with dispassion. The film calls out for audiences to engage with it, and to do so with critical indignation. Nonetheless, it is important to situate this classic film in the context in which it was produced and initially exhibited. The sociopolitical environment in which Griffith made *The Birth of a Nation* is reflected in the film itself. Ironically, this is most clear when looking at the way in which Griffith represented the past. In other words, we find the ideologies of race that informed the production of *The Birth of a Nation* in 1915 directing the story of the Civil War and Reconstruction (1861 to 1877) represented in the film. The history outside the film as well as the representation of history in the film comprise a key issue informing the significance of *The Birth of a Nation*.

The early twentieth century saw the growth of cinema as a popular form of entertainment. European immigrants followed their predecessors into nickelodeon theaters to discover the fictionalization of American democracy, and, in the process, they were encouraged to assimilate into the social order of things. At the same time, during this period the United States was dominated by a racial formation that positioned people of color as threats to whiteness. Although few citizens advocated a return to slavery as a means of controlling this perceived threat, Jim Crow discrimination was widespread and widely accepted. Racism was an openly supported fact of American social life.

The social reality of racism informed the development of filmmaking, facilitating a troubling yet persistent link between cinema and the politics of racism. *The Birth of a Nation* was the first film to be screened at the White House, and on seeing the classic, President Woodrow Wilson (1856–1924) reportedly proclaimed, "It is like writing history with lightning. And my only regret is that it is all so terribly true."[1] Wilson was a key proponent of the League of Nations, the forerunner to today's United Nations, and a past president of Princeton University. Before becoming president of the United States, he authored a popular nonfiction book, *A History of the American People,* which Griffith later used to help ground the story of *The Birth of a Nation* in history. Wilson was also an open and persistent supporter of segregation. Under his administration (1913–21), the U.S. government maintained "separate but equal" federal workplaces, bathrooms, and restaurants. A southern

---

[1] Although this quote is widely attributed to President Wilson, there is no direct evidence he actually said as much. In later years he claimed not to have said it, but only after he was publicly criticized for embracing the film.

Democrat, the first to be elected president since the Civil War, Wilson reportedly encouraged screenings of *The Birth of a Nation* for Congress and at various government agencies.

Griffith not only used Wilson's *A History of the American People* to legitimize his interpretation of the Civil War and Reconstruction, but also included in the film historical facsimile scenes of Robert E. Lee's surrender to General Grant and the assassination of President Abraham Lincoln at Ford's Theater in Washington, D.C. He also loosely based the senior patriarch of the Stoneman family, Austin Stoneman, on Representative Thaddeus Stevens (1792–1868), a Republican congressman who created the "forty acres and mule" proposal and advocated strongly for an integrated postwar society. Stoneman as Stevens comes off as a well-intentioned but terribly misguided politician who eventually understands the error of his integrationist ways. In the end, he reveals his loyalty to whiteness when he reacts in horror to the idea that Silas Lynch, his handpicked mulatto politician and model of integration, aspires to marry his daughter. Taking great liberties with the historical record, Griffith represents Northern politicians as wayward souls who ultimately end up supporting the purity of whiteness.

The historical references found in *The Birth of a Nation* have less to do with the film's plot than they do with the story of whiteness that it perpetuates, as the classic work is based less on past events than on a romantic discourse with the past—one that wraps the ideology of white supremacy in the flag of historical "accuracy." Capitalizing on both popular memory and political change, Griffith used historical references to legitimize the artistic decision to represent blackness as bestial or servile and whiteness as superior yet under threat. In this way, the representation of the past forms a key aspect of the film's complicated role in race relations, helping to ensure the film's and its director's place in history. In *The Birth of a Nation,* "Legend," notes Robert Lang, "rewrites history to conform to ideological imperatives" (4).

Griffith's commitment to white supremacy was legitimized by the rise of social Darwinism and the eugenics movement in the nineteenth century, two related scientific paradigms that divided "man" into biological subspecies that principally included Mongoloid, Negroid, and Caucasoid. The so-called Caucasoid race, particularly those of Aryan stock, was considered to be innately superior. Conversely, the Mongoloid and Negroid races were considered to be innately inferior and, as such, not quite worthy of the full rights of a democratic society. Coupled with socioeconomic systems supported by separate but overtly unequal civil rights, the science of race at this time worked to support the belief in and structure of whiteness. Although these scientific schools of thought are considered by current scientists to have been motivated by ideology rather than empirical evidence, as pointed out by, among others, Stephen J. Gould in *The Mismeasure of Man* (1981), they nonetheless helped shape the meaning of race that contemporaneous politicians and filmmakers used to support creative and legal decisions.

The influence of biological paradigms on *The Birth of a Nation* is illustrated in the scene, set in South Carolina, in which newly elected African American legislators during Reconstruction sit back in their chairs, shoeless feet perched on desks, eating chicken and leering at white women, apparently unable or unwilling to pay attention to the workings of democracy. In this interpretation of history, the story seems to be suggesting that African Americans are unable to think beyond primitive impulses. In the scene, blacks are represented as inherently unequal to whites. Scenes like this legitimize the South's efforts to deny African Americans the right to vote, which Griffith depicts at the end of the story, when the Ku Klux Klansmen stand guard, guns in hand, to supervise new elections and banish African Americans to the margins of the frame. This is a story about whiteness. Indeed, instead of showing the Klan committing acts of brutality and terrorism, which by the time Griffith made *The Birth of a Nation* was a matter of public record, he depicted them as heroes working to ensure a reunited white nation. As Hernan Vera and Andrew Gordon write, "In *The Birth of a Nation,* blacks simply do not matter: they are only counters in the struggle of a split white self to reunite" (20).

Griffith's representation of race in this way is linked directly to Dixon's novels. In Dixon's stories, the most treacherous and threatening characters are the mulattoes, people who are considered "half" white and "half" black. According to the social Darwinian paradigm, specifically its use in determining and supporting racial hierarchies, interracial relations improved the mind but not the morals of African Americans. For Dixon, this made mulattoes an even greater threat to white civilization. Although the racial order of things, or the socioeconomic structure of contemporaneous race relations, positioned African Americans as primitive and thus not too difficult to control, mulattoes were positioned as intelligent, crafty, manipulative, and immoral. They were more difficult to control, which is why interracial relationships had to be made illegal and socially unacceptable. Mulattoes were a visible sign that the riches of whiteness were being plundered by the treachery of blackness.

In *The Birth of a Nation,* we see Austin Stoneman's mulatto maid begin to tear apart her clothing at the thought of seducing the elder statesman. Her aspirations are lascivious, as she plots an improved social standing through sexual immorality. Moreover, Silas Lynch, Stoneman's mulatto politician, aspires not only to turn the South black but to marry his daughter, Elsie. His prurient aspirations are represented as vengeful and violent. "Lynch," an intertitle reads, "drunk with wine and power, orders his henchman to hurry preparations for a forced marriage." In the end, his attempt to force the white woman to wed is stopped—in the nick of time—by the Klan.

Cinematic Technique and the Story of Whiteness

Although Griffith relied on Dixon's historical fiction and Wilson's fictionalized history, the director had a long-lasting commitment to the ideology of whiteness. This history is evident in the films he made before *The Birth of a Nation*. The father of American cinema directed over 450 short films, each roughly ten minutes long, for the American Mutoscope and Biograph Company, also known as American Biograph, from 1908 to 1913. In these works, Griffith refined his technique for creating compelling stories on film. He developed a commitment to telling a story of white supremacy that included the depiction of people of color as inferior, savage, and unrestrained. For Griffith, Asians, Latinos, Native Americans, Gypsies, Jews, as well as African Americans, posed clear threats to the sanctity of whiteness. The director went as far as to use the titles of a number of his early works to market racism, including *The Greaser's Gauntlet* (1908), *Romance of a Jewess (1908), The Zulu's Heart* (1908), *The Mexican Sweethearts* (1909), *That Chink at Golden Gulch* (1910), and *The Heart of a Savage* (1911). As I have argued elsewhere, the racism in *The Birth of a Nation* can be traced to the director's Biograph work (104).

Griffith also made several Civil War films for American Biograph, including most notably *His Trust* (1911) and *His Trust Fulfilled* (1911). In these works, we see a sweeping battle scene, shots of slaves running wild as Northerners pillage Southern homes, close views that reveal the inner thoughts and emotions of characters, and compositions that feature recurring symbols of the Old South—including most prominently a Confederate officer's sword. Indeed, the sequel is based on the devotion a faithful soul has for his former Confederate master's sword long after the master has died in battle and the slaves have been freed. Griffith's camera work and plot structure seem to fetishize the Confederate sword, making it a symbol of white power and pride. And, as Michael Rogin notes in perhaps the most insightful essay written on Griffith's film, "The Sword Became a Flashing Vision," these same stylistic choices are all found, refined and coherent, in *The Birth of a Nation* (275).

Most of the stylistic innovations credited to *The Birth of a Nation* can be found in the director's earlier films. This is most clear in his development of chase-and-rescue scenes. Constructed through parallel editing, which is sometimes referred to as crosscutting or intercutting, chase-and-rescue scenes consist of shots of two or more separate but usually parallel locations interwoven to advance the film's plot. In one scene, we see the person(s) being chased. In another, we see the person(s) doing the chasing. The filmmaker cuts back and forth between the locations, sometimes increasing or decreasing the tempo of individual shots to further heighten suspense. He does this until the chaser either catches his victim or is interrupted by a hero. This is famously illustrated in one of Griffith's last yet most successful films, *Way Down East* (1920), where, at the end of the film and not a moment too soon, the hero saves the damsel in distress from crushing death as her body floats precariously toward a waterfall. We see this rescue through a series of parallel edits that serve to increase the tension caused by a woman heading perilously close to a gushing waterfall while casting a male as a savior. Griffith's stagings of chase-and-rescue scenes are always dramatic and intense, facilitating narrative suspense while emphasizing the plight of the characters. They also serve nicely to advance the story to a moral conclusion.

And yet Griffith did not develop chase scenes and parallel editing simply to advance causal events. In many of his films, including the earliest instances in which the technique is employed, the person being chased is a white woman, the chaser is a person of color, and the hero is a white male. In other words, Griffith developed the technique to support the tension surrounding interracial relations. This is perhaps best illustrated in *The Girls and Daddy* (1909). In this short work, a blackface brute is distracted from a burglary after coming upon two unsuspecting white girls. Griffith goes to great lengths to represent the girls as beautiful and innocent. Several shots show them playful in bed, hugging and kissing before they fall asleep. On seeing the young beauties, the blackface brute chases them from bedroom to living room to bedroom, only to be stopped by a white burglar who, at the risk of losing his loot and getting captured, elects to defend white purity and segregation and defend daddy's girls. The white burglar jumps on and pummels the blackface brute. Throughout the scene, Griffith employs cuts and even a panning shot, a rare technique at this point in film history, to both heighten the threat posed by blackness and to create a moral ending that reveals the innate heroics of whiteness.

This chase scene foreshadows the famous sequence in *The Birth of a Nation* in which Gus, another lustful blackface brute, chases Flora, a darling daughter of the Confederacy, to her death. As in *The Girls and Daddy,* Griffith cuts back and forth between Gus pursuing Flora with an obvious intent to rape and Flora either strolling ignorant of Gus or, realizing what Gus desires, running away from the "renegade Negro" in abject fear. "You see, I'm a Captain now—and I want to marry . . . ," an intertitle linked to Gus reads. Following the earlier scene of the legislature voting down antimiscegenation laws, the scene is constructed tautly in a forest; long shadows cast by looming trees divide natural lighting in ways that add a visual rhyme to the narrative context of the scene. Moreover, the pacing of the edits adds a degree of tension to the sequence, as Griffith initially lingers on shots of Flora. There is also a close-up of Gus with a menacing and prurient expression on his face. "Wait, missie, I won't hurt yeh," a provocative intertitle reads. In the meantime, Griffith cuts to a third location, where Ben Cameron searches in despair for the young Flora. In one of the most notorious scenes in film history, Flora elects to jump off a cliff to her death rather than be defiled by Gus. Ben is too late to save his Confederate sister, but not too late to organize and rally the Klan to track Gus down and bring him to justice. As punishment, Gus is castrated and lynched (the castration scene was later cut by Griffith in response to threats of censorship by local film-review boards). Although he doesn't save Flora from tragic death, Ben is a hero nonetheless for his creation and stewardship of the Klan.

Another brilliant parallel-editing scene is found at the end of the film, as the Klan rides to save otherwise helpless whites from threatening blacks. The end of the film actually includes two chase scenes, one following the other and both including the Klan as heroic. In one, we find a Northern father, held up with the elder Cameron in a cabin, holding his rifle butt over his child's head, poised to kill her lest she be attacked by the black brutes outside. The situation apparently calls for the same fate suffered by Flora. Griffith moves the camera into a closeup of the little girl's face, revealing simultaneously fear and innocence. In the other scene, we see Lynch and his henchman on the verge of forcing Elsie to marry the mulatto politician. She falls into his dark arms as he seemingly smiles in satisfaction. Both scenes are powerful, as Griffith has the camera follow the Klan's ride to the rescue along a winding forest road. The effect of this technique is that the shots of the Klan offer viewers a sense of impending heroism. In both scenes, the Klan indeed arrives in the nick of time, narrative tension at full pressure, restoring white supremacy once and for all. The blacks are subdued, and the Klan receives a parade and, ostensibly, applause. Constructed with artistry through parallel editing, a technique now commonly employed by filmmakers around the world, these final shots are among the most racist moments in American film history.

Refracting Whiteness

Disgusted by the negative images of African Americans and the positive images of the Klan in *The Birth of a Nation,* the National Association for the Advancement of Colored People (NAACP), as well as numerous other social and political organizations, called for protests and boycotts.

W. E. B. DuBois, one of America's leading intellectuals at the time, published poignant commentaries in *The Crisis,* the NAACP's journal. These actions resulted in exhibitions of the film being delayed, as well as local review boards, fearful of race riots, requiring minor changes. Even the Communist Party got involved, picketing the film as evidence of the Fascist failings of capitalism. As Janet Staiger, quoting Nickieann Fleener-Marzec, notes, "Between 1915 and 1973 the right to screen *The Birth of a Nation* was challenged at least 120 times" (199).

The famous director responded to the criticism of his film in an editorial published in the *New York Globe.* Claiming that his "associates" maintained a "dignified silence in the face of an organized attack" by "publicity seekers and fanatics," Griffith sought to ensure both the box-office success of the film and its place in film history:

> *Most well informed men know now that slavery was an economic mistake. The treatment of the Negroes during the days of Reconstruction is shown effectually and graphically in our picture. We show many phrases of the questions and we do pay particular attention to those faithful Negroes who stay with the former masters and were ready to give up their lives to protect their white friends. No characters in the story are applauded with greater fervor than the good Negroes whose devotion is so clearly shown. (Griffith 169)*

Griffith's response was clearly designed as a marketing ploy to further ensure the success of the film. As we have seen, it reveals also a key feature of the story. In *The Birth of a Nation,* there are "good" blacks, African Americans who remain faithful to whiteness and segregation, and "bad" blacks, African Americans who are bestial, lustful, untrustworthy, ignorant, and unfaithful to whiteness. This is a narrative pattern Griffith established during his days at American Biograph, as we have seen in *His Trust* and *His Trust Fulfilled,* and it remained throughout his career a preferred marketing strategy.

The controversy over *The Birth of a Nation* did not end with Griffith's deft use of the editorial pages of the *New York Globe,* and in fact continued through subsequent exhibitions of the film. Several scholars report race rioting in major cities after screenings of the film. Equally disturbing is the apparent fact that the Klan used the classic film as a recruiting tool. According to Michael Rogin, the Klan "screened the movie in the 1920s to build membership in the millions" (290). Other scholars have reported a rise in the number of lynchings of blacks by white vigilantes due to the film's depiction of African American men as rapists.

The impact of *The Birth of a Nation* was felt not only in the political and legal spheres of American life, but also in the specific experiences and protests of the African American community. In 1920, for example, African American independent filmmaker and novelist Oscar Micheaux addressed the film when he made *Within Our Gates.* In this classic, Micheaux's ending serves as a challenging homage to the end of *The Birth of a Nation.* We see the attempted rape of a black woman by a white man as her family is being lynched for a crime they did not commit. In this scene, which is not explicitly tied to a historical event but is nonetheless far more historically accurate than any image of blackness found in Griffith's classic, Micheaux exposes the representation of African Americans in *The Birth of a Nation* as a lie that masks the horrors of white supremacy during the era of slavery and Reconstruction. It must be remembered that, in reality, white slaveholders raped African American women in numbers that were both horrific and apparent to most people living in the South.

Despite protests and direct evidence that the Klan was violent in the extreme, Griffith remained stoic and even belligerent—refusing to acknowledge the film's racism or its culpability in advancing the agenda of the Klan. In 1930, upon the release of one of his last films, *Abraham Lincoln,* the southern director sat down with Walter Huston, the star of the Lincoln film, for an interview. In this filmed interview, which is included on the Kino International DVD *("The Birth of a Nation" and the Civil War Films of D. W. Griffith),* Huston presents Griffith with a Confederate officer's sword, an ironic recapitulation of the sword found in *His Trust, His Trust Fulfilled,* and *The Birth of a Nation.* Griffith is visibly touched by the gift, and goes on to defend his depiction of the Klan as honorable and justified. He even reminisces romantically about how Mother helped stitch their white robes as they rode in defense of the Old South.

Conclusion

Irrespective of Griffith's indifference to the history of the Klan, the controversy over the film illustrates the ways in which cinema is informed by and informs our approach to race relations. To this day, scholars continue to argue about how to situate the film in history: Should it be approached as art or as propaganda? Should it be condemned for advocating racism or for the censorship it provoked? It is not uncommon for contemporary scholars to sidestep the issue and either avoid teaching the film altogether or, on showing it, ignore the incestuous relationship between the development of cinematic style and the story of white supremacy.

The Birth of a Nation should remind film scholars of at least two critical imperatives. First, films do not simply reflect the context in which they are produced. They also inform the direction of both creative and social forces. Griffith's classic work certainly reflected the meaning of race dominating the early twentieth century, as this essay has tried to demonstrate. Yet it also refracted racial ideologies in ways that impacted the meaning of whiteness in the future. *The Birth of a Nation* greatly influenced the direction of the Hollywood style. Moreover, it prompted protests, censorship, and rigorous debate about the American color line. Scholars have linked screenings of the film to a dramatic rise in Klan membership, to lynchings, to riots, and to a vigorous national critique of stereotypes. As late as the 1940s, the NAACP organized groups to picket screenings of the film and to protest the negative stereotypes the film promotes. In response, the film was rereleased numerous times in attempts to edit, minimize, and excuse the film's racist message while maintaining its status as a classic. As KVC Entertainment advertises on the back cover of its video case, "Because the story was told from the South's point of view, *The Birth of a Nation* was denounced by various liberal and civil rights organizations, and banned by the NAACP. Yet, no film before, or ever since, has portrayed the most painful chapter of America's history with such profound realism."

A second critical imperative concerns a presumed distinction between art and ideology. *The Birth of a Nation* illustrates the fact that film can be at once stylistic and political, simultaneously imaginative, brilliant, reactionary, and racist. If *The Birth of a Nation* teaches us anything, it is the ways in which the art of cinema can construct white supremacy as history written with artistry. The innovations Griffith made in pursuit of a style of narrative filmmaking were not simply in the service of storytelling; they were in the service of white supremacy. Thus, the art of *The Birth of a Nation* is its racism, particularly its construction of whiteness through the lens of black stereotypes and the craft of cinematic technique. In *The Birth of a Nation,* art is ideological, form is content, and cinema is simultaneously moving, artistic, ugly, and painful.

Credits

United States, 1915, Epoch Producing Company

Director and Producer: D. W. Griffith
Screenplay: Thomas F. Dixon Jr. (novel and play), D. W. Griffith, Frank E. Woods, and Thomas F. Dixon Jr.
Cinematography: G. W. Bitzer
Art Direction: Cash Shockley, Joseph Stringer, and Frank Wortman
Music: Joseph Carl Breil and D. W. Griffith
Costume Design: Robert Godstein

CAST:

Elsie Stoneman	Lillian Gish
Flora Cameron	Mae Marsh
Col. Ben Cameron	Henry B. Walthall
Margaret Cameron	Miriam Cooper
Lydia Brown	Mary Alden
Austin Stoneman	Ralph Lewis
Silas Lynch	George Siegmann
Gus	Walter Long
Tod Stoneman	Robert Harron
Jeff (blacksmith)	Wallace Reid
Abraham Lincoln	Joseph Henabery
Phil Stoneman	Elmer Clifton
Mrs. Cameron	Josephine Crowell
Dr. Cameron	Spottiswoode Aitken
Wade Cameron	George Beranger
Duke Cameron	Maxfield Stanley
Mammy	Jennie Lee
Gen. Ulysses S. Grant	Donald Crisp
Gen. Robert E. Lee	Howard Gaye

Bibliography

Bernardi, Daniel. "The Voice of Whiteness: D. W. Griffith's Biograph (1908–1913)." *The Birth of Whiteness: Race and the Emergence of U.S. Cinema.* Ed. Daniel Bernardi. New Brunswick: Rutgers UP, 1996. 103–28.

Gould, Stephen J. *The Mismeasure of Man.* New York: Norton, 1996.

Griffith, D. W. "Reply to the *New York Globe.*" *New York Globe* 10 Apr. 1915. Rpt. in Lang, *"Birth of a Nation"* 168–70.

Lang, Robert, ed. *"The Birth of a Nation": D. W. Griffith.* New Brunswick: Rutgers UP, 1994.

Lang, Robert. *"The Birth of a Nation:* History, Ideology, Narrative Form." Lang, *"Birth of a Nation"* 3–24.

Rogin, Michael. "The Sword Became a Flashing Vision: D. W. Griffith's *The Birth of a Nation.*" Lang, *"Birth of a Nation"* 250–93.

Staiger, Janet. " 'The Birth of a Nation': Reconsidering Its History." Lang, *"Birth of a Nation" 195–213.*

Vera, Hernan, and Andrew Gordon. *Screen Saviors: Hollywood Fictions of Whiteness.* New York: Rowan, 2003.

The Birth of a Nation:
Reconsidering Its Reception

Janet Staiger

In August 1978, the Ku Klux Klan of Oxnard, California, exhibited *The Birth of Nation* as a fund-raiser and membership promotion. A militant communist splinter group, the Progressive Labor party, counterdemonstrated. And local Mexican-American and black associations protested against both camps. Tempers were hot and eventually violence broke out.[1] Once again, sixty-three years after its first turbulent showings, the 1915 film *The Birth of a Nation* had precipitated a ferocity and wrath sufficient to provoke men and women into a physical response.

One of my questions about the reception of *The Birth of a Nation* is why this film continues to outrage individuals. While the subject matter itself is probably sufficient as a solution to this problem, I would offer the thesis that *The Birth of a Nation* is encrusted with a history of responses and debates which make it a symbol of more than racist propaganda. At least for two decades, diatribes against it and defenses of its director play out major political battles in leftist politics as well as important debates in the history of film scholarship. Consequently, the continuing history of the reception of *The Birth of a Nation* can be considered as a nodal point for analyzing conditions of reception as they relate to evaluating subject matter and narrational techniques, positing effects of movies, and, ultimately, revealing racial attitudes and political positions of a film's opponents and defenders.

Specifically, although the 1915 reception of *The Birth of a Nation* can be organized around interpretations related to the question of racism—in which one can construct a complex continuum of reactions labeled by Joel Williamson as liberal to radical conservatism,[2] in the late 1930s, another continuum transforms the conditions for the film's subsequent reception. This second continuum can be associated with the contemporary political crisis of the European war for leftist radicals. Here the dynamics shift from, on the one hand, according to Communist party members, accusations of the film's complicity with capitalism's exploitation of workers and blacks to, on the other hand, defenses of the film by some leftists breaking from the party line. These defenses include attacking the film's critics as "totalitarians." Consequently, the race issue per se is reconfigured, intersecting with debates over the political economy and arguments about evaluating films and other cultural products of that political economy. The popular representation of the reception of a film becomes one of the conditions for its subsequent reception. First, a bit of context before I move to an analysis of the history of the film's reception.

The Historical Setting

Most film scholars are somewhat familiar with events surrounding the initial distribution of *The Birth of a Nation*. Thomas Cripps notes that the film appeared as conditions for African Americans were deteriorating. Despite its progressivism in some areas of social action, Woodrow Wilson's presidency was perceived by blacks as a resurgence of "Southern ideals"; black people were denied the ballot box; Jim Crow laws were expanding; and between 1898 and 1908, race riots occurred in Wilmington

(North Carolina), New York City, New Orleans, Atlanta, and Springfield (Illinois). However, African-American leadership and consciousness had also "sharpened."[3] Although from the mid-1890s, Booker T. Washington was assumed by many to represent the voice of African Americans, extensive violence by white racist extremists during the same time provoked alternative strategies. W.E.B. Du Bois specifically began to stand out after 1903, with his published attack on Washington's leadership. In 1905, Du Bois organized the Niagara Falls Conference, assaulting accommodationism and promoting a nascent "black is beautiful" campaign. In 1909, the Niagara movement and northern white liberals formed the National Association for the Advancement of Colored People (NAACP), which by 1914 had six thousand members in various cities.[4]

African Americans on the west coast began to protest against *The Birth of a Nation* once they were aware that the film was to be based on Thomas Dixon's play, *The Clansman*.[5] In 1905, Dixon combined two of his novels, *The Leopard's Spots* (1902) and *The Clansman* (1905), into dramatic form and began a theatrical road tour. At that time, however, Dixon's extreme racism was not widely acceptable, even in the South. Joel Williamson in *The Crucible of Race* argues that the recent race riots produced repercussions. For various reasons, including public safety, after 1906 few individuals encouraged representing blacks as beasts and advocating their deportation in order to achieve national unity and security—two extremely radical-conservative positions taken by Dixon.[6] Williamson argues that from 1880 through 1920, three "mentalities" exist in southern thinking about people of color. The "liberal" believed in the black's possibilities. Perhaps the oldest, the "conservative," presumed inferiority but was willing to permit these people in their "place." The "radical conservative" (which Williamson argues emerges in 1889 and appears through 1915 and in which category Williamson places Dixon) thought that the " 'new' negro" was regressing into savagery. For this mentality, the paranoia over interracial sex (through rape or marriage) was a fear of the possible "perverted" offspring. As Thomas Gassett expresses it, "If a black has white intermixture, he is especially dangerous. White intermixture, Dixon thought, improved the intellect of blacks without changing their morals."*[7] Dixon was not, however, unique in his opinions (and many may have held them more quietly). For example, in 1907, Benjamin R. Tillman, a U.S. senator from South Carolina, defended the South's repression of blacks by arguing that the evils of the Reconstruction era proved the inability of people of color to assume public roles, that they were inherently inferior, and that southern men needed to protect their women. Tillman claimed that black militiamen were overheard to say: "The President is our friend. The North is with us. We intend to kill all the white men, take the land, marry the white women, and then these white children will wait on us."[8] Nor was radical-conservative racism confined to the South. In 1916, New York City anthropologist Madison Grant in *The Passing of the Great Race* claimed that racial "hybrids" were suicidal for the American.*[9] Dixon's two novels and play dramatized these beliefs. In 1906 in Philadelphia, blacks rioted over the play, with the effect that public safety claims were used to block some openings.[10] *The Clansman,* however, did continue to tour through the end of the decade.

One month prior to *The Birth of a Nation*'s opening in New York City, the NAACP chose the strategy of a nationwide protest against the film, hoping to prevent its exhibition on similar grounds of threat to the peace. This tactical choice produced conflicts among the NAACP's supporters since many of the association's white backers also tended to oppose censorship.[11] Furthermore, the film's technical virtuosity became a compensating feature to rationalize exhibiting the movie. Thus, any individual (then or now) might have conflicting or overdetermined views about *The Birth of a Nation* depending on that person's attitudes toward and judgments of its representation, its technical presentation, and censorship.

The NAACP did manage to delay several showings of the film, and some film review boards required changes. Although violence—such as throwing eggs at the screen—occurred,*[12] public safety alarmists were disarmed by the protesters' recognizing the long-term disadvantage of violent tactics. In an effort to "soften" the content, the film was edited, several intertitles were added, and the short-lived Hampton Institute epilogue was tacked on. Aggressive defenses by Dixon and D. W. Griffith also blocked opponents.*[13] I will return to these arguments momentarily.

Between 1915 and 1973 the right to screen *The Birth of a Nation* "was challenged at least 120 times."[14] Indeed, the strategy of the NAACP was to continue its opposition to the film anytime someone tried to revive it. In 1921 the NAACP petitioned the Boston mayor not to show it "because it is a malicious misrepresentation of the colored people, depicting them as moral perverts," while five people were arrested for picketing and protesting in New York City.[15] When *The Birth of a Nation* was to be rereleased with a sound track in 1930, the NAACP and others appealed to Will Hays and the Motion Picture Producers and Distributors Association to censor it, as they controlled sexual and criminal content, but no equivalency for racism was made.[16]

A reinforcement to protesters was apparent proof from social scientists that the film created attitudinal changes. When one of the 1933 Payne Fund studies screened *The Birth of a Nation* to 434 middle and high school students in a predominantly white Illinois town, the researchers determined the "largest effect found in any of the experiments we conducted."[17] The children's "favorable" opinion of African Americans dropped from a mean of 7.46 on a scale of 11 to 0 to 5.93, down 1.48 points. Testing five months later suggested only a partial return to the original views.

But it was later in that decade when a radical transformation in the implications of the film's interpretation and evaluation occurred among a political subculture in the United States. One's view of *The Birth of a Nation* became not only a litmus test of one's attitudes or beliefs about races, censorship, and aesthetics but also about the contemporary international political scene. The film became encrusted with debates and accusations exchanged between party-line Communists and anti-Stalinists.

The Initial Reception of *The Birth of a Nation*

To clarify the complexities and ironies of positions that were to be taken in the late 1930s, when Communists appropriated the film as a symptom of fascist and monopoly capitalist ideologies, I want to summarize the debates of the midteens.*[18] The comparison between these periods valuably illuminates the complexities and contradictions that this transformation produces.

When *The Birth of a Nation* was originally exhibited, reviewers uniformly praised the presentation of the subject matter, separating off the narrational techniques (i.e., style) from what was being represented. (This "form/content" split is typical of reviewing of the period and is due most immediately to nineteenth-century aesthetics.) The writers then varied: some thought the representations were accurate; others were neutral; some ignored the issue; and the rest regretted or challenged what they saw. Numerous attacks on the subject matter were marshaled, but for the sake of brevity, five may be delineated as major themes. The most obvious indignity was that the film distorted and consequently falsified the history of the Reconstruction era. Within this theme were subroutines: the facts were inaccurate or the examples were not representative of the whole history. Second, and related to the fabrication of history attack, was the assertion that the film misrepresented the character of blacks both as individual people and as a race. In particular, reviewers noted that the only people of color shown were either bestial or subservient to whites. As the *Crisis* put it, "The Negro [is] represented either as an ignorant fool, a vicious rapist, a venal and unscrupulous politician or a faithful but doddering idiot."*[19]

A third theme was that the film glorified crime, specifically lynching. Writers pointed out ironies and contradictions following from that: pictures showing murder and robbery were routinely censored. Furthermore, whites were willing to suppress by law boxing pictures in which blacks beat whites, but they would not stop the exhibition of *The Birth of a Nation*. Specifically, the 1912 Sims act preventing interstate transportation of boxing films was enacted after the heavyweight champion, John Arthur "Jack" Johnson, who was black, kept beating white contenders. In 1910, when Johnson defeated Jim Jeffries, at least eighteen blacks were killed in the fight's aftermath, which reinforced sentiment for the passage of the federal bill.[20]

Fourth, opponents argued that the film incited prejudices against people of color, having an immoral effect or threatening public peace (as its predecessor *The Clansman* had done). Finally, *The Birth of a Nation* taught the doctrine that African Americans should be removed from the United States, a doctrine undemocratic, unchristian, and unlawful.

Defenders of *The Birth of a Nation* did not directly respond to all of the opponents' themes, and they introduced ones of their own. Griffith and Dixon both argued that the historical representation was accurate. Griffith wrote in 1915 that to show the history of the West one would have to "show the atrocities committed by the Indians against the whites."[21] Dixon appealed to the argument that historical accounts are variable since they are based on perspectives. At another point he claimed historical truth based on popular consensus: the film "expresses the passionate faith of the entire white population of the South. If I am wrong, they are wrong. The number of white people in the South who differ from my views of the history of Reconstruction could be housed on a half-acre lot [*sic*]."[22]

Regarding the accusation of a biased representation of blacks, Dixon, Griffith, and others claimed that the film authentically depicted the character of blacks during the Reconstruction era, if not now. Furthermore, the film not only portrayed bad people of color but also praised good ones who protected their former masters. Thus, the representation was balanced.

Defenders attacked their opponents in three ways. They argued that artistic and dramatic merit justified the film's exhibition, that their opposition was stifling free speech, and that those who wanted the film banned supported interracial marriages. This last theme was particularly promoted by Dixon, but even Griffith writes, "The attack of the organized opponents to this picture is centered upon that feature of it which they deem might become an influence against the intermarriage of blacks and whites."[23]

Among the approximately sixty reviews and articles studied, no extrinsic reasons for alignment with one position or another were discernible; for example, there were no consistencies from a regional perspective. Although Russell Merritt writes, "Most of the audience that came out of the [Boston] Tremont theatre that night in 1915 . . . believed Griffith's story was historically true,"[24] other northerners were not of that opinion, with many of them leading the attack on the film. Dixon claimed he presented "the passionate faith of the entire white population of the South."[25] This view is somewhat supported by John Hammond Moore's survey of South Carolina's reviews. Moore found that the state's papers about-faced from their 1905 denunciation of Dixon's *The Clansman*. When the play toured, reviewers took issue with the historical accuracy of the thesis, chastised the Ku Klux Klan for getting out of hand, and opposed the themes of blacks as beasts and the need to transport them out of the United States. *The Birth of a Nation* received no similar objections, with "almost unanimous approval" of the film.*[26] However, the white arrested for throwing eggs at the New York Liberty Theater presentation claimed, "1 am a Southerner and a libertarian, and I believe in the education and uplifting of the negro. It made my blood boil to see the play and I threw the eggs at the screen."[27]

The lack of a coherent regional response is scarcely surprising since racism occurs throughout the United States. While a more systematic analysis of opinions might reveal patterns associated with sectors of the nation, Williamson's observation of at least three southern "mentalities" (liberal, conservative, and radical-conservative) during the 1880–1920s seems reconfirmed by this study although these mentalities may be more national than regional. Furthermore, from today's perspective, even the 1880–1920s liberal mentality is scarcely a nonracist attitude.

For these 1915 spectators of *The Birth of a Nation*, besides the questions of causes or types of racism, it is important to consider the complications of assumptions about the possible effects of watching movies and social responses to that possibility. While turn-of-the-century reformers operated on the assumption that a scientific study of society and humans provided the basis for policymaking, many also steered away from overt censorship. The National Board of Review, the film industry's voluntary self-regulation system, merely advised film companies about subject matter (although local boards with legal powers could require changes). Confronted by this film, many opponents argued that portions of the film could have real behavioral effects, stimulating or changing preexistent attitudes in directions unfavorable to social harmony. On the basis of actual experiences following theatrical productions, they tried to argue that *The Birth of a Nation* was a threat to public peace. While defenders did not disagree with the position that films could be causal forces, they stressed First Amendment rights of free speech—a widely accepted discourse considered an idea fundamental to the preservation of the United States. As a constructed characteristic of the identity of "American," "free speech" serves as a centering notion against which non-American positions are positioned as dangerous. Opponents to *The Birth of a Nation* could only argue, *not* that the defenders were wrong, but that the film threatened public peace, which might be more important than free speech. This prediction of danger, however, was a hard claim to prove since violence was very local and sporadic.

Placing positions of free speech versus public safety in a continuum of political persuasions (liberal to conservative) is impossible, given the historical variations on this debate. Witness, for example, the 1989 U.S. Supreme Court decision that burning the American flag is acceptable as a form of political expression. Judges labeled in 1989 as "liberal" and "conservative" show up on both sides of the judgment, as do individuals in the subsequent furor over amending the Constitution to prohibit such an act. For the analysis of *The Birth of a Nation;* however, the implications of the differing positions need to be stressed, if not labeled. Everyone agreed that films had some type of effect, but not everyone concurred as to the relative merits of solutions in balance with possible compensating values (e.g., free speech and a widely accepted aesthetic quality). Legal actions related to society's needs were in conflict, but everyone recognized that this film pushed the question to a certain limit. That racist (from today's perspective) material was eventually tolerated is not indicative of a social decision that free speech overrides filmic effects. After all, legal and semilegal apparatus (mainstream industry agreements not to compete in subject areas that might provoke the retaliation of pressure groups) did censor subject matter related to certain types of criminal behavior and sexuality. Thus, one conclusion is that either racism was perceived as less menacing than that other subject matter, or it was in the interest of those in positions of authority to permit an amount of racist representation up to the borderline of the tolerable (relative to the counterthreat of suppression of opinion). However you understand these conditions, a significant factor in the reception of *The Birth of a Nation* in 1915 is the political and racist underpinnings of social policy in relation to the film's representation and effectivity.

Thus, the initial reception of *The Birth of a Nation* constitutes what might be called a generic reaction quite understandable within the contradictions of the period's social formation. While I might draw out numerous other discursive strands within the individual essays relating them to their historical contexts, the dominant points involve an agreement that subject matter and narrational procedures could be judged separately, but differences existed over evaluating subject matter and its potential effects on spectators. Here tacit race attitudes intersect with other beliefs—ones about what constitutes acceptable historiography; whether a film should be judged on the content or effects of its subject matter, narrational procedures, or some combination of them; and whether censorship of certain representations is more important than free speech. All three of these issues still concern scholars and citizens today, making these aspects of the reception of *The Birth of a Nation* constant across a stretch of seventy-five years.

A Transformation of the Reception of *The Birth of a Nation*

In the late 1930s, themes from the 1915 period would reoccur, but other revisions are indications of how historical change and political perspectives influence argumentation about films. As events in Europe and the Soviet Union altered the political strategies and alliances of the American radical Left, *The Birth of a Nation* continued to be an exemplary case in film studies for issues of socially acceptable representations of U.S. racial minorities, procedures of response against some subject matter, and systems of evaluating narrational procedures and possible audience effects.

In 1936 Richard Watts published in the leftist journal *New Theatre and Film* a commentary on Griffith that criticized *The Birth of a Nation*'s "cruel unfairness to the Negro." Three years later, Lewis Jacobs published his history *The Rise of the American Film,* concluding that "the film was a passionate and persuasive avowal of the inferiority of the Negro. In viewpoint it was, surely, narrow and prejudiced." But in December 1939, David Platt went further. Writing for the Communist party newspaper, the *Daily Worker,* Platt argued that *The Birth of a Nation*, "by creating racial prejudice, helped create the basis for war [World War I] propaganda." Furthermore, the resurrection of the

Ku Klux Klan, aided by the film, worked to harass African Americans to participate in the First World War effort.²⁸

Now, this argument may need some context. From the early 1930s, but particularly from 1939 until the end of the Hitler-Stalin pact, the *Daily Worker* took an antiwar stance. Part of that project was an appeal to individuals such as blacks to see the European events not from a nationalist perspective but from one of class. This was not their fight since it was not that of any member of the working class; neither capitalists in the United States nor fascists in Germany were the blacks' friends. In early 1940, the *Daily Worker* and its supporters participated with blacks in picketing theaters reviving *The Birth of a Nation.* *²⁹

Platt's act had a tradition in marxist aesthetic criticism: demonstrating the complicity of a film or literary text with capitalist goals was a well-established approach to art evaluation and the activation of political sensibilities. Furthermore, after 1915 *The Birth of a Nation* had been continually criticized for its racism by individuals not all of whom were particularly aligned with radical-Left politics. For instance, in 1938 in *Current History,* V. F. Calverton published an outstanding analysis of the historiographical problems of the film, pointing out "its inaccuracies, exaggerations, and historical indecencies and distortions."³⁰

In February 1940, Platt continued his assault, printing a series of seven articles reviewing the representation of blacks in Hollywood and painstakingly developing the thesis that Hollywood, in cooperation with capitalist interests, "deliberately and carefully fostered" prejudice to divide Negro and white and rule both." Citing the 1933 Payne Fund Studies and evidence of an increase in lynching in 1915, Platt implied that the film was directly responsible for changes in attitude and behavior.³¹

Whether because of a personal change in politics, a response to Platt's articles, or another cause, Seymour Stern took up in 1940 the defense of the film. Stern was to claim later that articles he wrote in 1940 "provoked a bitter reaction": "former friends and acquaintances ceased to be such." Writing for the socialist and, in his words, "anti-Stalinist" *New Leader,* Stern accused "Negro leaders and left-wing liberals" of attacking Griffith as being "anti-Negro." He went on to claim that after Platt's February *Daily Worker* articles, growing evidence indicated "a well-organized, underground boycott campaign against 'The Birth of a Nation,'" a "campaign of boycott and terrorism." "Several days [after Platt's articles], Communist Party agents and stooges from innocent-front organizations, who had gotten wind of the proposed revival [of *The Birth of a Nation*], visited the manager of the theatre and proceeded to terrorize him in much the same manner as the alleged clansmen in the picture terrorized Negroes."³² The *New Leader*'s editorial note accompanying Stern's essay said that the article was

> *the first of a short series on Communist activity in the movie business, [which] shows how, in accordance with the new Stalinite [sic] line on the Negroes, the caviar comrades are trying to suppress the showing of "The Birth of a Nation."... The next articles by Seymour Stern, who has spent more than a decade in Hollywood writing motion picture scenarios will reveal the Communist ramifications in the Museum of Modern Art Film Library and in the documentary [filmmaking] field.* *³³

The Dies Committee was already investigating Hollywood for communists when this invective appeared.

What is happening becomes, in retrospect, ironic and sad. For Stern *and* Platt, along with Lewis Jacobs and Harry Alan Potamkin, had started the 1930s on a high and cooperative note. In 1930, these four individuals were cofounders and editors of *Experimental Cinema,* an early progressive film journal.*³⁴ However, several factors during the decade were to split these people and their associates into bitter factions.

Among the most significant of these factors were debates by leftists over the connections between literature and social or political policy, the appropriate roles of artists concerning approved party aesthetic policies, and the analysis of subject matter and narrational procedures. The vicissitudes of radical progressive thought in the 1930s about these concerns are extensive and complex.

In only the most general terms, in the 1920s, marxists equated "good art with successful propaganda" but considered aesthetic experimentation permissible. Liberals such as Stark Young at the *New Republic* or Joseph Wood Krutch at the *Nation* dissented from that view, emphasizing internal structure and personal responses over content. This judgment reversed in the next decade. By the mid-1930s, splits among leftists developed over the artists' responsibilities to people, given the crisis of the depression. Could artists afford to detach themselves or their art from social communication? Richard Pells argues that Edmund Wilson's *Axel's Castle* (1931) participates in laying the groundwork for the need to communicate with people, developing the thesis that the symbolists and avant-gardists unconsciously absorbed the worst features of bourgeois individualism: intense subjectivity was inappropriate. Not all radicals agreed.[35]

Another factor, most important at the end of the decade and interpenetrating with aesthetic and cultural theory, was artists' increasing disenchantment with the Communist party as it changed policies during the 1930s. Darnel Aaron argues that the execution of Nicola Sacco and Bartolomeo Vanzetti in August 1927 mobilized many liberals into more radical politics. Furthermore, the depression deepened individuals' beliefs that capitalism was a bankrupt economic system. But after 1937, Stalinism began to seem as threatening as European fascism. The causes for this shift included the purges, dissatisfaction with party policies during the Spanish Civil War, and the blow of the Hitler-Stalin Pact on 23 August 1939, followed by Germany's invasion of Poland a week later. It should not be surprising that conservatives and even liberals attacked Bolshevik marxists at this point, but progressives such as socialists did as well. Max Nomad in the *New Leader* proceeded to redefine allies and enemies: " 'The Socialist system of collective ownership is compatible with totalitarianism,' " he wrote in January 1941.[36]

Experimental Cinema started publication in 1930. Its initial and consistent stance in favor of Soviet cinema was, as George Amberg put it, "in 1930, . . . implicitly involved [in] a taking of sides, if not a political commitment. The position adopted and advocated by *Experimental Cinema* was unequivocally socialist."*[37] However, in 1934 a "bitter dispute" among the journal's staff and supporters developed. The communist Workers' International Relief commissioned Stern and the editors of *Experimental Cinema* to make a film dealing with exploitation of Mexican migrant workers in Imperial Valley, California. Eighteen thousand feet of film were exposed, which the Workers' International Relief claimed publicly in the *Daily Worker* comprised mostly arty shots of cantaloupes. Stern responded that *Experimental Cinema* wanted an "artistic achievement as well as a piece of agitative propaganda." Furthermore, in the same (and to-be-last) issue of *Experimental Cinema* with Stern's justification appeared a tribute to Potamkin, who had recently died. Samuel Brody, writing in the *Daily Worker,* criticized *Experimental Cinema* for printing the tribute, since *Experimental Cinema* had disagreed with Potamkin's aesthetics. Brody wrote that in the previous three years divergent roads had been taken: "Potamkin Leftwards, E. C. to the Right."[38]

In early 1935, *Experimental Cinema*'s major support, the Workers Film and Photo League, broke up, and members adopted variant positions regarding politics and aesthetics. Jacobs remained independent in the far Left. Platt joined the *Daily Worker* as a staff writer, as well as working for other communist cultural publications. Stern continued on as a filmmaker and writer. His articles reflect his taking the position that judgments about aesthetics and narrational procedures were separable from those about subject matter and representation. Later, Stern became a strong anti-Stalinist while defending Griffith and *The Birth of a Nation*.

Given the political and personal context, Stern's 1940 vituperative response to Platt's strongly worded attack—Platt's charge that *The Birth of a Nation* as reactionary and racist—set off an escalation of charges and countercharges that would continue for the next fifteen years and beyond as Stern took on more critics of Griffith. Somewhere along the line Sergei Eisenstein's name must have been invoked, for in January 1941, Eisenstein telegraphed the *Daily Worker* to deny that he had praised *The Birth of a Nation*. His aesthetic choice was clear: "The disgraceful propaganda of racial hatred toward colored people which permeates this film cannot be redeemed by purely cinematographic effects in this production." Eisenstein also refers to his forthcoming article about "the interrelation between Soviet Cinema and the 'old man' of American films," most likely meaning his

"Dickens, Griffith, and the Film Today" (1944). There Eisenstein argues that narrational procedures are isomorphically related to ideological development.[39]

In 1946, Peter Noble published "A Note on an Idol" in *Sight and Sound*. Noble accused Griffith of being "a pioneer of prejudice," albeit he was also a pioneer of technique. Noble's reading of the film is extreme, exceeding any 1915 account that I found. He describes Silas Lynch as attempting to rape Elsie Stoneman, whereas initial spectators saw Lynch as violently forcing her to marry him. Additionally, Noble describes Gus as "frothy-mouthed" in his pursuit of Flora.[40] (Every 1915 review did assume though that Gus intended to rape Flora Cameron.)

In the following *Sight and Sound* issue, both Griffith and Stern reply. Griffith writes that "my attitude towards the Negroes has always been one of affection and brotherly feeling. I was partly raised by a lovable old Negress down in old Kentucky." He also claims that the film was historically accurate. Stern begins his response with what can only be considered Red-baiting, given the political climate at that time. He compares Noble's remarks to the pre–World War II "anti-Griffith libel issued periodically, and often in the identical phrases, from certain political publications in the U.S.A and the U.S.S.R." Stern then proceeds to argue and expand upon many of the themes that appeared in the 1915 defenses. *The Birth of a Nation* is historically accurate. In fact, Stern claims that it is based on Woodrow Wilson's *History of the American People*. He accuses Noble of basing his analysis on Jacobs's history of American film, a book filled with "errors, falsehoods and fanciful misinterpretations of American film in general and Griffith and his work in particular."[41]

The second theme is the representation of blacks. The villains in the movie are not "the uneducated and newly-freed Negroes but the *doctrines* of certain fanatical and vengeful Northern whites, who duped the Negroes with glittering promises of wealth and power."*[42] Moreover, the film shows good as well as bad African Americans: "In racial hatred, race is race, black is black, and there can be no exceptions."

Stern makes three additional observations. For one, he compares the South during the Reconstruction era to France and Norway during the Nazi occupation. Resorting to reading by allegory, Stern suggests that the South is rejecting the "totalitarianism" of northern radicals (e.g., Stoneman/Thadeus Stevens): "*The Birth of a Nation* exposes the ideology and tactics of a revolutionary movement; it dramatises the defeat of this movement by a counter-revolution, the leaders and protagonists of which are the people themselves." By paralleling northern carpetbagger politics to fascist totalitarianism and, eventually, to Stalinism, Stern makes *The Birth of a Nation* express liberal, democratic doctrines.

Additionally, Stern explains that it is communist propaganda to call Griffith a pioneer of prejudice:

> *[Noble] is, of course, merely echoing in strangely familiar accents and phrases the astounding falsehoods and unbelievable nonsense on the subject which already have poured in volume from the presses of the N.Y. "Daily Worker," the "New Masses," the defunct "Friday" and "New Theatre," or from such specious and shockingly misleading politico-economic tracts as "The Rise of the American Film."*

In this list, Stern ignores several decades of African-American protests. Finally, Stern counters the leftist claims that films have effects. He writes: "Surely Mr. Noble cannot but know that films do not start attitudes or trends in political or social relations; they merely *reflect* them."

The debates continued for several issues in *Sight and Sound*. In 1948 Noble published a monograph, *The Negro in Films*, only slightly modifying his stance. And in 1950, V. J. Jerome, considered a mainstream Communist, wrote *The Negro in Hollywood Films*—a sophisticated analysis of the ideology of racism in American films.[43]

Stern continued his defense of Griffith, admitting that the man's films had some faults but maintaining a spirited attack centered on communism and Stalinism as the source of Griffith's troubles. In 1949, as the U.S. Congress stepped up its repression of left-wing radicals and sent the Hollywood Ten to prison, Stern dates the " 'official' " start of the marxist attack on Griffith as 1940, when "the would-be cultural dictators of the Left—the new generation of Marxist film critics and self-styled film 'historians' " tried to destroy Griffith, who "stands in challenging and diametric opposition to contemporary Marxist-Stalinist ideological values." He expands this theme in 1956, publishing "The Cold War against David Wark Griffith," where he asserts that Communists also manipulate film scholarship: "Since the Communist movement is as much an ideological and cultural conspiracy as it is an economic, military and political one, it is not surprising Communists the world over devote considerable time and energy to influencing, and controlling, film criticism and history." Stern's position mellows somewhat in the 1965 number of *Film Culture,* in which Jonas Mekas gives over the issue to Stern's wealth of material about *The Birth of a Nation.*[44] If the film was not one already appropriated by Communists as a cause célèbre, Stern's attacks gave it to them.

Readings of *The Birth of a Nation*'s reception have traditionally been structured by the axes of region (North versus South) and racial attitude (liberal versus racist). This reconsideration has extended the film's reception into history, refusing to assume that the conditions for reception are restricted to the context of the film's original exhibition. I believe that historicizing the reception of *The Birth of a Nation* transforms the text's polysemy, for the political foundation underlying some of the historical debates becomes more apparent. In the film's later reception, racial attitudes are not autonomous effects; they relate to the political agendas of the debaters, causing strange alliances in which a former progressive defends the film using much of the rhetoric and arguments of 1915 radical conservatives. Additionally, complex theoretical questions such as the relation of subject matter and narrational procedures or possible effects of films and the consequences of those effects for social policy (censorship versus free speech) are lost to name-calling and a hardening of lines among the combatants. Consequently, this "encrustation" of the history of *The Birth of a Nation*'s reception has a double implication. For while the conditions for interpreting the film now include those years of political antagonisms, the "crust" that surrounds that interpretation also prevents a clear perception of what was once, and is still, at stake in the evaluation of the movie.

For *The Birth of a Nation* is not a simple problem. Its racism is obvious; its significance in the development of narrational procedures is also apparent. Following codes (or schemata) developed from the aesthetics of the nineteenth century, if not earlier, film histories have separated subject matter and narrational procedures, "content" and "form"; viewers have too.*[45] However, what aesthetic, social, and political theories vie in promoting or refusing to accept this separation? For these aesthetics have been sites of contestation. Additionally, how does social policy connect to this question? What are the merits of free-speech-versus-censorship debates?

Currently, these difficulties still face film scholars. Racism appears in numerous films (for example, the *Indiana Jones* and *Star Wars* series). So do all sorts of abhorrent representations of gender, sexual preference, ethnicity, nationality, and class. But the plea for free speech over censorship, the ambiguities of claims of effect, and the shifting vicissitudes of interpretation in relation to historical political contexts make any final evaluation difficult. Consequently, in any historical instance of the reception of a film, particularly ones not so obvious as *The Birth of a Nation,* some moments of that sequence of determining meaning and significance to an individual may be progressive; others, regressive; some may be subversive; others, reactionary. Labeling any single interpretive response as one thing or the other may be very difficult.

That a splinter group of the Communist party would protest the 1978 Ku Klux Klan screening of *The Birth of a Nation* is due to a forty-year history of progressive radicals' using that film as a nodal point for their argument that connections exist between racism and class exploitation and that the representations of films matter to social spectators. The act of defending the film's showing, however, does not automatically associate the proponent with the racists of 1915 or the Red-baiters of 1946, but defenders ought at least to be aware of that part of the encrustation surrounding *The Birth of a Nation.* Thus, the conditions for the continued reception of *The Birth of a Nation* are now very complicated.

Endnotes

This is a revision of a paper first presented at the Society for Cinema Studies Conference, Iowa City, Iowa, 12–16 April 1989.

1. Gladwin Hill, "Polyglot City Is in Shock after a Melee," *New York Times,* 3 August 1978, A-14.

2. Joel Williamson, *The Crucible of Race: Black-White Relations in the American South since Emancipation* (New York: Oxford University Press, 1984).

3. Thomas Cripps, *Slow Fade to Black: The Negro in American Film, 1900–1942* (London: Oxford University Press, 1977), pp. 41–43; Thomas R. Cripps, "The Reaction of the Negro to the Motion Picture 'Birth of a Nation' " (1963), rpt. in *Focus on "The Birth of a Nation,"* ed. Fred Silva (Englewood Cliffs, N.J.: Prentice Hall, 1971), p. 111 (hereafter *Focus).* Thomas F. Gassett describes how Wilson contributed to reasserting segregation; *Race: The History of an Idea in America* (Dallas: Southern Methodist University Press, 1963), p. 279.

4. James M. McPherson, "The Antislavery Legacy: From Reconstruction to the NAACP," in *Towards a New Past: Dissenting Essays in American History,* ed. J. Barton Bernstein (New York: Random House, 1967), pp. 126–57; Williamson, *The Crucible of Race,* pp. 70–78. Williamson's thesis for the deepening of antagonisms between whites and blacks extends C. Vann Woodward's economic and political determinations proposed in Woodward's *The Strange Career of Jim Crow* (1955) to include psychological and cultural factors. The deteriorating situation of the blacks was not isolated; racism extended to Jews and Asians as well, with segregation and discrimination particularly overt. The Anti-Defamation League of B'nai B'rith formed in 1913. See Oscar Handlin, ed., *Immigration as a Factor in American History* (Englewood Cliffs, N.J.: Prentice Hall, 1959), pp. 171–82. Also see Higham, *Strangers in the Land.*

5. Cripps, *Slow Fade,* pp. 52–64; "NAACP v. 'The Birth of a Nation': The Story of a 50-Year Fight," *Crisis 72,* no. 2 (February 1965): 96.

6. Williamson, *The Crucible of Race,* pp. 140–95.

7. Ibid., pp. 4–6. All of Williamson's "mentalities" are categorized from the position's view of the evolutionary potential of people of color, most likely a sensible system given the impact of social Darwinism on discourses of the period. Gassett, *Uncle Tom's Cabin and American Culture,* p. 346.

8. Quoted in Benjamin R. Tillman, *Congressional Record,* 59th Cong., 2d Sess. (21 January 1907): pp. 1140–44, rpt. in *Civil Rights and the American Negro: A Documentary History,* ed. Albert P. Blaustein and Robert L. Zangrando (New York: Washington Square Press, 1968), p. 319.

9. Grant worked at the American Museum of Natural History. His popular book counted as threatening Eastern and Southern Europeans as well as other groups of people. Handlin, *Immigration,* pp. 183–85. Also see material on this in my chapter 6.

10. Williamson, The Crucible of Race, pp. 140–48, 173–75; Gassett, *Uncle Tom's Cabin and American Culture,* p. 346; Cripps, *Slow Fade,* pp. 52–64.

11. "The Clansman," *Crisis* 10, no. 1 (May 1915): 33; "Fighting Race Calumny," *Crisis* 10, no. 1 (May 1915): 40–42, 87–88, rpt. in *Focus,* pp. 66–73. Later historical surveys of the events during this period include: "NAACP v. 'The Birth of a Nation,'" p. 96; Cripps, "Reaction," pp. 112–18; Goodwin Berquist and James Greenwood, "Protest against Racism: 'The Birth of a Nation' in Ohio," *Journal of the University Film Association* 26, no. 3 (1974): 39–44; Cripps, *Slow Fade,* pp. 52–64; Nickieann Fleener-Marzec, *D. W. Griffith's "The Birth of a Nation": Controversy, Suppression, and the First Amendment as It Applies to Filmic Expression, 1915–1973* (New York: Arno Press, 1980), p. 392–424; Richard Schickel, *D. W. Griffith: An American Life* (New York: Simon and Schuster, 1984), pp. 212–302.

12. In New York, the person who threw two eggs during the scene of "Little Sister" jumping off the cliff was a white, Howard Schaeffle. "Egg Negro Scenes in Liberty Film Play," *New York Times,* 15 April 1915, n.p.

13. For details on the alterations, besides the historical surveys (above), see "Films and Births and Censorship," *Survey,* 3 April 1915, 4–5; Seymour Stern, "The Birth of a Nation," *Cinemages,* special issue no. 1 (1955): 9. As Stern describes, among Griffith's deletions were some of the shots of blacks running through the streets of Piedmont, "flashes of screaming white girls being whisked by Negro rapists into doorways in back-alleys of the town," an epilogue "featuring, first Lincoln's forgotten letter to Staunton [sic], wherein Lincoln affirms that he does *not* believe in the equality of the black race with the white, and, finally, full-scale images of the deportation of masses of Negroes from New York Harbor to the (filmed) jungles of Liberia as a 'peaceable solution' for American and the Negroes." *Survey* (in 1915) describes an important insertion required by the National Board of Censorship in late March: "These [changes] are said to have been chiefly a substantial reduction in the details of the chase of the white girl by the renegade Negro, which in the original is said to have been the most dreadful portrayal of rape ever offered for public view; the insertion of various soothing captions, such as 'I won't hurt you, little Missy'; the entire excersion of a lynching; and a toning down of the scene in which the mulatto all but marries a white girl by force" ("Films and Births and Censorship," p. 4). "'Wid'" in "Films and Film Folk" (ca. 13 July 1915), *D. W. Griffith Papers,* 1897–1954 (Frederick, Md.: University Publications of America, microfilm) describes the Hampton Institute epilogue as a "shock," coming after *The Birth of a Nation*. Details on its production are in Nickie Fleener "Answering Film with Film: The Hampton Epilogue, a Positive Alternative to the Negative Stereotypes Presented in *The Birth of a Nation*," *Journal of Popular Film and Television* 7, no. 4 (1980): 400–425.

14. Fleener-Marzec, *D. W. Griffith's "The Birth of a Nation,"* p. 483.

15. "NAACP v. 'The Birth of a Nation,'" p. 97; "Negroes Oppose Film," *New York Times,* 7 May 1921.

16. "Movies Turn Deaf Ear to Colored Plea," *Christian Century* 47, no. 2 (24 September 1930): 1140–41.

17. Ruth C. Peterson and L. L. Thurstone, *Motion Pictures and the Social Attitudes of Children* (New York: Macmillan, 1933), p. 38.

18. Although Cripps, Berquist and Greenwood, Fleener-Marzec, and Schickel provide accounts of the reception of *The Birth of a Nation,* three other studies deserve special note. In 1961, Charles L. Hutchins surveyed much of the critical discussion to date in his master's thesis, "A Critical Evaluation of the Controversies Engendered by D. W. Griffith's *The Birth of a Nation*" (Master's thesis, University of Iowa). Hutchins's purpose was to outline and evaluate "major controversial issues which have grown up around *The Birth of a Nation*" (p. 3). Two stand out for him: Griffith's "treatment of the Negro" and the historical documentation regarding the "treatment of Thaddeus Stevens," the "role of the Negro in the Reconstructed South," and the "causes for the rise of the Ku Klux Klan" (p. 25). Hutchins's thesis is well-organized and useful (despite his evaluation procedures), but since he treats all responses as of the same time, determining patterns that might be considered historical is not possible. John Hammond Moore provides excellent information about the South Carolina press's negative reaction to Dixon's 1905 play but generally approving response for the 1915 film: "South Carolina's Reaction to the Photoplay *The Birth of a Nation*," *The Proceedings of the South Carolina Historical Association* (1963): 30–40. Russell Merritt studied the Boston events of April 1915, claiming that "most of the audience that came out of the Tremont theatre that night in 1915, for instance, believed Griffith's story was historically true, that *The Birth of a Nation* was a nostalgic, but essentially accurate description of the Civil War years and their aftermath" (p. 26). The evidence for this, however, is uncertain since certainly some Bostonians vehemently protested the film. (See below.) Merritt continues his essay, arguing that in comparison with Dixon, Griffith's representation of blacks is toned down. This approach to the film repeats one associated since 1915 with defenders of the film, "Dixon, Griffith, and the Southern Legend," *Cinema Journal* 12, no. 1 (Fall 1972): 26–45.

In chronological order, the period articles and reviews that I studied are: D. W. Griffith, "The Motion Picture and Witch Burners," n.d. (numerous papers in "Flickerings from Film Land by Kitty Kell" column), rpt. in *Focus,* pp. 16–99; D. W. Griffith, "The Future of the Two-Dollar Movie," n.d, (numerous papers), rpt. in *Focus,* pp. 99–101; Rev. Dr. Charles H. Parkhurst, " 'The Birth of a Nation,' " n.d. (review in numerous papers), rpt. in *Focus* pp. 102–3; " 'The Birth of a Nation,'" *New York Times,* 4 March 1915, 9; Hector Turnbull, "A Stirring Drama Shown," *New York Tribune,* 4 March 1915, 9; "Negroes Object to Film," *New York Times,* 7 March 1915, n.p.; "W," "The Birth of a Nation" *The New York Dramatic Mirror* 73, no. 1890 (10 March 1915): 28; Mark Vance, "The Birth of a Nation," *Variety,* 12 March 1915, rpt. in *Focus,* pp. 22–25; George D. Proctor, "The Birth of a Nation," *Motion Picture News* 11, no. 10 (13 March 1915): 40–50; W. Stephen Bush, "The Birth of a Nation," *Moving Picture World* 23 (13 March 1915): 1586–87, rpt. in *Focus,* pp. 25–28; Francis Hackett, "Brotherly Love," *New Republic* 2, no. 20 (20 March 1915): 185–86, rpt. in *Focus,* pp. 84–86; "A Reconstruction Story," *New York Times,* 21 March 1915, n.p.; "Moving Picture Justly Denounced by Jane Adams [sic]," *New York Evening Post,* 25 March 1915, n.p. (in D. W. Griffith Papers); "Protests on Photo Play," *New York Times,* 31 March 1915, n.p.; "Promise to Tone Down Two Scenes of Vicious Photo Play," *New York Age,* 1 April 1915, 1; James W. Johnson, "Views and Reviews," *New York Age,* 1 April 1915, 4; "Films and Births and Censorship" *Survey,* 3 April 1915, 4–5; "Capitalizing Race Hatred," *New York Globe,* 6 April 1915, n.p., rpt. in *Focus,* pp. 73–75; Thomas Dixon, "Reply to the *New York Globe,*" *New York Globe,* 10 April 1915, n.p., rpt. in *Focus,* pp. 75–77; D. W. Griffith, "Reply to the *New York Globe,*" *New York Globe,* 10 April 1915, n.p., rpt. in *Focus,* pp. 77–79; "Dixon on His Motive" (editorial), *New York Globe,* 8 April 1915 (in D. W. Griffith Papers); "What Some Globe Readers Have to Say," *New York Globe,* 9 April 1915 (in D. W. Griffith Papers); National Board of Review "Censoring Motion Pictures," *New Republic* 2, no. 23 (10 April 1915): 262–63; " 'The Birth of a Nation,' " *Outlook,* 14 April 1915, 854; "Egg Negro Scenes in Liberty Film Play," *New York Times,* 15 April 1915, n.p.; "Negroes Mob Photo Play," *New York Times,* 18 April 1915, n.p.; "Mass. Protests Vicious Movie" *New York Age,* 22 April 1915, 1; W. James Johnson; "Views and Reviews," *New York Age,* 22 April 1915, 4; "Censorship: The Curse of a Nation," *Boston Evening Transcript,* 23 April 1915, n.p., rpt. *Focus,* pp. 87–88; Thomas Dixon, "Fair Play for *The Birth of a Nation,*" *Boston Journal,* 26 April 1915, n.p., rpt. in *Focus,* pp. 90–95; D. W. Griffith, "Defense of *The Birth of A Nation* and Attack on the Sullivan Bill" *Boston Journal,* 26 April 1915, n.p., rpt. in *Focus,* pp. 88–90; "Tom Dixon's 'Clansman,'" *Crisis* 10, no. 1 (May 1915): 19–20; 'The Clansman," *Crisis* 10, no. 1 (May 1915): 33, rpt. as " 'The Birth of a Nation': An Editorial," in *Focus,* pp. 64–66; "Fighting Race Calumny," *Crisis* 10, no. 1 (May–June 1915): 40–42, 87–88, rpt. in *Focus,* pp. 66–73; "Chicago Prepares to Forestall 'Birth of a Nation,'" *Chicago Defender,* 1 May 1915, 3; "The Death of a Movie," *Chicago Defender,* 1 May 1915, 8; "Regulation of Films," *Nation* 100, no. 2601 (6 May 1915): 486–87; James W. Johnson, "Views and Reviews," *New York Age,* 6 May 1915, 4; "Mayor Thompson Bars 'Birth of Nation' from Chicago," *Chicago Defender,* 15 May 1915, 2; Rolfe Cobleigh, ["Why I Oppose *The Birth of a Nation*"], [26 May 1915], rpt. in *Fighting a Vicious Film: Protest against "The Birth of a Nation"* (Boston: Boston Branch of the National Association for the Advancement of Colored People, 1915), rpt. in *Focus,* pp. 80–83; "*Birth of a Nation* Case Dismissed," *New York Age,* 27 May 1915, 4; " 'The Birth of a Nation,'" *Crisis* 10, no. 2 (June 1915): 69–71; Helen Duey (?), *Woman's Home Companion,* 1 June 1915 (D. W. Griffith Papers); Charlotte Rumbold, "Against 'The Birth of a Nation,'" *New Republic* 3, no. 31 (5 June 1915): 125; "Progressive Protest Against Anti-Negro Film," *Survey,* 5 June 1915, 209–10; 'The Dirt of a Nation," *Chicago Defender,* 5 June 1915, 8; Henry MacMahon, "The Art of the Movies," *New York Times,* 6 June 1915, sect. 6, p. 8; "Meetings," *Crisis* 10, no. 3 (July 1915): 148–49; " 'Wid,'" Films and Film Folk" (ca. 13 July 1915) (D. W. Griffith Papers); Harlow Hare, *Boston American,* 18 July 1915, n.p., rpt. in *Focus,* pp. 36–40; " 'The Birth of a Nation,'" *Gazette* (Cleveland, Ohio), 11 September 1915, 2; " 'The Birth of a Nation,'" *Gazette,* 2 October 1915, [2]; Ward Greene, *Atlanta Journal,* 7 December 1915, n.p., rpt. in *Focus,* pp. 30–33; Ned McIntosh, *Atlanta Constitution,* 7 December 1915, n.p., rpt. in *Focus,* pp. 33–36; "The Attorney General's Broadside," *Advocate* (Cleveland, Ohio), 2, no. 37 (22 January 1916):

[4]; S.E.F. Rose, "The Ku Klux Klan and 'The Birth of a Nation,'" *Confederate Veteran* 24, no. 4 (April 1916): 157–59; Henry Stephen Gordon, 'The Story of David Wark Griffith," *Photoplay* 10, no. 5 (October 1916): 90–94; and Vachel Lindsay, *The Art of the Moving Picture* (1915) (1922; rpt., New York: Liveright, 1970), pp. 74–77.

19. The more irate reviewers already recognized the racism of "Uncle Tom" and "Sambo" characters. "'The Clansman,'" *Crisis* 10, no. 1 (May 1915): 65.

20. "The Dirt of a Nation," *Chicago Defender,* 5 June 1915, 8; Dan Streible, "A History of the Boxing Film, 1894–1915: Social Reform and Social Control in the Progressive Era" (Unpublished seminar paper, University of Texas at Austin, Spring 1989), pp. 13–22.

21. Griffith, "The Motion Picture and Witch Burners" (1915), rpt. in *Focus,* pp. 96–99.

22. Dixon, "Fair Play for *The Birth of a Nation*," *Boston Journal,* 26 April 1915, n.p., rpt. in *Focus,* pp. 90–95.

23. Griffith, "Reply to the *New York Globe*" (10 April 1915), rpt. in *Focus,* p. 79.

24. Merritt, "Dixon, Griffith, and the Southern Legend," p. 26.

25. Dixon, "Fair Play for *The Birth of a Nation*" (26 April 1915), pp. 90–95.

26. Moore, "South Carolina's Reaction," p. 40. Williamson argues in *The Crucible of Race* that the radical-conservative attribution of bestial qualities shifted from blacks to other minorities after 1906. Moore's information suggests otherwise.

27. "Egg Negro Scenes in Liberty Film Play," *New York Times,* 15 April 1915.

28. Richard Watts, Jr., "D. W. Griffith," *New Theater and Film* (November 1936), rpt. in *New Theater and Film, 1934 to 1937,* ed. Herbert Kline (San Diego, Calif.: Harcourt-Brace-Jovanovich, 1985), p. 238; Lewis Jacobs, "D. W. Griffith: *The Birth of a Nation*" (1939, from *The Rise of the American Film),* rpt. in *Focus,* p. 159; editor's note for David Platt, "Fanning the Flames of the War," *Daily Worker* (New York City), 20 December 1939, 7. This was one of four articles on prowar filmmaking in 1914–1918 published 18–21 December 1939. Films Platt considered possibly progressive were *Juarez* and *Mr. Smith Goes to Washington*; David Platt, "Will Film World Cave In as It Did in '14?" *Daily Worker,* 21 December 1939, 7.

29. A socialist newspaper, the *New Leader,* implied in 1940 that the Communist party chose particularly to "court" blacks because of defections due to the Hitler-Stalin pact. While the pact had serious repercussions in the party, direct approaches to blacks were at least a decade old. Ted Poston, "CP Purges Ford as Scapegoat for Failure among Negroes," *New Leader,* 30 March 1940, 4; Philip Taft, "Party Organizer (New York, 1927–1938)," in *The American Radical Press, 1880–1960,* vol. 1, ed. Joseph R. Conlin (Westport, Conn.: Greenwood Press 1974), p. 262; Cripps, *Slow Fade,* p. 68. Eugene Gordon, "'Yes, I Mean You Guys,' Barks Mr. Paglia," *Daily Worker* ca. 4 January 1940, n.p.; Seymour Stern "Suppression of Showing Marks 25th Year of 'Birth of a Nation,' " *New Leader*, 16 March 1940, 3.

30. Daniel Aaron, *Writers on the Left* (New York: Harcourt, 1961); Richard H. Pells, *Radical Visions and American Dreams: Culture and Social Thought in the Depression Years* (Middletown, Conn.: Wesleyan University Press, 1973). Additional criticisms and defenses of *The Birth of a Nation* through the 1930s include (in chronological order): Thomas Dixon, "Civil War Truth," *New York Times,* 8 May 1921; "[Griffith] Defends Film Production," *New York Times,* 9 May 1921; "Foes of Klan Fight 'Birth of a Nation,'" *New York Times,* 3 December 1922 5; "Movies Turn Deaf Ear to Colored Plea," *Christian Century* 47, no. 2 (24 September 1930): 1140–41; Barnet G. Braver-mann, "Griffith: The Pioneer," *Theatre Guild Magazine* 8 (February 1931): 28–31, 60–61 (Braver-mann would soon be an editor of *Experimental Cinema*; he writes: "It is thus clear that Griffith's background did not help him to develop a penetrative social outlook"); Seymour Stern, "Hollywood and Montage," *Experimental Cinema* 4 (1932): 47–52; Peterson and Thurstone, *Motion Pictures and the Social Attitudes of Children,* pp. 35–38, 60–61; Harry Alan Potamkin, *The Eyes of the Movie,* International Pamphlets, no. 38 (n.p., 1934); Seymour Stern, "Birthday of a Classic," *New York Times, 25* March 1935; Seymour Stern, "'The Birth of a Nation': In Retrospect," *International Photographer* 7

(April 1935): 4–5, 23–24; Richard Watts, Jr., "D. W. Griffith," *New Theater and Film* (November 1936), rpt. in *New Theater and Film* ed. Klein, pp. 237–40; Archer Winsten, "'The Birth of a Nation' Surprises Old Admirer," *New York Post,* 5 October 1937; Milton MacKaye, *"The Birth of a Nation," Scribner's Magazine* 102, no. 5 (November 1937): 40–46, 69; V. F. Calverton, "Cultural Barometer," *Current History* 49, no. 1 (September 1938): 45–47; Lewis Jacobs, "D. W. Griffith: *The Birth of a Nation*" (1939), rpt. in *Focus* pp. 154–68.

31. David Platt, "Negroes Barred from Hollywood Jobs, Slandered in Its Films," *Daily Worker,* 20 February 1940, 7. This is the second of the series that ran from 19 to 28 February 1940. On the 1933 Payne Fund studies, see Peterson and Thurstone, *Motion Pictures and the Social Attitudes of Children.*

32. Seymour Stern, "Griffith: I. *The Birth of a Nation,*" *Film Culture* 36 (Spring-Summer 1965): 36–37; Seymour Stern, "Suppression of Showing Marks 25th Year of 'Birth of a Nation,'" *New Leader,* 6 March 1940, 3. Stern's reference in 1965 is to his articles in the *New Leader* and the *New York Times.* However, the latter essay seems moderately harmless, with another essay in the *New York Herald Tribune* of possibly greater provocation. More likely, Stern's alienation from his colleagues develops from his second article in the *New Leader* in which he attacks Jay Leyda (see below). Seymour Stern, "'The Birth of a Nation' Marked an Industry's Coming of Age," *New York Herald Tribune,* 16 June 1940; Seymour Stern, "Pioneer of the Film Art," *New York Times Magazine,* 10 November 1940, 16–17.

33. "No Show," *New Leader,* 16 March 1940, 3. The following week Stern accused Jay Leyda, assistant curator at the Museum of Modern Art, of "depart[ing] from accepted canons of cinematic criticism, and substitut[ing] outright political propaganda" in Leyda's film notes for a retrospective of Soviet cinema. Seymour Stern, "Film Library Notes Build 'CP Liberators' Myth," *New Leader,* 23 March 1940, 3. Many people believe this article contributed to events that led to the request for Leyda's resignation from the museum.

34. The first issue (February 1930) of *Experimental Cinema* lists Platt and Jacobs as coeditors for the Cinema Crafters (Philadelphia), with Hollywood editor Stern and New York editor Potamkin.

35. Pells, *Radical Visions and American Dreams,* p. 34. Also see: Aaron, *Writers on the Left*; Ian H. Birchall, "Marxism and Literature," in *The Sociology of Literature,* ed. Routh and Wolff, pp. 92–108; and George Steiner, "Marxism and the Literary Critic," in *Sociology of Literature and Drama,* ed. Elizabeth and Tom Bums (Harmondsworth, England: Penguin Books, 1973), pp. 159–78.

36. Aaron, *Writers on the Left*; Pells, *Radical Visions and American Dreams,* pp. 342–46; Max Nomad, "1940 Saw Intellectuals Retreat from Leftist Traditional Orthodoxy," *New Leader,* 4 January 1941, 5. Nomad is citing Lewis Corey, in the *Nation* (1940).

37. George Amberg, "Introduction," *Experimental Cinema,* pp. iii–iv. Potamkin at least was already aligned with U.S. communists. Furthermore, as of issue number 3 (1931), *Experimental Cinema* was receiving support from the Workers Film and Photo League of America and The American Prolet-Kino. Issue 3 lists three coeditors: Jacobs, Platt, and Stern, with Potamkin dropping out because *Experimental Cinema* printed a criticism written by Samuel Brody of an essay that Potamkin had published in *Close Up.* Issue 4 (1932) has five coeditors: Jacobs, Platt, Stern, Alexander Brailovsky, and Barnet G. Braver-mann. The last issue, number 5 (1934) lists editors Jacobs, Stern, and Braver-mann, but Platt is not among the associate or corresponding editors. Platt *is* listed as teaching at the Harry Alan Potamkin Film School along with Jacobs, Brody, Ralph Steiner, Irving Lerner, and Leo Selzter (p. 54).

38. William Alexander, *Film on the Left: American Documentary Film from 1931 to 1942* (Princeton: Princeton University Press, 1981), pp. 46–47; Russell Campbell, *Cinema Strikes Back: Radical Filmmaking in the United States, 1930–1942* (Ann Arbor, Mich.: UMI Research Press, 1982), pp. 96, 329n.

39. "Eisenstein Attacks 'Birth of a Nation' / Protests Slanderous Use of His Name," *Daily Worker,* 14 January 1941, 7(?). Also see in this period: Paul Goodman, "Film Chronicle: Griffith and the Technical Innovations," *Partisan Review* 8, no. 3 (May–June 1941): 237–40; Barnet G. Bravermann, "D. W. G., The Creator of Film Form," *Theatre Arts 29* (April 1945): 240–50.

40. Peter Noble, "A Note on an Idol," *Sight and Sound* 15 no. 59 (Autumn 1946): 81–82.

41. D. W. Griffith, *"The Birth of a Nation," Sight and Sound* 16, no. 61 (Spring 1947): 32; Seymour Stern, "Griffith Not Anti-Negro," *Sight and Sound* 16, no. 61 (Spnng 1947): 32–35.

42. Italics in the original. This latter ploy comes from a 1921 defense by Griffith. "Defends Film Production," *New York Times,* 9 May 1921.

43. "Without Comment" (Museum of Modern Art pamphlet, ca. 1946, p. 3), rpt. in *Sight and Sound* 16, no. 61 (Spring 1947): 35; E. L. Cranstone, "'The Birth of a Nation' Controversy," *Sight and Sound* 16, no. 63 (Autumn 1947): 119 (Cranstone writes: "We have have heard it all before and know that red-baiting is a dangerous occupation" [p. 119]—an ironical observation given what was about to happen in the United States); Seymour Stern, "The Griffith Controversy," *Sight and Sound* 17, no. 65 (Spring 1948): 49–50; editor's note, *Sight and Sound* 17, no. 65. (Spring 148): 50; Peter Noble, "The Negro in *The Birth of a Nation,"* The Negro in Films (London: Skelton Robinson, 1948): 33–43, rpt. in *Focus,* pp. 125–32; V. J. Jerome, *The Negro in Hollywood Films* (New York: Masses and Mainstream, 1950). Also see: James Agee, "David Wark Griffith," *Nation* 167, no. 10 (4 September 1948): 264–65; James Mason Brown, "Wishful Banning," *Saturday Review* 32, no. 11 (12 March 1949): 24–26; Dore Schary, "Censorship and Stereotypes," *Saturday Review* 32, no. 18 (30 April 1949) : 9–10; Seymour Stern " 'The Birth of a Nation,'" *Cinemages,* special issue no. 1 (1955).

44. Seymour Stern, "D. W. Griffith and the Movies," *American Mercury* 68, no. 303 (March 1949): 308–19; Seymour Stern, "The Cold War against David Wark Griffith," *Films in Review* 7, no. 2 (February 1956): 49–59; Stern "Griffith: I. The Birth of a Nation," *Film Culture* 36 (Spring–Summer 1965): 1–210. Also see Seymour Stern, "The Soviet Directors' Debt to D. W. Griffith," *Films in Review 7,* no. 5 (May 1956): 202–9. For evidence that Stern's view has its current adherents, see Herbert C. Roseman, "Why the Wacko-Liberals Hate the Late Seymour Stern: The Most Authoritative of D. W. Griffith Scholars Long Ago Exposed Communists' Filmic Distortions," *Quirk's Reviews* (May 1985): 7 (in New York Public Library Performing Arts clipping file on Seymour Stern).

45. A recent exception to this pattern of separating form and content when discussing *The Birth of a Nation* is Michael Rogin's essay, "'The Sword Became a Flashing Vision': D. W. Griffith's *The Birth of a Nation,"* Representations 9 (Winter 1985): 150–95.

Reply to the New York Globe

D. W. Griffith

Editor of the Globe, Sir—In an editorial in your issue of April 6, 1915, under the heading: "Capitalizing Race Hatred," you undertake to label our picture *The Birth of a Nation* with alleged feelings of sectional difference between the North and South. You ask yourself questions and proceed to answer them in the same old way that the same things have been gone over and over again. Where I must take issue with you is that you intimate that these old differences have been raised and exhibited "for purely sordid reasons," to quote your own words.

In presenting this motion-picture story before the intelligent theater-goers of New York City, in a regular theater, which has been well advertised, I thought the moving drama told its own story. My associates have maintained a dignified silence in the face of an organized attack of letter writers, publicity seekers, and fanatics against our work. We have traced this attack to its source, and know the reasons for it. Without wishing to tell any newspaper its business, permit me to suggest that a cub reporter in one hour could find out that this attack is an organized effort to suppress a production which was brought forth to reveal the beautiful possibilities of the art of motion pictures and to tell a story which is based upon truth in every vital detail. Our story states, as plainly as the English language can express a fact, the reasons for this presentation. In our captions we reiterate that the events depicted upon the screen are not meant as a reflection upon any race or people of today.

I demand to know the authority upon which you base your intimation that this work of art has been exhibited "for purely sordid reasons." I further demand that failing to establish this authority you retract your statement in as prominent and direct manner as you have given publicity to the opinions of the writer of your editorial.

Our picture tells its own story and we are willing to stand upon the verdict of the New York public as to the fitness of this work of art to be judged as a drama of action based upon the authenticated history of the period covering the action of our plot.

The succeeding paragraphs of your editorial are political generalities which have nothing in common with the truths and purposes of the motion picture *The Birth of a Nation*. Our picture does show historic events which you undertake to use for an entirely different argument. We have contrasted the bad with the good and following the formula of the best dramas of the world we establish our ideals by revealing the victory of right over wrong.

I do not agree with your statements regarding the history of slavery and the Reconstruction period of this nation, but that is not a matter of importance in this connection. Most well-informed men know now that slavery was an economic mistake. The treatment of the Negroes during the days of Reconstruction is shown effectually and graphically in our picture. We show many phases of the question and we do pay particular attention to those faithful Negroes who stayed with their former masters and were ready to give up their lives to protect their white friends. No characters in the story are applauded with greater fervor than the good Negroes whose devotion is so clearly shown. If prejudiced witnesses do not see the message in this portion of the entire drama we are not to blame.

Your editorial is an insult to the intelligence and the human kindness of nearly 100,000 of the best people in New York City, who have viewed this picture from artistic interests and not through any depraved taste such as you try to indicate. Among those you have insulted are your contemporaries on the newspapers of New York, whose expert reviewers were unanimous in their praise of this work as an artistic achievement. Included in this list is your own able critic, Mr. Louis Sherwin, of the *Globe*.

We have received letters of the heartiest commendation from statesmen, writers, clergymen, artists, educators, and laymen. I have in my possession applications for reservations from the principals of ten schools, who having seen the picture, are desirous of bringing their pupils to view it for its historic truths.

The Rev. Dr. Charles H. Parkhurst, the Rev. Father John Talbot Smith, and the Rev. Thomas B. Gregory are among the clergy who have given us permission to use their names in approval of this picture in its entirety. Parents have asked us to make reservation for them that they may bring their children to see it. In every walk of life there are men and women of this city who have expressed their appreciation of this picture. Do you dare to intimate that these voluntary expressions of approval were voiced "for purely sordid reasons"?

The attack of the organized opponents to this picture is centered upon that feature of it which they deem might become an influence against the intermarriage of blacks and whites. The organizing opponents are white leaders of the National Association for the Advancement of the Colored People, including Oswald Garrison Villard and J. E. Spingarn, who hold official positions in this prointermarriage organization.

May I inquire if you desire to espouse the cause of a society which openly boasts in its official organ, *The Crisis,* that it has been able to throttle "anti-intermarriage legislation" in over ten states? Do you know what this society means by "anti-intermarriage legislation"? It means that they successfully opposed bills which were framed to prohibit the marriage of Negroes to whites.

Do you know that in their official organ, *The Crisis,* for March 1915, they brand 238 members of the Sixty-third Congress as "Negro baiters" because these Representatives voted to prohibit the marriage of Negroes to whites in the District of Columbia?

You close your editorial, in which by innuendo you link our picture to your own assertions, with this sentence:

> *"To make a few dirty dollars, men are willing to pander to depraved tastes and to foment a race antipathy that is the most sinister and dangerous feature of American life."*

That statement is obviously a generality, but it is printed at the end of an editorial which is a covert attack upon our picture, *The Birth of a Nation.* As the producer of that picture, I wish to say if the man who wrote it meant one iota of the sentence just quoted to apply to our picture he is a liar and a coward.

Whether this was the intent of the sentence quoted it could not fail to create an impression in the minds of your readers, damaging my reputation as a producer. Therefore, as a matter of justice, I ask that you publish my statement of the facts.

How I Made The Birth of a Nation

D. W. Griffith

When Mr. Woods[1] suggested *The Clansman*[2] to me as a subject it hit me hard; I hoped at once that it could be done, for the story of the South had been absorbed into the very fibre of my being.

Mr. Dixon wrote to me suggesting the project, and I reread the book at once.

There had been a picture made by another concern, but this had been a failure;[3] as the theme developed in my mind, it fascinated me until I arrived at the point where I had to make the picture; if I had known that the result would mean disaster I do not think it would have mattered to me; truly I never was sure that the result would be a success; that first night showing at the Auditorium,[4] if anyone had offered me just a shade over what it had cost, I would have taken the money just as quickly as I could reach for it.

There were several months lost in the negotiations for the rights, as by that time other producers had gained the same idea, like myself, undeterred by one failure having already been made.

As I studied the book, stronger and stronger came to work the traditions I had learned as a child; all that my father had told me. That sword I told you about became a flashing vision. Gradually came back to my memory the stories a cousin, one Thurston Griffith, had told me of the "Ku Klux Klan," and that regional impulse that comes to all men from the earth where they had their being stirred potently at my imagination.

But there was nothing of personal exhilaration required to make a picture out of that theme; few others like it in subject and power can be found, for it had all the deep incisive emotionalism of the highest patriotic sentiment.

I wouldn't say that the story part of that picture can ever be excelled, but as for the picture itself, there will be others made that will make it appear archaic in comparison.

For the feature picture has just begun to come into its own; my personal idea is that the minor pictures have had their day; the two- and three- and four-reel ones are passing, if not gone.

As I worked, the commercial side of the venture was lost to my view; I felt driven to tell the story—the truth about the South, touched by its eternal romance which I had learned to know so well.

I may be pardoned for saying that now I believe I did succeed in a measure in accomplishing that ambition.

---

[1] Frank E. Woods, film critic of *The Dramatic Mirror* and screenwriter for the Biograph Company.
[2] *The Clansman: An Historical Romance of the Ku Klux Klan,* by Thomas Dixon, Jr. (a novel). First published in 1905.
[3] Prior to 1912 the Kinemacolor Company of America began filming a version of the stage production of *The Clansman*. This film version was never completed, but one of the continuity writers for the production was Frank E. Woods who later suggested to DWG the idea of making a film of *The Clansman*.
[4] February 8, 1915, at Clune's Auditorium, Los Angeles, California. The film was then titled *The Clansman*. The title was changed to *The Birth of a Nation* for the New York premiere, Liberty Theatre, March 3, 1915. After the first New York showings, some 558 feet of film were removed by the censors, leaving 12,500 feet of the original release length of 13,058 feet.

It all grew as we went! I had no scenario, and never looked again at some few notes I made as I read the book, and which I read to my company before we began. Naturally the whole story was firmly in my mind, and possibly the personal exuberance of which I have told you enabled me to amplify and to implant in the scenes something of the deep feeling I experienced in that epoch that had meant everything, and then had left nothing to my nearest, my kin, and those about me.

There was not a stage star in my company; "Little Colonel" [Henry] Walthall had been out with Henry Miller, and had achieved some reputation; though by no means of stellar sort. Possibly he felt a bit of the impulse of locality, for his father was a Confederate colonel.

Miriam Cooper, the elder Cameron sister, was a perfect type of the beauty prevalent below the Mason and Dixon line, and Mae Marsh was from the same part of the Union, while Spottiswoode Aitken—"Dr. Cameron"—was related to a large group of distinguished Southern families.

These people were not picked because of place of birth or of their personal feeling about the story; still, it was a fortunate incident that they were what they were; it is hard to figure exactly how far what [is] bred in the bone will shine through the mind.

The casting frankly was all done by types; Miss Cooper, for instance, I kept in the company for all the months between the idea that I might make the picture until the work began, because I knew she would be an exact "Cameron" girl.

Everyone of the cast proved to be exactly what was required.

When I chose Lillian Gish as Stoneman's daughter, she seemed as ideal for the role as she actually proved to be in her acting. Mae Marsh had driven her quality so thoroughly into the estimation of the public in *The Escape* [1914; film made by DWG for Reliance-Majestic/Mutual] that I felt absolutely sure of her results. It was the same with Robert Harron and Elmer Clifton, for Stoneman's sons, and Ralph Lewis as Stoneman lived exactly up to what his personality promised when he was selected. And there was George Siegmann, the mulatto Lieutenant Governor, and Walter Long as the awful Negro Gus, and Mary Alden, Stoneman's mulatto housekeeper.

There has been question as to why I did not pick real Negroes or mulattos for those three roles.

That matter was given consideration, and on careful weighting of every detail concerned, the decision was to have no black blood among the principals; it was only in the legislative scene that Negroes were used, and then only as "extra people."

There were six weeks of rehearsals, before we really began. I think it took something like six months to make the picture—that is, the actual photography; but in all I put in a year and a half of work.

It was a big venture in numbers at that time; I suppose from the first to last we used from 30,000 to 35,000 people.

That seemed immense at that era, but now, in the piece we temporarily call *The Mother and the Law* [Mr. Griffith's huge new feature, just completed, and named *Intolerance*], we have used since the first of January about fifteen thousand people a month [this statement was made in the latter part of April 1916], and I cannot see even the beginning of the end as yet.

With *The Clansman* it was not alone the first expense, but the incessant fighting we had to do to keep the picture going, that cost.

We spent over $250,000 the first six months, combating stupid persecution brought against the picture by ill-minded censors and politicians who were playing for the Negro vote.

Lawyers had to be retained at every place we took the picture, and we paid out enough in rents for theaters where we were not allowed to show the picture to make an average film profitable.

But we finally won.

Now we are showing the picture with no hindrance, and most of those who opposed us at first, are now either admirers of the picture or quiescent.

While on this censorship, this drooling travesty of sense, I want to say something that I have said before, but which is essential to a right understanding of my purposes and work.

The foremost educators of the country have urged upon moving picture producers to put away the slapstick comedies, the ridiculous sentimental "mush" stories, the imitation of the fiction of the cheap magazines and go into the fields of history for our subjects.

They have told us repeatedly that the motion picture can impress upon a people as much of the truth of history in an evening as many months of study will accomplish. As one eminent divine said of pictures, "They teach history by lightning!"[5]

We would like very much to do this, but the very reason for the slapstick and the worst that is in pictures is censorship. Let those who tell us to uplift our art invest money in the production of a historic play of the life of Christ. They will find that this cannot be staged without incurring the wrath of a certain part of our people. "The Massacre of St. Bartholomew," if reproduced, will cut off the toes of another part of our people.[6]

I was considering the production in pictures of the history of the American people. This got into the papers. From all over the country I was strongly advised that this was not the time for a picture on the American Revolution,[7] because the English and their sympathizers would not take kindly to the part the English played in the wars of the American Revolution, and that the pro-Germans would not care to see the Hessians enact their harsh roles in the narrative of our freedom.

Bernard Shaw spoke fatefully and factually when he said: "The danger of the cinema is not the danger of immorality, but of morality; people, who, like myself, frequent the cinemas testify to their desolating romantic morality. . . ."

If I approach success in what I am trying to do in my coming picture, *Intolerance,* I expect a persecution even greater than that which met *The Birth of a Nation.*

---

[5]A comment attributed to Woodrow Wilson and said to be his reaction to seeing *The Birth of a Nation.*
[6]DWG is, of course, referring here to one of the four stories in *Intolerance.*
[7]DWG's film of the American Revolution was later made as *America* (1924).

The Rise and Fall of Free Speech In America

D.W. Griffith

Why Censor the Motion Picture—the Laboring Man's University?

Fortunes are spent every year in our country in teaching the truths of history, that we may learn from the mistakes of the past a better way for the present and future.

The truths of history today are restricted to the limited few attending our colleges and universities; the motion picture can carry these truths to the entire world, without cost, while at the same time bringing diversion to the masses.

As tolerance would thus be compelled to give way before knowledge and as the deadly monotony of the cheerless existence of millions would be brightened by this new art, two of the chief causes making war possible would be removed. The motion picture is war's greatest antidote,

Intolerance: The Root of All Censorship

Ours is a government of free speech and a free press.
Intelligent opposition to censorship in the beginning would have nipped the evil in the bud.
But the malignant pygmy has matured into a Caliban.
Muzzle the "Movies" and defeat the educational purpose of this graphic art.
Censorship demands of the picture makers a sugar-coated and false version of life's truths.
The moving picture is simply the pictorial press.
The pictorial press claims the same constitutional freedom as the printed press.

Freedom of speech and publication is guaranteed in the Constitution of the United States, and in the constitution of practically all the states. Unjustifiable speech or publication may be punished, but cannot be forbidden in advance. Mayor Gaynor, that great jurist who stood out from the ordinary gallery-playing, hypocritical type of politician as a white rose stands out from a field of sewer-fed weeds, said in vetoing a moving picture censorship ordinance in the city of New York:

> *Ours is a government of free speech and a free press. That is the cornerstone of free government. The phrase "The Press," includes all methods of expression by writing or pictures. . . . If this (moving picture) ordinance be legal, then a similar ordinance in respect to the newspapers and the theaters generally would be legal.*

Today the censorship of moving pictures, throughout the entire country, is seriously hampering the growth of the art. Had intelligent opposition to censorship been employed when it first made itself manifest it could have easily been overcome. But the pigmy child of that day has grown to be, not merely a man, but a giant, and I tell you who read this, whether you will or no, he is a giant whose forces of evil are so strong that he threatens that priceless heritage of our nation—freedom of expression.

The right of free speech has cost centuries upon centuries of untold sufferings and agonies; it has cost rivers of blood; it has taken as its toll uncounted fields littered with the carcasses of human beings—all this that there might come to live and survive that wonderful thing, the power of free speech. In our country it has taken some of the best blood of our forefathers. The Revolution itself was a fight in this direction—for the God-given, beautiful ideal of free speech.

Afterwards the first assault on the right of free speech, guaranteed by the Constitution, occurred in 1798, when Congress passed the Sedition Law, *which made it a crime for any newspaper or other printed publication to criticize the government.*

Partisan *prosecution of editors and publishers took place at the instance of the party in power,* and popular indignation was aroused against this abridgement of liberty to such an extent that Thomas Jefferson, the candidate of the opposition party for president, was triumphantly elected. And after that nothing more was heard of the Sedition Law, which expired by limitation in 1801.

The integrity of free speech and publication was *not again attacked* seriously in this country until the arrival of the *motion picture,* when this new art was seized by the powers of intolerance as an excuse for an assault on our liberties.

The motion picture is a medium of expression as clean and decent as any mankind has ever discovered. A people that would allow the suppression of this form of speech would unquestionably submit to the suppression of that which we all consider so highly, the printing press.

And yet we find all through the country, among all classes of people, the idea that the motion picture should be censored.

Now, the same reasons which make a censorship of the printed press unconstitutional and intolerable to Americans, make a censorship of the pictorial press unconstitutional and intolerable.

The theory of the constitutional guarantee, in brief, is this: Every American citizen has a constitutional right to publish anything he pleases, either by speech, or in writing, or in print, or in pictures, subject to his personal liability *after publication* to the penalties of violating any law, such as the law forbidding obscenity, libel, and other matter legally unfit for publication.

But the distinction between this theory and a censorship is that a censorship passes upon and forbids printing a picture *before publication,* and so directly controverts the most valuable of all our liberties under the Constitution, which our fathers established for our guidance and our protection.

If the pictorial press can be subjected to censorship by a mere act of Congress, then so can the printed press. And, of course, there would be an end, at once, to the freedom of *writing and printing.*

The constitutional and rightful manner in which to keep the moving pictures within proper bounds is simply to make and to enforce laws which will severely punish those persons who exhibit improper pictures.

As a matter of fact, there are laws now on the statute books which are ample to punish all who deserve punishment. It is simply a question of enforcement. So that the creation of Federal censorship is absolutely unnecessary.

It is said the motion picture tells its story more vividly than any other art. In other words, we are to be blamed for efficiency, for completeness. Is this justice? Is this common sense? We do not think so.

We have no wish to offend with indecencies or obscenities, but we do demand, as a right, the liberty to show the dark side of wrong, that we may illuminate the bright side of virtue—the same liberty that is conceded to the art of the written word—that art to which we owe the Bible and the works of Shakespeare.

LESSON THREE

Slapstick and the Silent Period

Pie and Chase: Gag, Spectacle and Narrative in Slapstick Comedy[1]

Donald Crafton

Whether judged by production statistics, contemporary critical acclaim, audience popularity or retrospective opinions, it is abundantly clear that the American silent film comedy was flourishing in the mid-twenties, rivaling drama as the dominant form of cinematic expression. My aim in this essay is to rethink the function of the gag in relation to the comic film as a classical system. I seek not to examine or catalog all the possible variations of the gag (as joke, as articulation of cinema space or as thematic permutations) but rather to examine its operation in the slapstick genre. [2]

Let us introduce the subject by way of an amusing account of a screening of Charlie Chaplin films in Accra (Ghana, Africa), reported in the *New York Times* in 1925:

> *It was a film from the remote antiquity of filmdom; a film from the utter dark ages of the cinematograph, so patched and pieced and repieced that all continuity was gone; a piebald hash chosen from the remains of various comedies and stuck together with no plot. Just slapstick. But Charlie had survived even that, and how they did love it!*[3]

The anecdote provides several insights into both the reception of films in a non-western culture and the status of film comedy in its "golden age." Most important for us, it expresses the opinion that this assemblage of Chaplin shorts is primitive, in the view of the reporter, because it lacks continuity. The writer intuitively distinguishes between linear aspects of film (plot, narrative, diegesis) and non-linear components (spectacle and gag). Take away the story and what do you have left? "Just slapstick."

Much criticism of silent film comedy still hinges on the dichotomy between narrative and gag. Gerald Mast remarks in *The Comic Mind* that Max Linder's film *Seven Years' Bad Luck* "is interested in a gag, not a story to contain the gags or a character to perform them," or that the plots of Sennett's Keystone films "are merely apparent structures, collections of literary formulas and clichés to hang the gags on."[4] In such statements, there is an implicit valorization of narrative over gags. These films are flawed because the elements of slapstick are not "integrated" with other elements (character, structure, vision, cinematic style—Mast's criteria).

In this reading of film comedy, slapstick is the bad element, an excessive tendency that narrative must contain. Accordingly the history of the genre is usually teleological, written as though the eventual replacement of the gag by narrativized comedy was natural, ameliorative or even predestined.

While viewing dozens of short comedies from the teens and twenties in preparation for the Slapstick Symposium, it became clear that there was no such selective process operating. On the contrary, slapstick Cinema seems to be ruled by the principle of accretion: gags, situations, costumes, characters and camera techniques are rehearsed and recycled in film after film, as though the modernist emphasis on originality and the unique text was unheard of. Unlike "mainstream" dramatic cinema, which progressed rapidly through styles, techniques and stories, nothing was discarded in slapstick. Camera tricks perfected by Méliès and Zecca are still in evidence a quarter-century later; music hall turns that were hoary when Chaplin, Linder and Keaton introduced them to cinema in the teens were still eliciting laughs by those clowns and others at the end of the silent period. We are forced to ask, if gags were so scorned, then why did the gag film linger on for so long, an important mode of cinematic discourse for at least forty years? And is there not something perverse about arguing that what is "wrong" with a film form is that which defines it to begin with?

The distinction between slapstick and narrative has been properly perceived, but incorrectly interpreted. I contend that it was never the aim of comic filmmakers to "integrate" the gag elements of their movies. I also doubt that viewers subordinated gags to narrative. In fact, the separation between the vertical domain of slapstick (the arena of spectacle I will represent by the metaphor of the thrown pie) and the horizontal domain of the story (the arena of the chase) was a calculated rupture, designed to keep the two elements antagonistically apart. In *Narration in the Fiction Film*, David Bordwell asks, "Is there anything in narrative film that is not narrational?"[5] My answer is yes: the gag.

If we examine typical Hal Roach two-reel comedies from 1925 and 1926, we find a laboratory for what some film analysts have described as the series of symmetries and blockages that define the systematicity of classical American cinema. At the same time, it is important to differentiate these films from the contemporaneous feature. While at first the narrative structures of the shorts may resemble condensations or abridgments (features with the boring bits taken out), the high concentration of gag and spectacle defines the genre as unique. Among other features, the frequent intrusions of spectacle produce a kind of narrative lurching that often makes the plots of slapstick comedies distinctively incoherent (and delightfully so).

The Pie

Let us first look more closely at those nonnarrative gag elements that the term slapstick usually encompasses. This usage is appropriate when we consider the origin of that word, referring to a circus prop consisting of two thin slats joined together, so that a loud clack is made when one clown hits another on the behind. The violent aural effect, the "slap," may be thought of as having the same kind of disruptive impact on the audience as its visual equivalent in the silent cinema, the pie in the face. In fact, very few comedies of the twenties really used pies, but nevertheless their humor in a general sense frequently depended on the same kind of emphatic, violent, embarrassing gesture.

The lack of linear integration that offends some slapstick commentators can trace its roots to popular spectacle. For example, in his 1915 home correspondence manual, Brett Page advised would-be vaudeville writers that their scripts must account for the actors' *business*. He meant the visual, nonverbal performance component, "done to drive the spoken words home, or to 'get over' a meaning without words."[6] His pupils learned that:

> *So large a part does the element of business play in the success of the two-act that the early examples of this vaudeville form were nearly all built out of bits of business. And the business was usually of the "slap-stick" kind. (p. 98)*

Page defined slapstick as physical gags, and consistently emphasized its nonverbal nature:

> *Every successful two-act, every entertainment-form of which acting is an element—the playlet and the full-evening play as well—prove beyond the shadow of a doubt that what audiences laugh at—what you and I laugh at—is not words, but actions and situations. (p. 108)*

Page easily generalized and shifted his focus from the nonverbal to the nonnarrative. About the vaudeville sketch he wrote,

> *The purpose of the sketch is not to leave a single impression of a single story. It points no moral, draws no conclusion, and sometimes it might end quite as effectively anywhere before the place in the action at which it does terminate. It is built*

> *for entertainment purposes only and furthermore, for entertainment purposes that end the moment the sketch ends. (p. 147)*

Recalling the African projection of the fragmented Chaplin films, the movie might have been incomprehensible as a narrative, but it worked fine as a filmic sketch, an assembly of nonverbal gags. Such an aesthetic of spectacle for its own sake is clearly inimical to the classical narrative feature, but not at all hostile to slapstick cinema of the teens and twenties.

Again, we can use this concept to discriminate between the comic shorts and the comic feature. The latter purposefully (and more or less successfully) sought to produce an "integrated" spectacle. Certainly *The General* and *The Gold Rush* are exemplary in their attempt to set the hero's struggles within a determinant Griffithesque historical fiction. But when one examines the two-reelers, even late in the twenties and well into the sound era one finds a preponderance of anarchistic non- and quasinarratives that pass for movie stories.

Generally, there is a simple plot which frames the gags, with an opening premise and a closing scene which provides a resolution. The gags may or may not be thematically related. Whether this is a narrative depends on how insistently one defines it. I argue that despite a weakly structured set of causes and effects, many of these films remain, at best, quasinarratives. Although the shorts emulate feature film narrative structures, the audience is scarcely aware of it, navigating the film from laugh to laugh as though enjoying a sketch. This is gag-driven cinema.

There can be no concrete definition of a gag because it is marked by affective response, not set forms or clear logic. Further, gag and slapstick are not synonymous. Slapstick is the generic term for these nonnarrative intrusions, while gags are specific forms of intrusions. Like verbal jokes, to which they are closely related, gags have their own loose structures, systems and "fuzzy" logic that exist independently of cinema. The gag may also contain its own microscopic narrative system that may be irrelevant to the larger narrative, may mirror it, or may even work against it as parody. "Sight gags," those that depend primarily on visual exposition, still have characteristic logical structures, the same that one finds in multipanel comic strips.[7] Think, for example, of the gag in *Jus' Passin' Through,* a Will Rogers film from 1923, produced by Hal Roach and directed by Charles Parrott (a.k.a. Charley Chase). We see a hobo checking the gates of houses for the special chalk tramp-sign that indicates whether there is a mean dog inside. One can easily see how the sequence could be presented effectively as a wordless comic strip. In the first two frames we would see images of the tramp eschewing those yards with the mark on the gate (the exposition of the nonhumorous part of the joke that vaudevillians would have called the "buildup"); in the penultimate panel we would see him fleeing a yard through an unmarked gate with a dog in hot pursuit; the final panel would show him adding his own beware-the-dog sign to the gate. Whether this corresponds to a "punch line" depends on how much visual/narrative information is perceived, and how the viewer's expectations are subverted.[8]

Other examples of "comic strip logic" might be mistaken identity gags (accomplished by fluid montage and parodic sight line constructions) such as the one that begins the Charley Chase film *Looking for Sally* (1925): from a ship's deck, the arriving hero waves to a girl on the dock whom he incorrectly assumes to be his fiancée; she waves back, not to Charley (as he thinks) but (as we see) to *her* friend on another deck. (See also Chaplin's *A Dog's Life* for the same gag.)

Also commonplace are camera tricks, for instance, double exposures and animation, that exploit the film medium's capability of disrupting the normal vision that the narrative depends on for its consistency and legibility. Manipulation of cause and effect—for example, when a little action produces a disproportionate reaction—is another form of cinematic excess characteristic of the sight gag. It is important to remember that the narrative content of the gag may be *nil*—for example the jarring close-ups of Ben Turpin's eyes. Such cases are illustrations of what Eisenstein called "attractions," elements of pure spectacle.

Writing in 1923, Eisenstein defined the "attraction" as: "every aggressive moment in [the theater], i.e. every element of it that brings to light in the spectator those senses or that psychology that influence his experience."[9] Eisenstein also referred to those moments as "emotional shocks," and insisted that they are always psychologically disruptive (for example, the gouging out of an eye). He contrasted the attraction to the lyrical, that being the part of the presentation readily assimilated by the spectator. Probably referring to *The Kid* (1921) he notes that the lyrical may coexist with the disruptive attraction, for example, the "specific mechanics of [Chaplin's] movement." In slapstick comedy, I am claiming, there is a variant of this concept: the "lyrical" is the narrative, functioning as the regulating component; the "attraction" is the gag or, again in Eisenstein's words, the "brake" that has to be applied to sharpened dramatic moments."[10] In another context, Tom Gunning has described early cinema (pre-1906) as a "cinema of attraction:"

> *Whatever differences one might find between Lumière and Méliès, they should not represent the opposition between narrative and nonnarrative filmmaking, at least as it is understood today. Rather, one can unite them in a conception that sees cinema less as a way of telling stories than as a way of presenting a series of views to an audience.... In other words, I believe that the relation to the spectator set up by the films of both Lumière and Méliès (and many other filmmakers before 1906) had a common basis, and one that differs from the primary spectator relations set up by narrative film after 1906.... Although different from the fascination in storytelling exploited by the cinema from the time of Griffith, it is not necessarily opposed to it. In fact the cinema of attraction does not disappear with the dominance of narrative, but rather goes underground, both into certain avant-garde practices and as a component of narrative films, more evident in some genres (e.g. the musical) than in others.[11]*

Gunning's observation is astute; the disruptive gags of slapstick can be regarded as an anachronistic manifestation of the cinema of attraction. I disagree, though, with his unwillingness to polarize the two components. While other genres work to contain their excesses, this opposition is fundamental to slapstick. Furthermore it is carefully constructed to remain an unbridgeable gap. In this sense it is *not* underground, but instead overt, flagrant and flamboyant.

The Chase

Let us look briefly at the other component, the Chase, or the narrative dimension of film comedy. Again, rather than examining specific narrative structures, it is enough for our purposes to say that the narrative is the propelling element, the fuel of the film that gives it its power to go from beginning to end. (To continue the automotive metaphor, one would say that the gags are the potholes, detours and flat tires encountered by the Tin Lizzie of the narrative on its way to the end of the film.) Film narrative has been the subject of considerable recent scholarly exposition, and rightly so. But its other, that is, those elements that block narrativity—the Pie—has been dismissed as textual excess, if it has been considered at all. Although, in the twenties, actual chases were more frequent than pie-throwings, I am also using the term Chase metaphorically, suggesting the linear trajectory of the narrative in general, not a specific instance. The term includes many characteristic twenties plots, such as pursuing a criminal, retrieving a lost object, restoring a family, and—most importantly—reuniting a separated couple in a presumed marriage. Of course the same themes predominate in dramatic films as well, and we should bear in mind that, as Gunning, Eileen Bowser, Andrew Horton and others have noted, the line between comedy and melodrama can be very fine.[12] One thinks, for example, of Anita Loos's claim that she tried to turn the screenplay of Griffith's *The Struggle* (based on *Ten Nights in a Barroom*) into a comic farce, while the film that Griffith made from the screenplay turned out to be a "serious" temperance melodrama. The disruptive elements, the parodic "attractions" concocted by Loos, were recuperated by Griffith's narrative priorities.

So Much for Theory...

When Steve Neale writes of "the emergence of terms like Fate, Chance and Destiny," or "a character's mistaken perception, or lack of knowledge,"[13] instead of melodrama, he could just as well be discussing *His Wooden Wedding,* a short produced in 1925 by Hal Roach, directed by Leo McCarey, and starring Charley Chase.[14]

Rich playboy Charley is marrying Katherine (Katherine Grant) on Friday the 13th. The date is a portent of the loss of stasis that is about to occur, and an explanation, couched in the uncanny, of several aspects of bad luck that will inevitably mar the wedding: the best man (unknown to Charley) is Katherine's rejected suitor, who is spiteful and, besides, would like to steal the diamond engagement ring. He plants false knowledge, in the form of a note to Charley informing him that his fiancée is not what she seems: "Beware! The girl you are about to marry has a wooden leg." By coincidence (extraordinary in life, but typical in fiction), Katherine sprains her ankle just before the wedding, causing her to limp down the aisle, apparently substantiating the outrageous rumor. Charley shouts "Stop! I've been engaged to a girl with a wooden leg—I must break it off." When he confronts Katherine in her room after the aborted wedding ceremony, he is unaware that he is actually speaking to a manikin. In the course of his explanation, her leg falls off and he walks out.

Drowning his sorrows in a bottle of wine, Charley then boards a cruise ship to forget Katherine's presumed treachery. On board he discovers the plot, recovers the diamond, and turns the boat around to meet Katherine, who has learned independently of the hoax and is following the ship on her father's yacht. When she arrives, Charley and the rival are struggling in the water. She strips down to her bathing suit to save Charley and, when the villain is hauled aboard, she displays her very real bare leg and uses it to kick him back into the water, thus cancelling the effects of his libelous false knowledge with this empirical demonstration of her corporeal integrity.

What is especially interesting, and also very typical of many shorts of the period, is the manner in which the apparent narrative closure, eliminating the villain, is not really final. There is a coda reunion scene as the lovers pose in an embrace. The formal tableau ending suggests that the symmetry of the narrative is insufficient by itself to properly close the film.

It is as though the narrative's validity must be confirmed by subsuming it into spectacle showing that the initial promise of order—the protagonists' marriage—will be fulfilled. To put it another way, the man and woman must be rejoined and visually wed before they can be wed in the later fiction, the one after the film ends, the one the spectator (not the filmmaker) creates.

Also typical of comedy as well as melodrama is the insistence on a woman's body as the site for restoring natural order through heterosexual coupling. In this reading, the imagery in Chase's film is essentially a castration nightmare: the revelation to the groom on his wedding day that his bride has a horrifying lack (a symbolic missing leg) and an intolerable replacement (the metonymic wooden member). Charley contemplates his future children and the family dog all sporting peg legs, as if the wound were a genetic flaw passed on by the wife. The woman is being projected as the scene of the man's fears and anxieties concerning familial responsibility and sexual performance. Only when the threat of the woman's repugnant phallic intrusion into their relationship, the despised wooden leg, is removed ("broken off") can the wedding—of flesh and not of wood—take place.

This film is an excellent example of how gag and narrative interact and regulate each other by means of a lively dialectic. One cannot help but compare the complex system of alternation of spectacle and diegesis to the same systems observable in Einstein's films of the period. While space does not allow a thorough analysis, we can point out some of the ways in which gags disturb the narrative.

The film's opening scenes of wedding preparations provide the armature for an "instant" narrative form, since viewers understand the protocol of such ceremonies. But expectations for a normal unfolding of events are soon derailed. Instead of providing background information on the story of characters, the intertitles make gratuitous jokes that interfere with our comprehension: "The happy bridegroom—So excited he telephoned the minister to bring along a shotgun and a good bird dog." The verbal content diverts the narrative rather than advancing it. The rival's note about the wooden leg similarly challenges the viewer to rationalize a motive for its effect. Why would the rival choose this particular lie (instead of the "usual" marital impediments: bigamy, secret lovers, dreaded diseases, racial taint, illegitimate children)? Would not even the most priggish of grooms already be aware of this physical trait of his fiancée? Would having a prosthesis really be sufficient grounds for halting a marriage? To "explain" Charley's motives, the viewer sees a subjective vision of Charley's family in the future; but what Charley imagines is biologically impossible. However improbable, it nevertheless convinces *him* to interrupt the wedding. The spectacle of the wooden-legged family also halts the deployment of the ready-made narrative of the wedding ceremony. In a trope that will be replayed several times in the film, a small action (the bogus note) prompts a massive and irrational overreaction (the cancellation).

But the disjunctive titles are inserted into a very ordinary *mise-en-scène* quite typical of any 1920s feature (complete with characteristic matchcuts, eyeline matches, and so on). The exception is when Charley looks at the camera and performs his signature "slow burn," for instance when the manikin (whom he has mistaken for Katherine) loses her leg.

The advancement of the wedding ceremony is frequently halted by Charley's inappropriate actions: he attempts to shake the hand of an old friend, he is distracted by the crying mother-in-law-to-be. And fate intervenes when Katherine sprains her ankle. When Charley exits the wedding, the restoration of the narrative commences by way of a triple pursuit structure. Katherine, learning of the hoax, follows Charley; the rival pursues Charley to get the diamond; and Charley seeks the diamond (and thence Katherine). These three motives are articulated in parallel montage sequences.

Each pursuit has its own trajectory, which is protracted by fate's intervention: The rival retrieves the diamond, but loses it to Charley in a hat mix-up; Katherine and her father pursue Charley but keep just missing him; Charley finds the diamond but loses it in a woman passenger's clothing.[16] Neale's description of melodrama structure is once again applicable here:

> *The constantly changing and apparently arbitrary course of events articulates and intensifies these vicissitudes, and, in turn, is motivated by them. Blockages, barriers and bars to the fulfillment of desire are constantly introduced as events change course.*[17]

There are running gags involving hats (thrown overboard, blown by wind, knocked off). There are sight gags (the manikin) and spatial gags (the double door keyhole in the woman's stateroom). An example of another kind of block is Charley's subjective insert, in which he fantasizes the "future," set in faraway 1934. While the viewer understands the diegetic time to be in the character's future, the diegetic tense is nevertheless the present. For, though it takes a few seconds to unfold on the screen, for Charley, the vision is an instantaneous flash of clairvoyance. The confusion of tense is something like the effect of the temporal lapses in musicals.

Special effects also break into the diegetic world. When the boat swerves there is a cut to a small model ship, hilarious in its obviousness. Similarly, the effect of the ship's turning is done simply by having the actors lean in one direction and fall over. A splice creates the effect of Charley picking up a full decanter of wine and setting down an empty one.

Many of the gags are based on inversions of normal logic. As mentioned, small actions that spark big reactions are a *leitmotif*. When Charley's servant tosses his suitcase out the window it destroys a parked car; the policeman tells Charley he cannot park his car on the quay, so he pushes it into the ocean. There is also the truncated syllogism. The joke is set up as a set of logical relations, but the expected conclusion does not follow. Charley throws his hat (with the diamond in it) over the ship's rail, and it returns three times. But when he throws the captain's hat it sails away. These subversions of logic undermine the viewer's ability to match effects with causes.

The most elaborate set piece occurs when Charley entices the woman passenger to dance the Charleston with him in the hopes of shaking loose the diamond. This important scene is semidiegetic; that is, it furthers the narrative in a crucial way—it produces the object of the chase, the diamond—but it is also predominantly a spectacle, and the sequence which provokes the most belly laughs in viewers. Again there is a humorous failure of logic. The dancers' contortions become more frenetic and gynmastic, causing the woman to shed first her watch, her powder puff, then her brassiere. This progression *ad absurdum* is anticlimactically cut short when the envelope containing the diamond falls out, and Charley strolls out without a word, as though the episode never took place.

The three pursuits wind down, but are again prolonged by inserting a spectacle—Katherine's exposed leg—and by the "business" of kicking the rival back into the water. By the time the final closure is achieved, sealed with a kiss between the betrothed, the audience experiences relief, but also a temporal waste, a *temps perdu* because the "story" has been set back to a time before the film began (the plans for a new wedding have to be made). All that transpired was "excess"—slapstick.[18]

"Pie"	"Chase"
Gag Titles	*Glance-object editing style*
Inappropriate actions (Charley recognizes old friend as he walks down the aisle)	*Expected chain of events* (structure of wedding ceremony)
Fate (sprained ankle)	*Triple pursuit:*
Mistaken perception (cane for leg)	• Katherine → Charley
Subjective insert (temporal confusion)	• Rival → diamond
	• Charley → diamond
	Motivating action (duplicitous note)
	Parallel action in different spaces
Attenuated reaction/direct address (long glance at camera when manikin's leg falls)	*Actions to restore order:*
Drunken gags	• Rival retrieves diamond
	• Diamond in Charley's hat
Running gags (e.g. hats)	• Katherine's father discovers note; she and he pursue Charley
Small action → large reaction	
	• Charley pursues his hat, finds diamond, hides it on old maid
Repeated action (car destructions)	• Charley wins old maid's admiration and tricks rival (keyhole)
Inappropriate action	
Truncated syllogism (hat over rail)	• Charley tries to recover ring
Sight gags	*Closures*
Spatial gags	• Charley retrieves diamond
Semidiegetic insert (dance scene)	• Katherine intercepts ship; Charley turns boat around; jumps into ocean (with rival)
Progression ad absurdum (dance scene)	
Exaggerated reaction (boat turning → dancers falling)	• Katherine kicks rival with "real" leg
Special effects (obvious model boat)	
Revelation (display of "real" leg)	
Final tableau (apotheosis)	

In his response to this paper in its original version, reprinted following this essay, Tom Gunning made some valuable criticism that I should address briefly. First, he drew attention to the two-dimensionality of my picture of the "forces that disrupt and the forces that contain," and insisted on the complexity of the relationship. I agree. But I disagree that the narrative is always a complex "process of integration in which smaller units are absorbed into a larger overarching pattern and process of containment," or that gags are "an excess that is necessary to the film's process of containment." This may be an accurate description of other genres, but slapstick seems to actively construct this "failure" of containment and to resist bourgeois legibility and rationality.

Gunning cites the dance sequence as an example of the recovery of gags by narrativization. True, the purpose served by the scene is to retrieve the engagement ring from the "virgin wilderness of the old maid's underclothes," but at what lack of economy! The same function would have been satisfied by Charley's finding the ring on the deck. Instead the woman is presented in such a way as to reward the audience's desire to see an old maid making a shimmying spectacle of herself. The abruptness of Charley's desertion after he gets the ring is funny in part because his offhand gesture points up the irrelevance of the ring to the narrative; it's a MacGuffin. It is the diegetic content of the scene (ring as object of the chase) that becomes the excessive part of the elaborate joke.

Gunning also rightly notes that my chart contains several elements (such as truncated syllogisms) that, as inversions, are possible only through the gag's deceptive assimilation of narrative form. He points out that parodies of narratives are still narratives "in which narrative logic is not so much ignored as laid bare."

No one will argue that *His Wooden Wedding* is lacking in parody. Charley's "courting" of the old maid, for example, is a parody of his court ship with Katherine and its vicissitudes (the woman's agility contrasting with Katherine's lameness). But again, I maintain that in these instances, the tail *really is* wagging the dog! To say that the gags' assimilation of narrative structure is laying bare the illusionist invisibility of the fictional mechanism is simply another way of saying that spectacle is here "containing" narrative, and not the other way around. The "message" of this and other slapstick films is that the seeming hegemony of narrative in the classical cinema is being assaulted by the militant forces of spectacle. The film's multiple narrative closures are overly redundant, even by classical standards. The obstacles mounted by fate are overcome, but not at the cost of annihilating the impact of the gags. It is the *non sequitur* components of the humor that we recall best—as in one of Brett Page's ideal sketches. Like the wedding of the title, the absorption of all the disruptive elements by the narrative never takes place.

If there is a controversy here, it may be resolved simply by asserting that while films generally are not all-or-nothing, spectacle-versus-narrative propositions, there are certain cases that encourage the viewer to see them in just this binary fashion. *Don Key, Son of Burro* (Roach, 1926) is a good illustration of the slapstick genre's awareness of its own ambivalent attitude toward narrative containment.

The "story" of the film is minimal: a movie writer enters a producer's office to pitch his screenplay. As he speaks, the actions of his screenplay appear as a series of vignettes, separated from the main narrative by conventional dissolves. These usually denote another narrative level (dream, fantasy, and so on), but in this case, the vignettes show us the writer's fiction.

The joke is that the writer's "story" is only a succession of sight gags and business that ultimately fail the test of a narrative: there is no cause and effect, no consistent pattern or development of the represented events. The "episodes" vary from the surrealistically strange to the hilariously funny. In one sequence the leading lady's boyfriend is getting a shave. Every time the barber applies the razor, a dog runs up to the chair as though begging for a bone. The barber explains, "He's such an optimist. Once he got an ear."[19]

As best as can be reconstructed, the writer's "story" begins with a boy who has a chimp as a babysitter. They live next to a den of lions. An old, ugly playboy (Jimmy Finlayson) is spying on the girl and her boyfriend. There is a bank robbery, and a sheriff who chases the bandits over railroad tracks and fields. The chimp runs away with the boy, and the playboy falls into the lion's den. All this is punctuated with numerous "pie" elements: Finlayson's constant mannerism of looking at the camera; the chimp's victimization by a pesky duck; Finlayson's kissing the chimp instead of the girl; and extensive animated effects: Finlayson's beating heart, the robbers' car careening around a curve on a cliff; a strange car that bucks off the passengers.

As the writer tells his incomprehensible tale, we cut back to the reactions of the producer and his flunkies. His assistants appear with a sledgehammer, a bomb, and a bow and arrow and ask their boss, "Now?" The producer replies, "Not yet," and finally dismisses the writer. (He shoots the next writer who walks in without even listening to his screenplay.)

The film recounts vividly the antagonism between slapstick business and the institutional drive to subdue it to the demands of Hollywood. By showing plural interpretations of the "screenplay," the film exploits the viewer's conflicting associations. On the one hand, the writer's gags are truly funny, his sight gags successfully crafted; on the other, his film will never be produced (existing only as an unrealized fiction). For the writer it works, for the producer it fails, but we can see it both ways: successful as a comic spectacle; a flop as a movie melodrama.

We can see it binocularly because we know the parameters of film narrative. Our *de facto* orientation is that of the producer. But unlike him and his yes-men, we do not reject the writer's proposal because of its nonconformity; we relish it precisely because it flaunts conventions of Hollywood storytelling. Certainly this is parody. And the film finally "recuperates" Hollywood by throwing out the writer. But like inadmissible evidence at a trial, the point of the film was understood, and lingers subversively in the minds of the viewers. Slapstick gags are more effective than melodramatic tears.

Conclusion

It may be that the tendency to suppress the antinarrative elements of film history results from a hasty overclassicism of actual Hollywood output in the 1920s. Richard Koszarski has reminded us that cinema in the twenties was *an evening's* entertainment.[20] The slapstick short took its place among the travelogues, cartoons, 3-D novelties, sing-alongs, live prologues and musical performances. Like these expressive forms, spectacle "attraction" was the primary characteristic; narrative was greatly diminished, if present at all. Some features—*The General* is a good example—even contained color sequences that were narratively expendable, but contributed visual novelty.

One way to look at narrative is to see it as a system for providing the spectator with sufficient knowledge to make causal links between represented events.[21] According to this view, the gag's status as an irreconcilable difference becomes clear. Rather than providing knowledge, slapstick misdirects the viewer's attention, and obfuscates the linearity of cause-effect relations. Gags provide the opposite of epistemological comprehension by the spectator. They are atemporal bursts of violence and/or hedonism that are as ephemeral and as gratifying as the sight of someone's pie-smitten face.

Endnotes

1. This somewhat grizzled text requires a bit of explanation. In early 1985, Eileen Bowser proposed a "Slapstick Symposium," which would be held in conjunction with a congress of FIAF (The International Federation of Film Archives). Those of us in the New York vicinity were able to preview a selection of films at the Museum of Modern Art. Ms. Bowser's concept, original and elegantly simple, was that each presentation would be not just a paper, but rather a running commentary integrated with projections of complete films. This was spectacularly successful as live performance at the symposium, which took place May 2–3, 1985, but proved nettlesome when the time came to produce written papers. Besides the shift from an informal verbal mode to written discourse, the presenters/authors had to cope with the inaccessibility of the films for many of the readers.

    Meanwhile I was asked to re-present the talk at the Columbia University Seminars at the Museum of Modern Art. I was fortunate to have Tom Gunning, who had participated in the Slapstick Symposium, as my respondent on November 14, 1985. His reactions, suggestions and criticisms, as well as those of others at the symposium and the seminars, were incorporated into the 1988 publication of the proceedings.

    Since 1985, of course, the slippery banana peel has been the subject of much serious study, and likewise the study of narrative and narration in cinema has developed. Although I considered writing a completely updated revision for the present anthology, I ultimately rejected the idea. Nevertheless, I have made some changes of emphasis which I believe will clarify some murkiness in the original.

    I would like to dedicate this essay to Eileen Bowser, on the occasion of her retirement from the Museum of Modern Art in 1993.

2. See for example, Dan Kamin's chapter "The Magician," in *Charlie Chaplin's One-Man Show* (Metuchen: Scarecrow Press, 1984), pp. 37–55; David Madden, *Harlequin's Stick, Charlie's*

Cane: A Comparative Study of Commedia dell' Arte and Silent Slapstick Comedy (Bowling Green, OH: Popular Press, 1975); François Mars, *Le Gag* (Paris: Editions du Cerf, 1964); Jean-Paul Simon and Daniel Percheron, "Gag," in Jean Collet, et al., eds., *Lectures du film* (Paris: Editions Albatros, 1980), pp. 104–107.

Other useful works include Andrew Horton's anthology, *Comedy/Cinema/Theory* (Berkeley: University of California Press, 1991); Steve Seidman, *Comedian Comedy: A Tradition in Hollywood Film* (Ann Arbor, MI.: UMI Research Press, 1981); Gerald Weales, *Canned Goods as Caviar: American Film Comedy of the 1930's* (Chicago: University of Chicago Press, 1985); Steve Neale and Frank Krutnik, *Popular Film and Television Comedy* (London; New York: Routledge, 1990); and Henry Jenkins, *What Made Pistachio Nuts?* (New York: Columbia University Press, 1992).

3. "Charlie's Gold Coast Triumph," *New York Times,* quoted in *Film Daily Yearbook* 1926, p. 15.
4. Gerald Mast, *The Comic Mind: Comedy and the Movies* (Indianapolis: Bobbs-Merill, 1973), pp. 39, 53.
5. David Bordwell, *Narration in the Fiction Film* (Madison: University of Wisconsin Press, 1985), p. 53. Bordwell's answer is also yes, but qualified. Such elements are "excess" (citing Kristin Thompson's analysis of *Ivan the Terrible*) and "whatever its suggestiveness as a critical concept, excess lies outside my concern here."
6. Brett Page, *Writing for Vaudeville* (Springfield, MA: The Home Correspondence School, 1915), p. 98 fn. Thanks to Henry Jenkins for bringing this book to my attention.
7. Noël Carroll's six categories of sight gags are a useful catalogue ("Notes on the Sightgag," in Horton, ed., *Comedy/Cinema/Theory*, 25–42). His defining principle is based on the construction of conflicting interpretations in the visual organization of a scene.
8. Carroll's distinction between verbal and visual jokes ("Notes on the Sightgag") is generally, but not always, valid. He argues: "Sight gags differ from verbal jokes. Verbal jokes generally culminate in a punchline that at first glace is incongruous by virtue of its appearing to be nonsense. . . . One is initially stymied by the incongruity of the punchline, which leads to a *re*interpretation of the joke material that makes it comprehensible. Sight gags also involve a play of interpretations. But with sight gags, the play of interpretation is often visually available to the audience simultaneously throughout the gag: the audience *need not* await something akin to the punchline in a verbal joke to put the interpretive play in motion" (p. 27). There are many examples of gags that deliver just such a "punch" due to a surprise cut or change in *mise-en-scène,* prompting a reinterpretation analogous to the one Carroll describes in verbal humor.
9. Sergei Eisenstein, "Montage of Attractions," in Jay Leyda, ed., *The Film Sense* (New York: Harcourt, 1947), pp. 230–231.
10. Eisenstein, "The Unexpected," in Leyda, ed., *Film Form* (New York: Harcourt, 1949), p. 23.
11. Tom Gunning, "The Cinema of Attraction: Early Film, Its Spectator and the Avant-Garde," *Wide Angle* 8, 3/4, 1986, p. 64.
12. Andrew Horton states succinctly, "No plot is inherently funny. Put another way . . . any plot is potentially comic, melodramatic, or tragic, perhaps all three at once" ("Introduction," *Cinema/Comedy/Theory,* p. 1).
13. Steve Neale, "Melodrama and Tears," *Screen* 27,6, November–December 1986, p. 7.
14. *His Wooden Wedding* is available from Blackhawk Films. Other players are Gale Henry, Fred deSilva, John Cossar. Photographed by Glen R. Carrier. Edited by Richard Currier. Running time: 24 minutes at 24fps. Released December 20, 1925.
15. The throwaway function of marriage in this film is another good way to distinguish the short from the feature. In *His Wooden Wedding* it is a perfunctory motive, almost a gag in itself; in Keaton's *Seven Chances* it is a "narrativized" orchestration of delays that build in intensity. Horton notes that "Most screen comedy concerns romance . . . of one form or another, and romance requires personal compromise and social integration, as traditionally represented in

the final marriage" ("Introduction," *Comedy/Cinema/Theory,* p. 11). The lack of character development, a hallmark of the slapstick short, precludes all but the most brusque references to social integration, whereas the feature foregrounds character development.

16. The passenger is a stereotypically sexist "old maid" character.
17. Neale, "Melodrama and Tears," p. 12.
18. In a melodrama—or in an "integrated" comedy feature like *City Lights*—the "lost time" of the story is not wasted, because there has been some intangible gain. For example, a character may have gained maturity, or self-knowledge, or may have survived a rite of passage, or two people's affection may have grown into love. In slapstick the characters are cartoonlike and the plots too shallow to encourage the kind of empathy that leads to melodramatic recuperation. In slapstick shorts, lost time is seldom recovered.
19. Thanks to Peter Demetz for translating the Czech titles on the print back into English for me.
20. Richard Koszarski, *An Evening's Entertainment: The Age of the Silent Feature Picture 1915-1928* (New York: Charles Scribner's Sons, 1990).
21. "Narration refers not to what is told, but rather to the conditions of telling—to the overall regulation and distribution of knowledge in a text. . . ." (Edward Branigan, "Diegesis and Authorship in Film," *IRIS* 7, 2nd semester 1986, p. 38).

Response to "Pie and Chase"

Tom Gunning

The term "narrative" has been something of a dirty word in film studies for the last few decades. It was assumed that telling stories was the most simple and boring thing a film could do. Narrative was associated with "content" or "thematics," and understood as clearly a less sexy thing for a film theorist to be involved with than form or style. When Truffaut said that he loved the moments in film when the narrative stops, he seemed to announce a whole generation's preoccupation with the contingent and nonnarrative elements of film practice.

The recent refocusing on narrative has somewhat redressed the balance, calling attention to what we might term the structural aspects of narrative, seeing story not as content but as a structuring force. However, narrative seems to still carry an ambivalent reaction, a taint of ideological conformity and containment. The Bellour-Heathian view of narrative which Don Crafton cites may announce narrative as a respectable topic for investigation, but still approaches it with a lingering suspicion. Narrative, in this view, is a dynamic process which charts, as Crafton puts it, a disruption of an original stasis and a consequent process of containment that seeks to limit the violence of disruption and regain the original equilibrium.

The usefulness of the description is obvious, and although there may be doubts about its universality, its range of application is certainly broad in commercial narrative films. However, what needs to be emphasized is that this view sees two elements to narrative: the forces that disrupt and the forces that contain. While most narratives operate so that containment dominates disruption, thus providing closure, it should be emphasized that the forces of disruption *are essential* to even the most conventional narrative.

I think that Crafton's paper is fairly clear on this point, but the relation between the disruptive elements of narrative and the "pie" elements of pure nonnarrative spectacle is complex. Like the disruptive elements, gags are, as he puts it, the potholes, detours and flat tires of narrative, that which Barthes and the Russian Formalists would call the "delays" of narrative.

This is not at all to deny that slapstick comedies (along with a number of other popular genres, most obviously the musical) involve an interrelation of narrative and nonnarrative elements. I like very much the relation Crafton draws between gags and Eisenstein's concept of theatrical attractions, a relation which I have also made dealing with elements in pre-1907 films. However I believe that Crafton opens here a subject for further analysis. The interrelation of these nonnarrative and narrative features is quite complex, precisely because narrative acts as a system of regulation which ultimately absorbs nonnarrative elements into its pendulum sways.

Ben Brewster recently pointed out to me the limitations to our conception of narrative as linear. Useful as this two-dimensional metaphor may be in describing the goal-directed aspect of many narratives and narrative's own rush to containment, it also makes narrative appear more simple than I think it is in practice. Rather, we could think of narrative as a process of integration in which smaller units are absorbed into a larger overarching pattern and process of containment.

Crafton underestimates the interplay between the pie and the chase. First, gags become absorbed into the narrative economy of most films, marking perhaps an excess, but an excess that is necessary to the film's process of containment. The dancing sequence in *His Wooden Wedding* is a good example. This is, as Crafton notes, a progression *ad absurdum*. However, along with the delightful absurdity, we also get an important progression in the narrative: Chase's regaining of the diamond lost in the virgin wilderness of the old maid's underclothes.

But only the most boring of semioticians could feel that the regaining of the diamond was the *point* of this sequence. It is, rather, its excuse. But it is important to maintain this double vision: the excess of the gags and their recovery by narrativization.

The most important aspect which this double view allows is the realization that, in their contact with narrative, gags do not simply lose their independence, but precisely subvert the narrative itself. This is done not through their nonnarrative excess, their detouring of narrative concerns into pure attraction, but precisely through their integration with narrative, their adoption of narrative's form of logical anticipation, and then their subversion of it.

For instance, in Crafton's excellent list of gags from *His Wooden Wedding,* a number are quite correctly described as inversion in narrative logic ("inappropriate action," "truncated syllogism," "small action–large reaction"). The point here is that such inversions are possible only through the gag's deceptive assimilation of narrative form. It is by seeming to resemble certain narrative situations that narrative anticipation is subverted. This is not simply an issue of two separate forms, but of a dialectical interrelation. It is in fact the process of parody, in which narrative logic is not so much ignored, as laid bare.

When, as in *Don Key, Son of Burro,* the pie in the face (or its equivalent) is repeatedly delayed, it takes on one of the basic aspects of narrative. And when narrative situations are repeatedly rendered absurd by laying bare their devices, this subversion brings them close to gags. Eisenstein called, of course, for a *montage* of attraction, and noted that, in this structure, elements of narrative could be introduced in such a way as to lose their usual claim to coherence and diegetic realism. Slapstick comedy takes us not simply into the realm of the pie, but into the land of carnival, where narrative reveals the absurdity of its principle of integration, as legs transform from flesh to wood and back again, and pies end up in the face rather than the mouth.

Interview with Marion Mack

Raymond Rohauer

The first performance of THE GENERAL with Marion Mack appearing in person with Raymond Rohauer and talking to the audience took place in Toronto, Canada, on December 18, 1972. With the ovations still ringing in our ears, we recorded the following reminiscences:

RAYMOND ROHAUER: Well, Marion, how do you feel now that you've heard the people out there?

MARION MACK: I still can't believe it. They treated me as if I was Gloria Swanson. I'm really glad now that you found me and brought me out here, although to tell you the truth, at first I thought you were some kind of nut. But only for a little while!

RR: I'm glad we did it, too. But I must say you were one of the most elusive ladies I ever had to pursue.

MM: You know, I still wonder how you actually tracked me down. I wasn't listed anywhere, and practically nobody had my address.

RR: Yes, I know, I tried everything: *Variety,* the Screen Actors Guild, the Academy of Motion Picture Arts and Sciences—nothing! At MGM, they only knew that up to 1940, your husband was producing shorts for them. This made me realize you might be traceable under your husband's name, but what threw me there is that I was looking for Marion, and you were using your real first name, Joey.

MM: Yes, I thought that would be safe enough. And it was, for all these years. You know when you finally got me on the phone and asked me if I was Marion Mack, I was so shocked I couldn't answer you for a while. And when I'm at a loss for words, that's something!

RR: Do you know how I finally got to you? I just simply looked up the name Lewyn in the Los Angeles phone book. Of course, there was neither Marion nor Louis listed, but there was another Lewyn, and I called up and they said they didn't know themselves, but that a member of their family who happened to be living in Switzerland was a distant relative of yours. So, as I was just then on my way to France to attend the Avignon film festival, I contacted the lady in Switzerland while I was there, and once she said you lived in Costa Mesa I called you up at once.

MM: Yes, that was part of what threw me. All these years no one knew about me, and then you call me from Paris and right off the bat say: "Are you Marion Mack?" I thought someone was playing a practical joke on me again, as Buster used to do.

RR: Marion, I wonder if you would mind going over some of the things you were just talking about with your fans out there, so that we could get it on the record, so to speak. By the way, is this the first time you made a personal appearance with the film?

MM: Oh yes, it is. You know back in 1927 neither Buster nor the producers thought much of the picture. It was a routine comedy, and they didn't make any big fuss about opening it, no personal appearances or anything. And also, by that time I had other interests, and in fact I was practically out of the picture business when the film opened—at least out of the acting stage of the business. So tonight is my very first personal promotion with the film. In fact, this is the first time I ever saw THE GENERAL and didn't have to pay!

RR: You mean you had to buy a ticket to see your own performance?

MM: And not just once, either. My husband and I attended the opening of the picture, but purely as spectators. We both liked it, of course, but we were surprised when it took off as it did. It was the audiences that made it such a hit, the studio never realized what a gem they had on their hands until the money started rolling in. And in later years, every once in a while I used to go to one of the revival theaters when THE GENERAL was showing. At first I used to tell them I was the co-star, but I think they either didn't believe me, or it meant nothing to them. I was sort of hoping one of the managers would let me in free, but they used to say something like "Oh, really?" or "That's nice," and then they would politely show me where the box office was. You see what fun it is to be a famous movie star!

RR: Don't give it a second thought, Marion. Back in the early fifties, when I ran a theater in Los Angeles, Buster Keaton himself used to come and buy a ticket like anyone else, because none of my ticket takers recognized him. Anyway, Marion, could we have a little of your background—such as, how did you ever come to Hollywood in the first place?

MM: Well, Raymond, believe it or not, I just wrote a letter to Mack Sennett, and that's all there was to it. I was just a high school girl from Mammoth, Utah, and I said I wanted to be in the movies and enclosed a few snapshots, and they were real polite and Sennett's manager wrote back they would be happy to interview me if I ever came to Hollywood. It sounds like fiction but it's true. You see, this was in 1920 and it could still happen like this.

RR: Did they just say you should come right out to Hollywood?

MM: Not just like that, I had to be properly chaperoned. Now it so happened my father was married for the second time, and my step-mother was only about 24, and I was 18. So she agreed to help me, and we went to Hollywood.

RR: So you went in and just got a job at the first studio you contacted?

MM: Would you believe it, Raymond, that I got not one but two offers? You see, at about the same time, there was a beauty contest at the Ince Studio, and so I entered it, too. That is, I sent in my picture and that was it. They would let me know, one of those things. So naturally, I thought nothing more of it, and went over to Sennett's Studio and saw Jack Waldron, that was Sennett's manager, and I got hired at $25 a week. And then about a week later, there was my picture in the paper that I won the contest at Ince's. Now they wanted me, and I told them I was already working for Sennett, and Ince's publicity man got a little mad at me. Hans Sternberg, I think his name was.

RR: So how did you finally solve the problem?

MM: Well, I didn't want to work for Ince because I already had a job with Sennett, and in those days Sennett was the king. But Sternberg insisted that I must at least pose for some Ince publicity, at the Billion Dollar Theater I believe, and so I thought that's the least I could do. And the funny thing is, when those publicity pictures got back to Sternberg, he showed them to Louis Lewyn, who later became my husband, and Lou said: "What a lemon! How did you ever pick her?"

RR: Oh, really? Then how did you and Mr. Lewyn get together?

MM: Well, some time later Lou came over to the Sennett lot to take some publicity pictures of some of the girls. And all of a sudden he saw me, and either I looked better in make-up or those Ince photos must have been really bad, because now he didn't recognize me as a lemon but actually asked me to pose for some pictures for him separately from the other girls. And after the posing, he kept asking me if he could bring me home. I told him my father wouldn't let me date, but he insisted and so I let him take me to my house and on the way he asked how I got in the movies. So I said: "There was this contest at the Ince Studio and I won it," and he nearly fainted. And then I learned the whole story of what he thought of me at first, but I finally married him, anyway, and it worked out fine.

RR: That's quite a story, Marion. But tell me, what did you think of Mack Sennett?

MM: I was a little scared of him at first. He sounded a little rough, you know. But in those days I looked a little like Mabel Normand, who was Sennett's sweetheart, so I guess he liked me.

RR: How did you get your screen name? Did Sennett give it to you?

MM: No. At Sennett's, they called me Joanne McGuire. Later, when I went to work for the Little Mermaid and Sunshine Comedies, they wanted me to take another name, so I just took the middle part of my real name. I was born Joey Marion McCreery, so I clipped off Joey on one side and Creery on the other, and what was left was Marion Mc. All I had to do was spell out the "Mc." Marion Mack.

RR: All right, you say you left Sennett. Why was that?

MM: Well, I wanted to do a little more than just stand around in a bathing suit, so I took the first good offer that came along. By about 1922 I was making feature films, and then in 1923 Lou and I were married, and as you know he became later quite a big producer, and right from the start he let me write some of the scripts for the films he was doing, and I liked that. In this way, I made MARY OF THE MOVIES with my husband in 1923, and then THE CARNIVAL GIRL in 1926.

RR: Now tell me, Marion, how did you get to work with Keaton on his most important film?

MM: Buster was looking for an old-fashioned girl, with long curly hair, for the character of Annabelle Lee, because they wanted everything to look just right for the Civil War period. Well, Percy Westmore, who was making up Norma Talmadge for some picture, heard this from her, and of course she knew it because her sister, Natalie, was married to Keaton. And Percy mentioned that he knew a girl with just the right hair, because he had been my make-up man on CARNIVAL GIRL. And Norma said to Percy he should try to find out if I was available, and he called me and first thing he said was: "I hope you still have those long curls you had in CARNIVAL GIRL!" Well, Raymond, this was the year everyone was bobbing their hair, and so only about a couple of days before I cut my hair short, too, and I told it to Percy and he said, "Don't worry, we'll give you a fall or something."

RR: A what?

MM: A fall, you know, a wig. So that's what I wore to the interview with Buster Keaton.

RR: Who was present there? Was Keaton personally in on the interview?

MM: Yes, he was there, but he didn't say much. The guys who really talked to me were Lou Anger, the studio manager, and Clyde Bruckman. And then they sort of looked at Buster, and Buster said he thought I would do, and so I was hired right then and there.

RR: Up to this time, had you ever met Keaton?

MM: No, this was the first time. But, of course, everybody in town knew about him, he was well known, but he didn't get around to many of the smart parties and places, and stuck pretty much to his own pals.

RR: Now, let's take up the story of THE GENERAL. How long did it take to shoot the picture?

MM: We were six months on it. Actually, we went up to Oregon twice. First in the spring, around April, we stayed for about four months. Then we went back to Hollywood in September to do the studio scenes, and in October we went back to Cottage Grove for some more outdoor shooting.

RR: How was it set up on location?

MM: We all stayed at the Cottage Grove Hotel, and every morning we took that little train which you can see in the picture, and we rode out to location. It took about an hour. Buster had his own chef with him, Willy his name was, and he prepared hot lunch on location so that we could stay there all day.

RR: How did they shoot the picture? Was there a script?

MM: They used what I think today would be called just an outline. Not a real script as we now know it. I mean, they told you what the scene was, but you were expected to make up your own bits of business, and if anybody had an idea they would try it and see how it played. Like when I have the scene where I'm getting on the train Buster is driving, and I'm still supposed to be mad at him for not enlisting, I made a big business out of admiring the medal my brother was wearing, and polishing his uniform buttons, just to show how much I admired him, because of course I know that Buster is looking at me. And this was not in any script, but they said it looked cute and so it stayed in.

RR: Can you think of other incidents like that where you improvised right on camera?

MM: Oh yes, we did that all the time. You know the scene on the engine where I'm supposed to feed the fire, I'm supposed to be a little dumb about it. So somebody said I should get hold of a log with a knothole in it, and throw it away. I did that, but I didn't think the audience would understand it, and then I saw a very small piece of wood, and I picked it up and threw it in. Buster liked it, so right away he built it up; I mean he picked up an even smaller piece, just a splinter really, to see if I would be dumb enough to use that, too. And of course I did, and so he jumped on me as if he was going to choke me, but at the last moment he really gave me a little peck on the cheek. I think I got that kiss more for thinking of the gag than for anything else. And none of this was in written form at all.

RR: Did you get to know Keaton very well as a person?

MM: Buster was really a shy person. Some people said he was aloof, but his aloofness was mostly just shyness, I think. He wasn't easy to know very closely. Off screen, he always had his friends to play baseball with; why, sometimes they stopped the train when they saw a place to play baseball, and everything would be delayed by a couple of hours. And also, he had Natalie with him there, so there wasn't much socializing, actually. I had never worked with a leading man like that before, I can tell you, usually they were outgoing and chummy, but Buster just stuck to the job and to his little clique, and that was all. At first I felt a little bit, I'd say, ignored or slighted, but then he got a bit more friendly as he lost some of his shyness, and he turned out to be a very nice and warm person. And a very humble one, too, that's the surprising part.

RR: When did you feel that the ice was broken?

MM: I guess when he started playing jokes on me. In his book, when he made you the butt of some practical joke, that meant you were OK. Funny you should mention breaking ice, one of the first gags he ever played on me was to have a couple of the guys grab me from behind and hang me upside down over a cake of ice as we were on the way to location on the train. I already had my make-up on, which took about an hour to do, and all of it got ruined and I was very uncomfortable, so as soon as they put me down again I went and punched Buster in the eye. It gave him such a shiner they had to stop shooting for a week. This was before I understood that he meant no harm. He'd go to any length to get a laugh, but there was no malice in his practical jokes.

RR: So he kept it up even after you hit him in the eye?

MM: Oh boy, he sure did. Like the time he found out that sometimes I used to like to take my bike and go up about three miles from Cottage Grove to a spot on the river that was nice and secluded, and there I would swim. So he and a couple of his buddies sneaked up after me one day, and found where I left my clothes and tied them up in such knots that I couldn't unravel them. And so I had to pedal back to Cottage Grove in my bathing suit, and this was quite a shocking thing to do in 1926, you simply didn't ride a bike in your bathing suit in those days, and a wet one at that!

RR: Did Buster play any tricks on you in front of the camera?

MM: Yes, he did. You know, I was told at the beginning that there would be a double to do all the stunts, and a girl was actually hired and was standing by, so I was satisfied. But then, as Buster got to know me better I guess he decided I was a good sport, and would you believe it, they never used that girl once as far as I know. Like in the scene where I'm in the sack and Buster is supposed to step all over me. He told me to get in the sack, and then they would cut and let the other girl replace me for the rough stuff. But next thing I knew, he was stepping all over me, and the cameras were grinding. But I didn't get mad at him that time, I must say he knew just how to do it so it wouldn't hurt me. I guess it was his vaudeville training.

RR: Is that you in the scene on top of the box car where you are drenched from the water tank?

MM: That was another time when Buster said all I had to do was help set up the scene, and then they would cut and the extra would get the soaking. Now, as soon as we're up there Buster grabs the big spout and it comes off accidentally the wrong way, and we get all wet. Right away, Buster realized it was probably funny, and so now he puts the spout in the right way but also pulls the wire that releases the water, and I got soaked the second time. So I got it twice, and both times I didn't know it was coming, so the surprise you see on my face up there is for real. Boy, I sure was as wet as a drowned rat that time. But it would never have looked so good if it hadn't really happened by accident the first time, and if Buster hadn't helped a little the second time. He had all his crew trained to keep the cameras running even if something unexpected happened, you never knew what was going to turn out good when you saw it on the screen.

RR: Do you remember the scene where you're climbing through a small opening in one of the cars? Was it really as hard as it looked?

MM: Buster wanted it to look as if we were having a hard time, so I had to put out one leg first and pretend I couldn't quite make it, and then try it the other way. Actually, with those long skirts it was a bit awkward, and also the train was actually moving, so there was some danger. I'm sure they would never do it today with the real stars, they'd have stunt men or they'd fake the train motion in some way by back projection. But in those days we never gave it a second thought, we just did it.

RR: When you get into the sack the first time, there in the woods when Buster is supposed to pick you up, was that really you in there when he lifts it?
MM: Yes, again, like I told you, he was supposed to let the other girl get in, she was about ten pounds lighter, anyway, and so I didn't think Buster would be too anxious to lug me around. But, as I told you, by now I think he got used to me, and so he always found a way to keep me in the scene. But you know, in this scene another accident happened which they left in; he is supposed to empty the sack which is full of Army boots, and when he did it his own shoes came off and for a while he couldn't find the right ones among all the other shoes. It was never planned but since it looked funny, they kept it in the picture. And then he gets me in the sack and all of a sudden I feel he's picking me up, but he was stronger than I thought, and it never fazed him a bit. And that's really my hand you see uncoupling the wagons from inside the sack later.
RR: Which scenes were done in the studio in Hollywood?
MM: Very few, really. The one that gave us the most trouble was the night scene when Buster and I are running away from the cottage. We were three weeks doing that, and even here in the studio he wanted to do it as true to life as possible, and so we did it on the back lot at night, with rain and wind machines. We came in every night at about 7, and stayed until maybe one a.m., and this went on for three weeks, and each night we got soaked to the skin, it's a wonder we didn't catch pneumonia. But as I said, we just never thought much about it. It had to be done, so we did it.
RR: What other scenes did you do in Hollywood?
MM: The indoor scenes, but as you know there were only a few. Some of the supposed indoor scenes, like the one with Buster in the recruiting office, these were actually done in Cottage Grove outdoors, with fake walls but no ceiling. Also the scene at the beginning, where Buster comes to call on me and I sort of play a trick on him and follow him to my house, that was all done up on location.
RR: How many times did you usually run through a scene?
MM: Most of them Buster okayed after one or two takes. The only ones that had to be timed to precision were the gags, and they sometimes took five or six tries. But they also shot quite a few whole scenes which were never used in the finished picture, because Buster was a perfectionist and he only used the best scenes. That's why the whole film is so tightly edited, he took out all the scenes which would have dragged it out.
RR: Well, now, I hope you don't mind telling us, Marion, why is it that you never made another picture after THE GENERAL. Surely, with the film being such an enormous success, you could have had your pick of directors and films?
MM: Well, Raymond, I was really an old-fashioned girl at heart. And when Lou told me he didn't like me to be away on location so long, I realized we would always have friction if I stayed in the business. Besides, he needed me to help him write the short films he was now producing for Paramount, and I truly enjoyed that side of it even more than I liked acting. Since my marriage meant more to me than anything else, I just refused all offers, and finally they stopped asking me. And you see, it worked, Lou and I stayed married even when everyone in Hollywood was always getting divorced, and we were only about two years away from our golden anniversary when he passed away.
RR: Did you see Keaton anymore after the filming?
MM: Yes, we remained friends and saw him off and on. I remember one time, right after we finished THE GENERAL, we were invited to a New Year's Eve party in Caliente, at a night club owned by Joe Schenck, and Buster was there, and he did one of his famous slides. As I told you, he would go anywhere for a laugh, and he did one of the bits he learned on stage, slid on his stomach right across the whole dance floor. And the reason he did it, he saw Peggy Joyce, she was one of the supposed glamour girls with more jewelry than anyone in the world, sitting there across the floor, so he did the slide and pretended to get all mixed up and accidentally on purpose he tipped over her chair and spilled her all over the floor. I guess he just wanted to take her down a peg.
RR: There was a lot of publicity about Buster's drinking problem. Did you ever witness any excessive drinking?
MM: No, that all came later. He certainly never drank while working, at least not so that it would affect him, or I'm sure I would have noticed. This was still when he was in top form. Later, his marriage went

on the rocks, and they wouldn't let him make films the way he wanted to make them, and I felt really sorry for him. That's what I think drove him to drink. But by then we had drifted apart, anyway, and we saw him very seldom. I prefer to remember him when he was at his best, when we were playing little jokes on each other up in Cottage Grove on our little train. That was the real Buster: Funny as hell on the screen and a true friend off the screen. They just don't make them like that anymore.

RR: They never did even then, Marion. He was unique.

MM: You said it, Raymond. He was the best of them all.

Fourteen

Charlie Chaplin

At the end of the Mutual contract I was anxious to get started with First National, but we had no studio. I decided to buy land in Hollywood and build one. The site was the corner of Sunset and La Brea and had a very fine ten-roomed house and five acres of lemon, orange and peach trees. We built a perfect unit, complete with developing plant, cutting-rooms and offices.

During the studio's construction, I took a trip to Honolulu with Edna Purviance, for a month's rest. Hawaii was a beautiful island in those days. Yet the thought of living there, two thousand miles from the mainland, was depressing; in spite of its effulgent beauty, its pineapples, sugar-cane, exotic fruits and flowers, I was glad to return, for I felt a subtle claustrophobia, as if imprisoned inside a lily.

It was inevitable that the propinquity of a beautiful girl like Edna Purviance would eventually involve my heart. When we first came to work in Los Angeles, Edna rented an apartment near the Athletic Club, and almost every night I would bring her there for dinner. We were serious about each other, and at the back of my mind I had an idea that some day we might marry, but I had reservations about Edna. I was uncertain of her, and for that matter uncertain of myself.

In 1916 we were inseparable and went to all the Red Cross fêtes and galas. At these affairs Edna would get jealous and had a gentle and insidious way of showing it. If someone paid too much attention to me, Edna would disappear and a message would come that she had fainted and was asking for me, and of course I would go and stay with her for the rest of the evening. On one occasion a pretty hostess, who was giving a garden fête in my honour, pranced me about from one society belle to another and eventually led me into an alcove, again the message came that Edna had fainted. Although I was flattered that such a beautiful girl always asked for me after she came to, the habit was becoming a little annoying.

The dénouement came at Fanny Ward's party, where there was a galaxy of pretty girls and handsome young men. Again Edna fainted. But when she came to, she asked for Thomas Meighan, the tall, handsome leading man of Paramount. I knew nothing about it at the time. It was Fanny Ward who told me the next day; knowing my feelings for Edna, she did not wish to see me being made a fool of.

I could not believe it. My pride was hurt; I was outraged. If it were true it would be the end of our relationship. Yet I could not give her up so suddenly. The void would be too much. A resurgence of all that we had been to each other came over me.

The day after the incident I could not work. Towards afternoon I telephoned her for an explanation, intending to fume and fuss; but instead my ego took over and I became sarcastic. I even joked lightly about the matter: 'I understand you called for the wrong man at Fanny Ward's party—you must be losing your memory!'

She laughed and I detected a tinge of embarrassment. 'What are you talking about?' she said.

I was hoping she would fervently deny it. Instead she acted cleverly; she asked who had been telling me all this nonsense.

'What difference does it make who told me? But I think I should mean more to you than that you should openly make a fool of me.'

She was very calm, and insisted that I had been listening to a lot of lies.

I wanted to hurt her by a show of indifference. 'You don't have to make any pretence with me,' I said. 'You're free to do whatever you like. You're not married to me; so long as you're conscientious in your work, that's all that matters.'

To all this Edna was amiably in agreement, and wanted nothing to interfere with our working together. We could always be good friends, she said, which made me all the more desperately miserable.

I talked for an hour on the phone nervous and upset, wanting some excuse for a reconciliation. As is usual in such circumstances, I took a renewed and passionate interest in her, and the conversation tapered off by my asking her to dinner that evening on the pretext of talking over the situation.

She hesitated, but I insisted, in fact I pleaded and implored, all my pride and defences slipping away from me. Eventually she consented. . . . That night the two of us dined on ham and eggs, which she cooked in her apartment.

There was a reconciliation of a sort and I became less perturbed. At least I was able to work the next day. Nevertheless, there lingered a forlorn anguish and self-reproach. I blamed myself for having neglected her at times. I was cast into a dilemma. Should I completely break with her or not? Perhaps the story about Meighan was not true?

About three weeks later she called at the studio to get her cheque. As she was leaving I happened to bump into her. She was with a friend. 'You know Tommy Meighan?' she said blandly. I was somewhat shocked. In that brief moment Edna became a stranger as though I had just met her for the first time. 'Of course,' I said. 'How are you, Tommy?' He was a little embarrassed. We shook hands, and after we had exchanged one or two pleasantries they left the studio together.

However, life is another word for conflict which gives us little surcease. If it is not the problem of love it is something else. Success was wonderful, but with it grew the strain of trying to keep pace with that inconstant nymph, popularity. Nevertheless, my consolation was in work.

But writing, acting and directing fifty-two weeks in the year was strenuous, requiring an exorbitant expenditure of nervous energy. At the completion of a picture I would be left depressed and exhausted, so that I would have to rest in bed for a day.

Towards evening I would get up and go for a quiet walk. Feeling remote and melancholy, I would wander around town, looking vacantly into shop windows. I never tried to think on these occasions; my brain was numbed. But I was quick to recuperate. Usually the following morning, driving to the studio, my excitement would return and my mind would get activated again.

With a bare notion I would order sets, and during the building of them the art director would come to me for details, and I would bluff and give him particulars about where I wanted doors and archways. In this desperate way I started many a comedy.

Sometimes, my mind would tighten like a twisted cord and would need some form of loosening. At this juncture a night out was efficacious. I never cared much for alcoholic stimulus. In fact, when working, I had a superstition that the slightest stimulus of any kind affected one's perspicacity. Nothing demanded more alertness of mind than contriving and directing comedy.

As for sex, most of it went in my work. When it did rear its delightful head, life was so inopportune that it was either a glut on the market or a serious shortage. However, I was a disciplinarian and took my work seriously. Like Balzac, who believed that a night of sex meant the loss of a good page of his novel, so I believed it meant the loss of a good day's work at the studio.

*

A well-known lady novelist, hearing I was writing my autobiography, said: 'I hope you have the courage to tell the truth.' I thought she meant politically, but she was referring to my sex-life. I suppose a dissertation on one's libido is expected in an autobiography, although I do not know why. To me it contributes little to the understanding or revealing of character. Unlike Freud, I do not believe sex is the most important element in the complexity of behaviour. Cold, hunger and the shame of poverty are more likely to affect one's psychology.

Like everybody else's my sex-life went in cycles. Sometimes I was potent, other times disappointing. But it was not the all-absorbing interest in my life. I had creative interests which were just as all-absorbing. However, in this book I do not intend to give a blow-by-blow description of a sex bout: I find them inartistic, clinical and unpoetic. The circumstances that lead up to sex I find more interesting.

Apropos of that subject, a delightful impromptu occurred to me at the Alexandria Hotel the first night I arrived back in Los Angeles from New York. I had retired early to my room and started undressing, humming to myself one of the latest New York songs. Occasionally I paused, lost in thought, and when I did so a feminine voice from the next room took up the tune where I had left off. Then I took up where she left off, and so it became a joke. Eventually we finished the tune this way. Should I get acquainted? It was risky. Besides, I had no idea what she looked like. I whistled the tune again, and again the same thing happened. 'Ha, ha, ha! that's funny!' I laughed, tempering my intonation so that it could be addressed to her or to myself.

A voice came from the other room: 'I beg your pardon?'

Then I whispered through the key-hole: 'Evidently you have just arrived from New York.'

'I can't hear you,' she said.

'Then open the door,' I answered.

'I'll open it a little, but don't you dare come in.'

'I promise.'

She opened the door about four inches, and the most ravishing young blonde peered at me. I do not know exactly how she was dressed, but she was all silky negligée and the effect was dreamy.

'Don't come in or I'll beat you up!' she said charmingly, showing her pretty white teeth.

'How do you do,' I whispered, and introduced myself. She knew already who I was and that I had the room next door to hers.

Later that night she told me that under no circumstances was I to acknowledge her in public, or even nod if we passed each other in the hotel lobby. That was all she ever told me about herself.

The second night when I came to my room she frankly tapped on the door, and once more we embarked nocturnally. The third night I was getting rather weary; besides, I had work and a career to think about. So on the fourth night I surreptitiously opened my door and tiptoed into my room, hoping to get to bed unnoticed; but she had heard me, and began tapping on the door. This time I paid no attention and went straight to bed. Next day, when she passed me in the hotel lobby it was with an icy stare.

The following night she did not knock, but the handle of the door creaked and I saw it turning slowly. I had, however, locked it from my side. She turned the handle violently, then knocked impatiently. The next morning I thought it advisable to leave the hotel, so again I took up quarters at the Athletic Club.

*

My first picture in my new studio was *A Dog's Life*. The story had an element of satire, parallelling the life of a dog with that of a tramp. This leitmotif was the structure upon which I built sundry gags and slapstick routines. I was beginning to think of comedy in a structural sense, and to become conscious of its architectural form. Each sequence implied the next sequence, all of them relating to the whole.

The first sequence was rescuing a dog from a fight with other dogs. The next was rescuing a girl in a dance-hall who was also leading 'a dog's life'. There were many other sequences, all of which followed in a logical concatenation of events. As simple and obvious as these slapstick comedies were, a great deal of thought and invention went into them. If a gag interfered with the logic of events, no matter how funny it was, I would not use it.

In the Keystone days the tramp had been freer and less confined to plot. His brain was seldom active then—only his instincts, which were concerned with the basic essentials: food, warmth and shelter. But with each succeeding comedy the tramp was growing more complex. Sentiment was beginning to percolate through the character. This became a problem because he was bound by the limits of slapstick. This may sound pretentious, but slapstick demands a most exacting psychology.

The solution came when I thought of the tramp as a sort of Pierrot. With this conception I was freer to express and embellish the comedy with touches of sentiment. But logically it was difficult to get a beautiful girl interested in a tramp. This has always been a problem in my films. In *The Gold Rush* the girl's interest in the tramp started by her playing a joke on him, which later moves her to pity, which he mistakes for love. The girl in *City Lights* is blind. In this relationship he was romantic and wonderful to her until her sight is restored.

As my skill in story construction developed, so it restricted my comedy freedom. As a fan who preferred my early Keystone comedies to the more recent ones wrote to me: 'Then the public was your slave; now you are the public's slave.'

Even in those early comedies I strove for a mood; usually music created it. An old song called *Mrs Grundy* created the mood for *The Immigrant.* The tune had a wistful tenderness that suggested two lonely derelicts getting married on a doleful, rainy day.

The story shows Charlot en route to America. In the steerage he meets a girl and her mother who are as derelict as himself. When they arrive in New York they separate. Eventually he meets the girl again, but she is alone, and like himself is a failure. While they sit talking, she inadvertently uses a black-edged handkerchief, conveying the fact that her mother has passed on. And, of course, in the end they marry on a doleful, rainy day.

Simple little tunes gave me the image for other comedies. In one called *Twenty Minutes of Love,* full of rough stuff and nonsense in parks, with policemen and nursemaids, I weaved in and out of situations to the tune of *Too Much Mustard,* a popular two-step in 1914. The song *Violetera* set the mood for *City Lights,* and *Auld Lang Syne* the mood for *The Gold Rush.*

As far back as 1916 I had many ideas for feature pictures. One was a trip to the moon, a comic spectacle showing the Olympic Games there and the possibilities of playing about with the laws of gravity. It would have been a satire on progress. I thought of a feeding machine, and also a radio-electric hat that could register one's thoughts; and the trouble I get into when I put it on my head and am introduced to the moon-man's sexy wife. The feeding machine I eventually used in *Modern Times.*

Interviewers have asked me how I get ideas for pictures and to this day I am not able to answer satisfactorily. Over the years I have discovered that ideas come through an intense desire for them; continually desiring, the mind becomes a watch-tower on the look-out for incidents that may excite the imagination—music, a sunset, may give image to an idea.

I would say, pick a subject that will stimulate you, elaborate it and involve it, then, if you can't develop it further, discard it and pick another. Elimination from accumulation is the process of finding what you want.

How does one get ideas? By sheer perseverance to the point of madness. One must have a capacity to suffer anguish and sustain enthusiasm over a long period of time. Perhaps it's easier for some people than others, but I doubt it.

Of course every budding comic goes through philosophical generalizing about comedy. 'The element of surprise and suspense' was a phrase dropped every other day on the Keystone lot.

I will not attempt to sound the depths of psycho-analysis to explain human behaviour, which is as inexplicable as life itself. More than sex or infantile aberrations, I believe that most of our ideational compulsions stem from atavistic causes—however, I did not have to read books to know that the theme of life is conflict and pain. Instinctively, all my clowning was based on this. My means of contriving comedy plot was simple. It was the process of getting people in and out of trouble.

But humour is different and more subtle. Max Eastman analysed it in his book *A Sense of Humour.* He sums it up as being derived from playful pain. He writes that *Homo sapiens* is masochistic, enjoying pain in many forms and that the audience like to suffer vicariously—as children do when playing Indians; they enjoy being shot and going through the death throes.

With all this I agree. But it is more an analysis of drama than humour, although they are almost the same. But my own concept of humour is slightly different: it is the subtle discrepancy we discern in what appears to be normal behaviour. In other words, through humour we see in what seems rational, the irrational; in what seems important, the unimportant. It also heightens our sense of survival and preserves our sanity. Because of humour we are less overwhelmed by the vicissitudes of life. It activates our sense of proportion and reveals to us that in an over-statement of seriousness lurks the absurd.

For instance, at a funeral where friends and relatives are gathered in hushed reverence around the bier of the departed, a late arrival enters just as the service is about to begin and hurriedly tiptoes to his seat, where one of the mourners has left his top hat. In his hurry, the late arrival accidentally sits on it, then with a solemn look of mute apology, he hands it crushed to its owner, who takes it with mute annoyance and continues listening to the service. And the solemnity of the moment becomes ridiculous.

The Studio Era

LESSON FOUR

The Production Code

The Fallen Woman Film and the Impetus for Censorship

Lea Jacobs

The important thing is to leave the audience with the definite conclusion that immorality is not justifiable, that society is not wrong in demanding certain standards of its women, and that the guilty woman, through realization of her error, does not tempt other women in the audience to follow her course.

Jason Joy, *industry censor*

In this advice, written to Columbia's Harry Cohn, the MPPDA official Jason Joy anticipated and sought to forestall some of the objections typically raised against Hollywood movies in the thirties.[1] Reformers argued that films exercised a pernicious influence upon women. Hollywood was held to be in violation of what one reformer called "the current moral code," to undermine normative definitions of femininity and to promote crime or promiscuity.

Present-day histories of film censorship typically allude to this controversy by using the example of Mae West. Notorious for wisecracks and sexual innuendo, West is said to have generated negative publicity for Hollywood and contributed to the institution of stricter mechanisms of film censorship in the mid-thirties.[2] But the publicity which surrounded West's films and persona formed only one part of a more general discussion about how films might possibly affect sexual mores and conduct. In my view, the pressure on the industry to regulate representations of sexuality is best understood as a function of a set of assumptions about spectatorship, specifically female spectatorship, current in the thirties. I will argue that these assumptions were brought to the forefront of public debate by a particular genre—the fallen woman film.

The criticism of Hollywood framed in terms of how films might affect women began as early as the teens, and varied according to the manner in which spectatorship itself was conceptualized. At the most literal level, newspapers and magazines depicted Hollywood as a cause and potential site of female delinquency—luring girls away from their homes and into a tenuous and morally suspect profession. A number of news stories about the "movie-struck girl" circulated in the popular press in the teens. The stories, often written in the form of a warning to the reader, described the fate of young women who left home and went to Hollywood to pursue an acting career. Unable to find work, encountering only indifference from the studios, or worse, a producer of dubious morals, hundreds of girls were supposedly stranded in Los Angeles.[3] *Photoplay* regularly ran features advising fans of the difficulty of obtaining work in Hollywood and on the daunting skills required to be an actress or film extra.[4]

Most of the films of the twenties adopt a cautionary tone similar to the print media in dealing with the stereotype of the movie-struck girl. An early example of the type is Maurice Tourneur's *A Girl's Folly* (1917). An innocent country girl is encouraged to break into the movies by a handsome matinee idol. She leaves home in expectation of finding work at the movie studio, but fails her screen test and is left without any source of income. Only the appearance of her mother saves her from ruin at the hands of the star. The *American Film Institute Catalog* of feature films from the twenties lists several other examples of melodramas in which a girl goes to Hollywood to seek her fortune, only to become vulnerable to the attentions of an unscrupulous actor, producer, or "sheik." Examples include *Mary of the Movies* (Columbia Productions, 1923), *Broken Hearts of Hol-*

lywood (Warner Brothers, 1926), and *Stranded* (Sterling Pictures, 1927). In a more comic vein, the heroine of *Are Parents People?* (1925) attempts to reunite her estranged parents by pretending to be "movie-mad" and to run away with a sheik, star of "The Love Brute." In *Ella Cinders* (1926), the eponymous heroine escapes from the tyranny of her mother and sisters by winning an acting contest and going off to Hollywood. No job is waiting for her at the studio, and she inadvertently causes mayhem on several sets, but eventually she is given a chance and becomes a star. Even when these films exculpate Hollywood as an industry, they indicate that the film producers felt the need to respond to public anxiety about the movie-struck girl. Indeed, the film industry trade association, the MPPDA, was so concerned about this issue that in 1925, in association with the YWCA, it organized a residence for young women seeking work as film actresses.[5]

The rather sensationalized stories about the fate of women in Hollywood were paralleled by a more abstract, and scientifically respectable, discourse on the psychological effects and social consequences of film viewing. The Payne Fund Studies, published in 1933, provide a good example of this kind of analysis of media effects. Although most of the studies dealt with the effects of film viewing on young children, one monograph focused upon male and female adolescents. This study, Herbert Blumer and Philip M. Hauser's *Movies, Delinquency and Crime,* explicitly linked the gangster film with the problem of violent crime among boys in the urban tenements, and the "sex picture"—stories about gold diggers, flappers, and vamps—with delinquency and various forms of prostitution among young women.[6] The following question, part of a survey administered by Blumer and Hauser to girls in reform school, indicates some of the assumptions they made about the effects of film viewing: "Did the movies suggest to you any of the following ideas of making easy money? By getting a job and working. By shoplifting. By 'gold-digging men.' By gambling. By sexual delinquency with men. By living with a man and letting him support you."[7] The responses charted out for girls in this survey question recapitulate many of the complaints about the movies which were being made by other reform groups in the period. Women's clubs, educators, and even some newspaper editors considered the movies a possible cause of "vice."[8]

While reformers and social scientists did not usually describe films in any detail, their discussions of female spectatorship frequently made reference to a genre which I call the fallen woman film.[9] While the genre is not popular with present-day audiences, it was a staple of Hollywood melodrama. Precisely because it was already recognized as a type, however loosely defined, it functioned as a lightning rod, channeling reformers' more general anxieties about Hollywood's effect on sexual mores. Moreover, because the fallen woman story turned upon an act of seduction or adultery, it thematized many of the reformers' own concerns about sexual deviance among female spectators. An overview of these recognized genre conventions will help to make clear how the films came to be perceived as transgressive.

Literary Antecedents

The story of the fallen woman derives from a set of nineteenth-century narrative and iconographic conventions which were themselves in flux in the twenties and early thirties. Traditional renderings of the story, in which the erring woman was irredeemably punished, had begun to seem outdated, at least for some sectors of the audience. For example, in a review of the 1929 version of *Madame X, Variety* warned its readers that the film might not appeal to urban audiences nor to younger viewers: " 'Madame X' should show other than in the metropolises and the keys before it is determined by the film buyers if there is mass appeal in it. The younger element nowadays doesn't want this kind of sex, for the sex angle here is of the sordid sort, the thorough-bred woman going down the line to become an absinthe wretch."[10] Hollywood both solicited and helped to construct the change in audience tastes to which *Variety* refers. The fallen woman story underwent decided transformations early in the postwar period, transformations which were sometimes foregrounded in films about changing sexual mores. In *Wine of Youth* (1924), for example, a young flapper's rather wild and free-wheeling style of courtship is misconstrued by her conservative father as a sign of her "ruin." I will argue that the resistance to the fallen woman film on the part of censors and reformers largely centered upon such new permutations of the genre. That is, I will explain the hostile reception of the films in terms of their deviations from the traditions of nineteenth-century melodrama.

The stereotype of the fallen woman pervaded nineteenth-century popular culture, appearing in fiction, stage melodrama, opera, and narrative painting, in British, American, and European contexts. A prototypical example is a set of three paintings by Augustus Egg exhibited in 1858 without titles and now known as *Past and Present*.[11] The first painting is set in a well-appointed drawing room. The accused woman lies prostrate before her husband; in the background two girls are playing, building a house of cards. The second painting is set in a poor and rather bare apartment. The children of the absent mother, now older and alone, stare out the window at the moon and a wisp of cloud. In the last painting, the repetition of the moon and clouds indicates that the scene is simultaneous with the previous one. The woman is beneath the arches of a bridge, an icon traditionally connected to the moment of the fallen woman's isolation and suicide.[12] She is poorly dressed and alone except for a baby (by convention illegitimate) which is barely visible in the frame. Her fall is enacted in this movement from the bourgeois drawing room to the bridge by the river, implying a loss of both class and familial status.

Another variant of the fall concentrates on a young servant, seamstress or uneducated village girl who is seduced by an upper-class man. In examples of this type, which include works as diverse as Elizabeth Gaskell's *Ruth* (1853), and Thomas Hardy's *Tess of the d'Urbervilles* (1891), class difference highlights the woman's defenselessness, her status as victim in a system she does not control.[13] Typically, she does not actively desire the rake who pursues her and is unaware of his designs.

In England, stories about errant mothers separated from their children or innocent servant girls seduced and abandoned were a commonplace of both serialized magazine fiction and the novel between 1835 and 1880.[14] Authors of domestic novels such as Elizabeth Inchbald, Amelia Opie, and Elizabeth Helm[15] dealt with the fallen woman, as did many of the major novelists of the period: Anthony Trollope (*Can You Forgive Her?* 1865; *The Vicar of Bullhampton*, 1870), George Eliot (*Adam Bede,* 1859), Wilkie Collins *(The Fallen Leaves,* 1879; *The New Magdalen,* 1873), and George Moore (*Esther Waters,* 1894). In America, two early domestic novels, Susanna Rowson's *Charlotte Temple* (1794) and Hannah Webster Forster's *The Coquette* (1797) treat the type.[16] The fallen woman also plays a central role in Eugène Sue's *Les Mystères de Paris* (1842–43), and, in a more realistic mode, Gustave Flaubert's *Madame Bovary* (1857). The courtesan, a more cynical and knowing version of the type, goes back at least as far as Abbé Prévost's *Manon Lescaut* (1753), but acquired particular notoriety with Zola's *Nana* (1879). The courtesan is redeemed by love in Balzac's *Splendeurs et misères des courtisanes,* in *La Comédie humaine* (1846), and Alexandre Dumas's play *La Dame aux camélias* (1852) from his novel of the same name.

The fallen woman story also provided source material for many well-known opera libretti and stage melodramas. Giuseppi Verdi's *La Traviata* (1853) derives from *La Dame aux camélias,* and Jules Massenet's *Manon* (1885) and Giacomo Puccini's *Manon Lescaut* (1893) from the Prévost novel. There were three stage versions of Mrs. Henry Wood's best-selling novel about an errant mother, *East Lynne* (1861). The play consistently attracted large audiences, becoming one of the standbys to which stock companies reverted when theater revenues were down.[17]

Despite its popularity, the fallen woman story attracted controversy throughout the nineteenth century and was subject to various forms of censorship. Lord Chief Justice Campbell urged enactment of the Obscene Publications Act in England in 1857 after becoming incensed by the English translation of Dumas's *La Dame aux camélias*.[18] In the mid-Victorian period, novels such as Mrs. Gaskell's *Ruth* engendered debate insofar as they represented rape or seduction in a popular medium which found its way into the home.[19] Mudie's circulating library, one of the major distributors of three-volume novels, refused to carry Eliot's *Adam Bede* and Hardy's *Tess of the d'Urbervilles*.[20] Perhaps the most notorious instance of censorship is the attempted prosecution of Gustave Flaubert in 1857 on the grounds that *Madame Bovary* was offensive to public morals.[21] While not the object of official censure, the second half of *Nana* had to be bowdlerized for serial publication in the journal *Le Voltaire*.[22]

The fallen woman genre consistently offended nineteenth-century readers because plot conventions ran afoul of normative definitions of femininity. Although there has recently been some question about the degree to which individuals adhered to the norm of chastity in practice, as an ideal, purity was central to the Victorian conception of womanhood, at least for the middle class.[23] The genre became problematic insofar as the sympathetic portrayal of the heroine seemed to undermine the distinction between chaste and unchaste women.

The controversies around the genre intensified toward the end of the nineteenth century under the impetus of a number of works which explicitly questioned the moral value of purity. These works, considered daring by contemporary readers, prepared the way for the updated variants of the fallen woman plot which became popular in film and fiction after World War I. In George Moore's *Esther Waters* (1894), the heroine denounces characters who condemn her for having an illegitimate child and struggles to raise her son on meager earnings as a domestic. She finally returns to live with the attractive gambler who seduced her rather than marry a minister. George Bernard Shaw's play *Mrs. Warren's Profession* (1894) also inverts traditional moral categories. A madam justifies her chosen profession as a way out of poverty, and argues that prostitution is a rational alternative for working-class women under capitalism. Theodore Dreiser's *Sister Carrie* (1900), written under the influence of naturalism, focuses upon the social circumstances and psychological pressures which make chastity difficult for the heroine. After having lost her job, and a berth in her older sister's household, Carrie drifts into a life as a kept woman. She is driven as much by a desire to buy pretty clothes and enjoy the nightlife of the city as by her desperate financial straits.

At the turn of the century, the works by Moore, Shaw, and Dreiser which debunked the ideal of female purity were subjected to lengthy censorship disputes. Both Mudie's and W. H. Smith, a circulating library and bookstore chain, refused to carry *Esther Waters*.[24] *Mrs. Warren's Profession*, though written in 1894, could not be performed until 1902 thanks to a ban by the Lord Chamberlain's Examiner of Plays.[25] The publisher of *Sister Carrie* required heavy emendations of the original manuscript, and even then was reluctant to publish the book.[26]

In the early years of the twentieth century, however, censorship pressures lessened, and popular fiction began to echo the representations of female sexuality found in Moore, Dreiser, and other naturalists. David Graham Phillips' *Susan Lenox: Her Fall and Rise,* completed prior to the author's death in 1911 and published in 1917, is in the vein of *Sister Carrie*. The heroine prostitutes herself in order to escape from the miseries of life in the tenements and the brutalizing effects of factory labor. As Elizabeth Janeway has pointed out in an analysis of the novel, Susan's fall is presented in Nietzschean terms, as an act of strength and self-affirmation.[27] In response to a sermon by a Salvation Army preacher, she asserts that "the wages of sin is sometimes a house on Fifth Avenue."[28] Like *Susan Lenox, Rain,* the 1922 play by John Colton and Clemence Randolph adapted from a short story by W. Somerset Maugham, repudiates the terms of the moral discourse directed at the fallen woman. The play focuses on a missionary worker who attempts to reform the prostitute Sadie Thompson. The missionary's treatment of Sadie is shown to be both hard-hearted—he proposes to deport her from Pago Pago to face jail in the United States—and a denial of his own sexuality. In the last act of the play, his own unconscious desire for Sadie drives him to rape and suicide. Sexuality is thus posed as an instinctual force which defies moral judgment and argument.

Although certainly not in the naturalist tradition of *Susan Lenox* or *Rain,* Anita Loos's comic best-seller *Gentlemen Prefer Blondes* (1926) takes to an extreme their cynicism about the ideal of purity. Written as a diary from the point of view of Lorelei, a kept woman, *Gentlemen Prefer Blondes* neither condemns nor justifies her sexual status. In a real departure from genre conventions, Lorelei does not even find herself in desperate circumstances; the overriding motivation for her actions is her frank and unabashed pursuit of diamonds.

The Fallen Woman Film

In the postwar period, there is a pronounced disparity between the reformers' treatment of the fallen woman genre in film and its literary counterparts. By the twenties, attempts to censor the fallen woman story in drama and popular fiction had largely abated. Of the examples cited above, censorship was attempted in only one case, that of *Susan Lenox* in 1917.[29] By the early thirties, one finds only isolated attempts to suppress fallen woman novels, such as Donald Henderson Clarke's *Female*.[30] In contrast, agitation for film censorship in this period often centered upon complaints about the "sex picture." The films became more notorious, and were eventually more closely regulated, than the literary sources from which they drew. The disparity in the treatment of film versus popular fiction derives from the ways in which censors and reformers regarded the audience for these two media. Reformers and MPPDA officials were often at pains to distinguish film from literature, and they argued that the cinema necessitated relatively stronger forms of control. In the Formula, a set of policies adopted in 1924 to govern the acquisition of literary properties by the studios, the MPPDA aimed to prevent "the prevalent type of book and play from becoming the prevalent type of picture."[31] The industry's Production Code, adopted in 1930, explained the logic of this distinction between film and literature:

> *Most arts appeal to the mature. This art appeals at once to every class, mature, immature, developed, undeveloped, law abiding, criminal. Music has its grades for different classes; so has literature and drama. This art of the motion picture, combining as it does the two fundamental appeals of looking at a picture and listening to a story, at once reached [sic] every class of society. [Thus] it is difficult to produce films intended for only certain classes of people.... Films, unlike books and music, can with difficulty be confined to certain selected groups.[32]*

The controversy around the fallen woman film clearly illustrates the special standards applied to the cinema as a mass medium. Versions of the story already current within the domain of popular fiction were deemed inappropriate for an audience which included children, teenage girls, and other groups defined as potentially "deviant," such as second-generation immigrants.

Much of the debate around the fallen woman genre attached to updated variants of the plot which criticized or trivialized traditional ideals of female purity. It should be noted, however, that while Hollywood was certainly influenced by contemporary literary treatments of the type, it drew material from the span of the genre's history, including nineteenth-century works from both Europe and America.[33] Adaptations from nineteenth-century sources included versions of *Anna Karenina* made in 1915, 1927 (as *Love*), and 1935; *La Dame aux camélias*, made in 1915, 1917, 1921, 1927, and 1936; and *East Lynne*, made in 1916, 1921, 1925, and 1931. In some cases even the traditional iconography of the genre was transferred to film. In *Waterloo Bridge* (1931, 1940), as in the Augustus Egg triptych described above, the bridge is the site of the fallen woman's despair and suicide. D. W. Griffith's *Way Down East* (1920), adapted from Lottie Blair Parker's popular play, contains a classic scene in which the heroine is cast out into the snow, forced to leave her domestic haven because of a past transgression. These older forms of the genre were complemented by adaptations from contemporary American literary sources. *Gentlemen Prefer Blondes* appeared in 1928. There were two versions of *Rain: Sadie Thompson* in 1928, and a second, under the original title, in 1932. MGM produced a version of *Susan Lenox: Her Fall and Rise* released in 1931, although the film softens the cynicism of the novel.

The influence of contemporary literary treatments of the genre went well beyond the specific works selected for adaptation. In a whole body of films devoted to working-class girls in an urban milieu, the stereotype of the injured innocent or world-weary demimondaine gave way to any one of a series of self-consciously "modern" American types: flappers, gold diggers, chorines, wisecracking shopgirls. While the heroine could be a kept woman, a trickster, or simply out to marry a millionaire, the stories revolved around the problem of obtaining furs, automobiles, diamonds, and clothes from men. Thus, the downward trajectory of the fall was replaced by a rise in class. Examples of this plot, dubbed the "Cinderella story" within the industry,[34] include *Manhandled* (1924), *Orchids and Ermine* (1927), *Possessed* (1931), *Bed of Roses* (1933), and *Baby Face* (1933).

The films dealing with class rise helped attract the attention of censors and reformers to the genre as a whole. While all of the variants of the fallen woman film were eventually subject to censorship by the MPPDA, the versions in which she came to a less than unhappy end made the representation of illicit sexuality especially problematic. The trajectory of the fall set the pattern for most nineteenth-century versions of the story, even given a liberal treatment of the figure of the prostitute. She was sympathetic precisely because, and to the degree that, she experienced remorse, and suffered a pronounced degradation and decline. The Hollywood films which played up the motif of class rise violated the structural underpinnings of this familiar nineteenth-century melodrama. Like the literary works from which they drew, the films undercut the narrative logic of sin, guilt, and redemption.

There is some question about when the tendency to invert or attenuate the trajectory of the fall was initiated in Hollywood films. The vamp, a figure common in the films of the teens, often got rich at the expense of her male victims. Considered from the point of view of genre conventions, however, the vamp film seems relatively conservative. The vamp's importance lay in the dilemma which she posed for the male hero: *A Fool There Was* (1914) set up an opposition between the Theda Bara character and the hero's virtuous wife. The film turned upon the man's inability to resist the vamp's overtures, and his attendant financial and moral ruin. In contrast, films such as *Susan Lenox* or *Possessed* centered upon the difficulties of women living alone in the city; they emphasized the *heroine's* financial predicament, and her ambition and success, often in amoral terms.

Apart from the vamp film, critics have discussed the emergence of stories about class rise almost entirely with reference to the Depression. For example, according to Richard Griffith, the fallen woman cycle of the thirties addressed the wishes or fantasies of women denied material goods.[35] The aggressive heroine and the motif of class rise predate 1929, however, and in my view are better explained as a function of the transformation of melodrama in the postwar era. The earliest use of the term "gold digger" I have found is the 1919 play *The Gold Diggers*, upon which the 1923 Warner Brothers film of the same name is based. The term appears in a film of 1928, *That Certain Thing*, applied to a poor girl from the tenements who is accused of tricking a rich boy into marriage. In both *Classified* (1925) and *Manhandled* (1924), the heroine accepts clothes and other favors from a wealthy man and is tempted to become a kept woman, although she ends up married to a man of her own class. Following an oft-repeated plot formula, in *It* (1927), the heroine, a sexually aggressive flapper, pursues and finally marries her upper-class boss. The outlines of the Cinderella story are thus well codified by the mid-twenties.

The maternal melodrama, one of the largest subcategories of the fallen woman genre, raises questions of periodization akin to those of the Cinderella films. This plot concerns an errant mother who comes back into contact with her child after many years and conceals her true identity for fear of her evil past. In a lengthy discussion of the type, Christian Viviani makes a distinction between older European forms of the story and more modern, American ones.[36] He claims that the heroine's decline is less protracted in the American versions and that a happy ending, in which she is reunited with her child, more common. Viviani explains this relatively upbeat variant of the story as a New Deal parable in which the heroine is "redeemed" by work and, with her illegitimate child, comes to represent the hope of a new society. Certainly there are instances of the maternal melodrama such as La Cava's *Gallant Lady* (1933) which seem to invoke a rhetoric of unity and hope characteristic of the New Deal. But I would argue that what Viviani terms "Americanized" variants of the plot are more frequently typified by a tendency to downplay the heroine's degradation and decline in favor of upward mobility. Further, this motif predates the Depression films.

In the case of the maternal melodrama, the heroine's rise can be motivated by any one of a number of plot devices—by work or marriage. As in the Cinderella story, the alteration of the heroine's class status is marked by the acquisition of clothes, automobiles, and new living accommodations. *The Goose Woman* (1925) opens with the mother already fallen. Once a famous diva, she has become a rude and scurrilous drunkard. A clever district attorney requires her testimony at a murder trial. In order to make her presentable in court, he has her bathed, coiffed, and elegantly dressed. Admired and treated with dignity once again, she is able to overcome her past and is reconciled with her son.

The films of the thirties continue to highlight the beauty of the mother's clothes and new surroundings as a means of representing her reintegration into society. In *Gallant Lady*, the heroine becomes an interior decorator and tastefully redesigns the mansion of the man she eventually marries. In *Rockabye* (1932), the heroine, a woman of dubious reputation, has become wealthy as an actress. Although forced to renounce her adopted child and later her lover, she never abandons her upper-class lifestyle. She wears a succession of furs and sequined gowns throughout the film. Her house includes a formal garden and a particularly elegant black and white kitchen. Moreover, in one sequence, she ventures back to a rowdy saloon in a poor part of the city, as various characters point out how far she has risen above her origins "in the gutter." Thus, in terms of both story and mise-en-scène, the mother's redemption is symbolized, and to a degree motivated, by the attainment of upper-class status.

The examples of the Cinderella story and the maternal melodrama give some indication of how the fallen woman plot was updated in the context of Hollywood in the twenties and early thirties. Although the films do not entirely abandon nineteenth-century narrative and iconographic conventions, a new emphasis on social mobility, and hence female aggressivity, overlays traditional plots and modes of characterization. Moreover, the heroine appears in increasingly lavish and exotic settings, greatly attenuating the severity of the fall. It is as if Eve were admitted to the Garden of Eden *after* having tasted the apple.

The Impetus for Censorship

In the thirties, the permutations of genre conventions I have described were acknowledged, and criticized, in terms of the films' putative effects upon real women. There was much discussion of the heroine's sexual trespasses and in particular violations of the ideal of female chastity. Consider a column by the film critic of the *Nation* entitled "Virtue in 1933":

> *It happens that the climaxes of the two pictures seen this week, one at New York's largest theater and the other at one of its smallest, hinge on the same problem of conduct in a young girl's mind. The problem, of course, is not a particularly new one. Long ago there was a picture called "Way Down East" in which Miss Lillian Gish was to be seen grappling with it. . . . The only reason that one calls attention to its recurrence as a major theme at this time is that it may serve to illustrate the profound change that has come over movie producers and audiences alike in their attitude towards this and similar problems. No longer is there a certain risk of sympathy in showing the hero in the arms of his mistress, the heroine having a child by someone other than her husband, the ingenue making a few mistakes before settling down to a closer observance of conventions.*[37]

The Nation, a liberal magazine, takes a "moderate" view: both the industry and the public participate in a general transformation of sexual mores. But other sources, more critical of the industry, argued that this type of film affirmed and promulgated undesirable changes in sexual mores. For example, in *The Content of Motion Pictures,* one of the Payne Fund Studies, Edgar Dale noted: "Colorful and attractive stars are commonly given roles depicting women who lose their virtue, who are ruined by men, lead profligate lives."[38] Dale found this a "dangerous situation" because the use of stars in such roles made the violation of the "current moral code . . . desirable or attractive."[39] Thus, the films were criticized insofar as Hollywood was presumed to promote sex outside of marriage for women.

While commentary was directed at the representation of sexuality within the cycle, there were also complaints about the representation of money. One finds references to films which show kept women "living in luxury" or what was rather vaguely identified as "glamour." Here, for example, is a letter of complaint sent to Will Hays from Alice Ames Winter, a former chairwoman of the General Federation of Women's Clubs who worked for the MPPDA representing the interests of women:

> *Recent pictures from [So] This is Africa, through Temple Drake, Baby Face, etc. down to Constance Bennett's latest [*Bed of Roses*], which I saw the day I got back home, and which again is the story of a criminal prostitute's methods of*

wangling luxury out of rich men . . . the constant flow of these pictures leaves me with mental nausea. . . .[40]

An article in *Photoplay* also bemoaned the trend with an article entitled "Charm? No! No! You Must Have Glamour."[41] The main objection to this aspect of the cycle was that the films encouraged prostitution by the representation of luxury. One newspaper columnist referred to the "flourishing crop of loose ladies on the screen," suggesting that such films constituted a temptation for women in that the heroine got rich, "practical lessons in sin."[42]

The point was discussed in an academic context in one of the Payne Fund Studies already noted, Blumer and Hauser's *Movies, Delinquency and Crime*. Blumer and Hauser's analysis of delinquency extended beyond representations of violence and criminality to include what researchers described as scenes of luxury, wealth, and ease. In analyzing the film preferences of delinquent youth, Blumer and Hauser called attention to films which they claimed stimulated a desire for money, stylish clothes, goods, and cars. Here is how they explained the potential effect of the movies on adolescent girls:

> *We have noted the influence of the motion pictures in instilling desires for clothes, automobiles, wealth, and ease in boys and young men and in suggesting the idea of easily attaining them. Among girls and young women this influence of the movies seems even more pronounced, for a greater premium seems to be placed on fine clothes, appearance, and a life of ease in the case of women. . . . In many cases the desire for luxury expresses itself in a smarter and more fashionable selection of clothes, house furnishings, etc., within the financial means of the girl; but, on the other hand, many of the girls and young women studied grow dissatisfied with their own clothes and manner of living and in their efforts to achieve motion picture standards frequently get into trouble.*[43]

Blumer and Hauser argued further that the girl's desire for represented objects could exacerbate the process of identification with sexually delinquent female characters. The researchers also noted, without the faintest trace of irony, that the allure of Hollywood's ideal of consumption was enhanced for those from "areas of high delinquency [where] the absence of wealth is generally greatest, and the opportunities of getting it legitimately are fewest. . . ."[44]

The Payne Fund Studies thus evoked the fallen woman film in the course of an attempt to analyze the possible deleterious consequences of film viewing, especially for working-class and immigrant women. More broadly, in the popular discourse on the films, the genre served as a privileged example of the kind of sexual license that reformers objected to within the Hollywood cinema as a whole.

The Model of Self-Regulation

There is every indication that the MPPDA was aware of the nature and extent of the criticisms being directed at Hollywood. For example, writing of the film *Red Headed Woman* in 1932, an industry censor compared the figure of the gold digger and that of the gangster, and noted that in each case complaints centered upon the problem of glamour:

> *There is a striking similarity between the treatment of this character and the earlier treatment of the gangster character. . . . Because he was the central figure, because he achieved power and money and a certain notoriety, our critics claimed that an inevitable attractiveness resulted. And that was what they objected to in gangster pictures. They said we killed him off but that we made him glamorous before we shot him. This is what you are apt to be charged with in this case. While the Red Headed Woman is a common little creature from over the tracks who steals other women's husbands and uses her sex attractiveness to do it, she is the central figure and it will be contended that a certain glamour surrounds her.*[45]

Writing in 1933, another industry censor noted:

> [This] is undoubtably an unfortunate time to bring the kept woman on the screen again and we are doing our best to make the studio heads conscious of the fact that the piling up of sex stories at the present time may bring about a situation where it will be necessary to get the studio heads together and make an agreement to lay off this type of story such as occurred when the gangster films got too numerous.[46]

At issue, then, for the MPPDA and for the industry, was how to enact the conventions of the genre given the complaints about rich, attractive, and loose-living heroines.

But how did the presuppositions and concerns of the reform movement inflect the censorship of specific films? In what forms, and by what mechanisms, did public debate and criticism of the industry impinge upon the production process? The most extensive description of the MPPDA's policy and procedure is Raymond Moley's *The Hays Office,* published in 1945.[47] Moley, who wrote a number of books and articles on behalf of the MPPDA in the forties, had access to primary materials which until recently have not been available to researchers. As his arguments have been widely accepted, they are worth summarizing in some detail. Moley focuses on the Production Code, a statement of industry policy proposed by the MPPDA and adopted by the industry in 1930. Moley's explanation of the function of the Code adopts what may be considered a legal model of self-regulation. Like a law, the Code is thought to provide a series of prohibitions or constraints on production (with a list of topics to be avoided as well as a "Reasons" section justifying regulation as such). According to Moley, these prohibitions could not be "enforced" prior to 1934. By an agreement reached in 1930, the studios were not to release any feature that did not meet with the Studio Relations Committee's approval. When a disagreement would arise between the committee and a producer, however, an appeal would be made to a panel composed of other producers—the so-called Hollywood Jury. Since the Jury usually decided in favor of its fellow producers, the recommendations of the Studio Relations Committee were easy to ignore.

The situation changed following the events of 1933–34. The Payne Fund Studies, widely quoted and discussed in the popular press, gave rise to much negative publicity for the film industry. The Catholic Legion of Decency's widely broadcast threat of a boycott of the cinema in April of 1934 augmented this negative publicity. Moley argues that as a result of this public pressure, the MPPDA made changes in the administrative mechanisms of censorship. Hays was able to negotiate concessions from producers which made it possible to "enforce" the Code. The Studio Relations Committee was reconstituted as the Production Code Administration under Joseph Breen and the Hollywood Jury eliminated. Moley claims that as of 1934 the Production Code Administration had the power to bar a film from exhibition in any theater owned by or affiliated with any member company of the MPPDA. During this period and up until 1948, Paramount, Warners, RKO, MGM, and 20th Century-Fox, all members of the MPPDA, owned 77 percent of the important first-run theaters in the United States.[48] The Code could be enforced, then, because in the final instance a producer could not get access to the major, first-run release outlets without the approval or "seal" of the Production Code Administration.

Moley's argument hinges upon the idea that censorship had a power almost comparable to that of the legal notion of prior restraint. But it seems unlikely that the Code was simply "enforced" in the manner of a law, through the exercise of such power. This argument runs counter to evidence which has become available to us since the publication of Moley's book in 1945: the MPPDA case files; the memoirs of a Hollywood censor, *See No Evil;* and an unpublished oral history conducted with Geoffrey Shurlock, a member of the Production Code Administration.[49] Further, considered as a model, it seems to me that the quasi-legal conception of censorship does not do justice to the peculiarities, the *specificity* of the system of self-regulation.

There is no evidence that industry censors were ever in a position routinely to block the exhibition of a film produced by one of the major studios. In direct opposition to Moley's argument,

Geoffrey Shurlock, who worked under Breen in the Production Code Administration, claims that censors could not refuse to pass a film (withhold a "seal"):

> *No, we never refused seals. We were in the business of granting seals. The whole purpose of our existence was to arrange pictures so that we could give seals. You had to give a seal.*[50]

Shurlock's remarks make sense if one considers the economics of industry self-regulation. The MPPDA, charged with protecting the long-run interests of the industry, would hardly consider it desirable to damage profits by disturbing the regular issue of films.[51] Thus, it is not likely that withholding completed films from exhibition was adopted as a matter of standard MPPDA procedure.

I am interested not in exposing the "errors" in Moley's history but in demonstrating the difficulties inherent in explaining MPPDA policy and procedures along quasi-legal lines. The powers of and limits on self-regulation differ markedly from those of state or civil censorship bodies. It is important to distinguish between the two if we are to account for the specificity of self-regulation as a process. State censors, who were independent of the film industry, were in a position to prevent exhibition. Short of banning a film, they could alter its editing at will by excising segments from a final print. In contrast, the censors for the MPPDA exercised more power while films were in the planning stages than in the review of completed features. This description of the Production Code Administration's operating procedure by Jack Vizzard, who worked under Breen, gives a sense of the importance of preproduction:

> *"Huddle" was the heart of the Code operation. . . . It started at ten o'clock sharp, like assembly call. It was nothing more or less than a story conference, in which the staff members reported on the scripts they had read on the previous day. It was during the huddle that decisions were made and lines of strategy were drawn up as to how this problem would be met, or that riddle dealt with. After the huddle, the staff members scattered and went their separate ways, some to studios for knock-down-drag-out fights with producers, some to write letters on scripts they had covered, and some to plunge into yet another script. Keeping up with the endless flow of scripts that poured through the office was like trying to run up a hill of sand. While the main body of the work was done on the scripts before the productions reached the sound stages, the right was always reserved to see the picture also. . . .*[52]

Vizzard's description of the daily meeting of the Production Code Administration as a "story conference" points to one of the basic differences between self-regulation and state censorship. Self-regulation was an integrated part of film production under the studio system. Industry censors were in a position to request revisions in scripts and, in consultation with writers, directors, and producers, to effect changes in narratives. I take this to be Shurlock's meaning when he says, "The whole purpose of our existence was to *arrange pictures* so that we could give seals" (italics mine). This is very different from a power of restraint—blocking exhibition or "cutting things out" of films. Censors participated in the decision-making process by which the studio hierarchy orchestrated and controlled production. They achieved their ends, within this hierarchy, by means of more or less successful negotiations, what Vizzard refers to as "knock-down-drag-out fights with producers."

It remains unclear, however, how the various social forces confronting the industry influenced the process of negotiation concerning specific films. If we abandon the idea that the Production Code Administration simply "enforced" the Code through the power to restrain exhibition, then it becomes necessary to propose an alternate explanation of how the social relations between the MPPDA and external groups determined censorship, especially during the tense years of 1933 and 1934. It is possible to take account of this social context if we assume that censorship sought to restructure specific films which posed some threat to the industry's political and economic interests. The process of self-regulation may then be described in terms of two distinct but related stages. The first stage—evaluation—consisted in the isolation of films or elements within films likely to offend reform groups or provoke action by government regulatory agencies. The case files indicate that the MPPDA employed a number of procedures for anticipating how external agencies might react to films. Its employees gathered information on the reception of films both domestically and abroad, and rendered expert opinions about what was likely to be found offensive. It regularly collected data on material cut by state and foreign censorship boards and reviewed letters of complaint from reform groups.

The second stage of censorship consisted in negotiations between the MPPDA and film producers. The MPPDA's object in these negotiations was to find some way of forestalling the anticipated complaints and minimizing the cuts that would be required by the state censorship boards. As a rule, however, producers did not want their films altered. They sought to retain potentially offensive genre elements which presumably had already "proven" their appeal at the box office. Thus this stage of censorship may be characterized as an attempt to compromise between the aims of the MPPDA (to eliminate potentially offensive material) and the aims of producers (to preserve this supposedly profitable material).

This account of the process of regulation does not posit a direct relationship between the demands of external agencies and the form assumed by censorship in any given case. In particular, I dispute the claim, advanced in some film histories, that after 1934 censorship reflected the values and beliefs espoused by the Catholic Legion of Decency.[53] To be sure, the MPPDA was particularly moved to respond to the Legion in this period, but, in terms of the model proposed here, regulation did not entail the simple assimilation of the demands of this or any other pressure group. In any given case the MPPDA employed devices for anticipating or projecting what would offend external agencies. Theoretically it could be, and in fact it sometimes was, wrong in this anticipation. Even after 1934 the MPPDA released films which offended the Catholic Legion of Decency and were given a "Condemned" rating.[54] Further, even if the MPPDA correctly anticipated the demands of external agencies, censorship proper consisted in a series of compromises between it and producers. The utopian ideal of self-regulation was to forestall criticism while at the same time allowing the producer maximal use of his original material. In practice there was continual tension, a kind of push-pull, between conflicting aims or tendencies. Thus censorship as an institutional process did not simply reflect social pressures; it articulated a strategic response to them. And this strategy was worked out on a case-by-case basis, before films went into production.

The usefulness of strategy as a concept for analyzing censorship is that it explains the logic of determination in terms of a dynamic interplay of aims and interests, rather than a cause—the Catholic Legion of Decency—which unilaterally produces an effect—the enforcement of the Code. The model allows for, indeed leads us to expect, a certain variation from film to film, since there would be some latitude in defining problems and arriving at compromises. Yet this model can also account for broader changes in the administration of censorship following the publication of the Payne Fund Studies and the Catholic Legion of Decency campaign.

Consider a problem which censors identified relatively frequently: "adultery is made attractive." As a matter of routine, sometimes with reference to previous cases in which adultery had been a question, censors and producers would work out a compromise which permitted some representation of this act. Certain compromises would thus become institutionalized, repeated, with slight variation, from film to film. These routines were altered following the events of 1934. In the face of escalating public criticism of the industry, censors were in a position to negotiate relatively more extensive revisions of films and scripts. Breen was particularly careful to refine the definition of what was acceptable under the Code. So producers needed to devise and employ a new set of representational strategies in order to justify or defend what censors deemed potentially offensive. There was a more far-reaching transformation, a different narrative elaboration, of offensive material.

This study thus posits censorship as a constructive force, in the sense that it helped to shape film form and narrative.[55] Making comparisons between the MPPDA's treatment of films before and after 1934, it seeks to ascertain differences in the representation of illicit sexuality, money, and class rise in these two periods. It is my contention that the rules censors developed for the treatment of the fallen woman film were primarily concerned with the *structures* of narrative—the nature of endings, motivation of action, patterns of narration. I seek to describe the development of these narrative strategies of censorship and to delineate their implications for Hollywood's representations of female sexuality and its construction of sexual difference.

Before 1934, negotiations between producers and industry censors involved discrete and localized elements of the text. Shots or lines of dialogue which censors deemed offensive might be eliminated or transformed. Frequently, a scene would be added in which the fallen woman's actions were denounced, or emphasis would be placed on her (the film's) unhappy end. After 1934, censors were able to negotiate relatively more systematic alterations of narrative. When evaluating scripts, censors routinely suggested alterations in plot—in the way in which the films motivated the fall and in the consequences which could follow from sexual transgression. A number of narrative strategies could delay or redirect the trajectory of class rise. Often the films stressed the heroine's abasement or punishment rather than her acquisition of wealth. In some cases, the films used some form of narration such as voice-over, opening titles, or a character telling a story in flashback, all of which more or less ambiguously proposed criticisms of the fallen woman's sexual transgressions and her aspirations to wealth.

Self-regulation was not, however, a smooth or completely successful operation. The public response to the fallen woman film, as well as the many disputes between the MPPDA and film producers, suggest that in many cases the MPPDA did not succeed in its efforts to alleviate causes for complaint. One must then explain not only how censorship affected narrative, but also the gaps or inconsistencies in its routines.

This question touches on an area of debate concerning what has been called the subversive or progressive text. Seeking to theorize the relationship between the classical Hollywood text and ideology, a number of critics, most prominently the collective associated with the *Cahiers du Cinéma* in the seventies, have proposed that certain films depart from the transparency and narrative closure typical of the classical text, thereby revealing the ideological presuppositions which underlie it.[56] Feminist critics such as Claire Johnston have been interested in the idea of such "readings against the grain" and have sought to identify mainstream Hollywood films which critique the dominant cinema from within the terms of its mode of address.[57] It is tempting to argue that at least certain examples of the fallen woman cycle constitute subversive texts in Johnston's sense of the term. This is to suggest not that the films directly set out to challenge the values of marriage, hard work, and female chastity, but rather that in their terms of address and enactment of narrative conventions the films inadvertently destabilize the moral and sexual categories which censorship sought to reinforce.

The very notion of a subversive text must be approached with caution, however. This mode of analysis has been criticized as anachronistic and historically untenable. For example, Richard Maltby argues that the process of finding subversive meanings is unbounded, "restrained only by the subjectivity of the critic," and thus necessarily ahistorical.[58] The problem is the status of textual analysis as evidence, that is, finding viable ways to delimit and contextualize the process of interpretation.

Because industry self-regulation functioned as a sort of machine for registering and internalizing social conflict, it provides an extraordinarily fruitful means of contextualizing film analysis. In the case studies presented here, I have sought to examine films through the grid of the MPPDA's concerns. Archival materials such as production and story files and the case files of the MPPDA have served as a basis for identifying what was considered offensive, morally repugnant, or politically dangerous.

I have chosen six representative cases for analysis out of an initial sample of one hundred titles. The sample includes films made between 1929, when the MPPDA first began to monitor scripts on the West Coast on a regular basis, and 1942, when the system of self-regulation becomes complicated by the Office of War Information's attempt to monitor scripts through its Bureau of Motion Pictures.[59] There were two criteria for selecting a film for close analysis. First, that film had to have occasioned a statement of MPPDA policy. In some cases, the files contain correspondence between industry censors and Will Hays concerning how a particular type of problem was to be handled. Such instances are instructive because they permit some generalizations about MPPDA routine. A second criterion for selecting a case was that it had to indicate some of the social constraints which had an impact on the formulation of policy. The data compiled by the MPPDA show that some films were heavily censored by external agencies. In several cases, films were banned outright by the New York state board and had to be reedited before their release. Other files contain letters of complaint or clippings of newspaper articles which report low or "condemned" ratings by the Catholic Legion of Decency. Thus, I have been able to single out films which we know in fact went beyond the bounds of the acceptable. These lapses or failures of self-regulation are important for they illuminate the social forces which motivated censorship. In a very real sense, such limit cases defined what was not permissible within the range of films which composed the cycle.

I have used the MPPDA case files not only as a basis for the selection of films, but also as a guide in the process of analysis. The files contain letters and memos in which censors discuss their objections to a script and provide suggestions for revisions. These documents call attention to specific moments of difficulty or stress. Further, by correlating the MPPDA correspondence, the successive drafts of the screenplay, and the completed film, I have charted how material deemed unacceptable came to be represented. Thus as a methodological principle, all of the extant written materials—drafts of screenplays, memos in which censors rewrote scenes or proposed readings of scripts—are placed at the same level of importance as the film itself. The object of study is, in effect, expanded to include not only the film as such but the entire process of revision. The analysis is concerned with the strategic logic which underlies this process: for example, it seeks to determine if the completed film emphasizes moral questions in a different way than the first draft of the screenplay, or if the events of the plot have been reordered to eliminate a potentially offensive scene from the completed feature,

This approach provides a sense of the *mechanisms* by which social conflicts impinged on a given text—that is, through the protracted negotiations and disputes between the MPPDA and the studios. Further, through sources such as the MPPDA case files it becomes possible to document, with some precision, the *way these conflicts surfaced in representation*—that is, as choices among various versions of the script. Analyzing the differences between these versions permits us to reconstruct the complex network of explicit rules and implicit narrative constraints which determined what was deemed aberrant or acceptable. Further, textual analysis, particularly a discussion of film style, suggests some of the ways these constraints could be circumvented or displaced. Finally, by comparing films across the decade, one can begin to get a sense of how the constraints imposed on representation changed over time. Thus, it becomes possible to delineate what was deviant or unusual within the films of the early thirties in relation to a clearly specified norm—the later versions of the cycle which were approved by the MPPDA.

Notes

1. Jason Joy to Harry Cohn, January 16, 1932, *Shopworn*, MPPDA Case Files, Academy Library.
2. For a recent instance of this argument see Leonard J. Leff and Jerold L. Simmons, *The Dame in the Kimono: Hollywood, Censorship, and the Production Code from the 1920s to the 1960s* (New York: Grove Weidenfeld, 1990), 19–32.
3. Robert Sklar, *Movie-Made America: How the Movies Changed American Life* (New York: Random House, 1975), 74–76, discusses this news story in connection with the star scandals of the teens; the phrase "movie struck girl" derives from William A. Page, "The Movie Struck Girl," *Women's Home Companion* 45 (June 1918): 18, cited in Sklar.
4. These examples are culled from a random selection of issues from the early thirties: Roland Francis, "The New Extra Girl," *Photoplay* (December 1929): 44–45, 122; Reginald Taviner, "Is It Easy Money?" *Photoplay* (March 1931): 52–53, 123–25; Jeanne North, "Do You Want a Job in the Studios?" *Photoplay* (May 1931): 68–70, 116–20; for a short story dealing with the same themes see Vesta Wills Hancock, "Ambitious Baby," *Photoplay* (May 1930): 58-59, 152–55.
5. Will Hays, *Memoirs* (New York: Doubleday, 1955), 380.
6. For references to the gangster film and the fantasy of being a criminal, see Herbert Blumer and Philip M. Hauser, *Movies, Delinquency, and Crime* (New York: Macmillan, 1933), 2, 46–59. In discussing the influence of movies on delinquent girls, Blumer and Hauser do not use the

term "sex picture" (the term is employed in industry journals such as *Variety),* but cf. the discussion of the representation of a "wild life" outside of the context of the family (87); the reference to the figure of the gold digger (100); and the discussion of films in which the sexually deviant heroine is "punished" by disease, illegitimate children, and social ostracism (117). I discuss the model of spectatorship inherent in the Payne Fund Studies in "Reformers and Spectators: The Film Education Movement in the Thirties," *Camera Obscura* 22 (Jan. 1990): 29–49.

7. Blumer and Hauser, *Movies, Delinquency, and Crime* 208.

8. Please see the objections to the fallen woman film, 15–17.

9. Film critics have proposed several names for this type of film: the confession tale (Richard Griffith), the maternal melodrama (Christian Viviani), and the fallen woman cycle (Marilyn Campbell, Betsy McLane). See Marilyn Campbell, "RKO's Fallen Women, 1930–1933," *Velvet Light Trap* 10 (Fall 1973): 13–16; Richard Griffith, "Cycles and Genres," from "The Film Since Then," an additional section of the book *The Film Till Now* by Paul Rotha (London: Vision Press, 1949); Betsy Ann McLane, "Hollywood's Fallen Women Features," Masters Thesis, University of Southern California, 1978; Christian Viviani "Who Is without Sin?: The Maternal Melodrama in American Film, 1930–1939," *Wide Angle* 4, no. 2 (1980): 4–17. I have decided to retain the name fallen woman cycle in order to emphasize the continuities between the films and their literary antecedents.

10. Review of *Madame X, Variety,* May I, 1929.

11. The trilogy, which has probably been mistitled *Past and Present,* is discussed in Nina Auerbach, *Woman and the Demon: The Life of a Victorian Myth* (Cambridge: Harvard University Press, 1982), 154–59; Linda Nochlin, "Lost and *Found:* Once More the Fallen Woman," *Art Bulletin* 60 (1978): 141–44; Raymond Lister, *Victorian Narrative Painting* (New York: C. N. Potter, 1966), 54–59.

12. Linda Noddin, ("Lost and *Found")* discusses this icon in connection with George Frederic Watts's *Found Drowned* (c. 1848-50), in which the fallen woman's body appears under the arch of a bridge.

13. For an interesting discussion of the woman's seduction/rape by an upper-class man as a figuration of class conflict, see Thomas Elsaesser, "Tales of Sound and Fury: Observations on the Family Melodrama," *Monogram* 4 (1972), reprinted in *Home Is Where the Heart Is: Studies in Melodrama and the Woman's Film,* ed. Christine Gledhill (London: British Film Institute, 1987), 45–46.

14. Sally Mitchell, *The Fallen Angel: Chastity, Class, and Women's Reading, 1835–1880* (Bowling Green, Ohio: Bowling Green University Popular Press, 1981); George Watt, *The Fallen Woman in the Nineteenth-Century Novel* (Totowa, N.J.: Barnes and Noble, 1984).

15. See Mitchell, *Fallen Angel* 8.

16. Nina Baym, *Women's Fiction: A Guide to Novels by and about Women in America, 1820–1870* (Ithaca: Cornell University Press, 1978), 51. Baym claims that relatively few American domestic novels represent women as the sexual prey of men (26), but she does not take account of the fact that British domestic novels, among them fallen woman stories, were widely read in America. See Dee Garrison, "Immoral Fiction in the Late Victorian Library" *American Quarterly* 28, no. 1 (Spring 1976): 74.

17. Sally Mitchell, Introduction, *East Lynne* (New Brunswick, N.J.: Rutgers University Press, 1984), vii and xiii.

18. Anne Lyon Haight, *Banned Books: 387 B.C. to 1978 A.D.,* updated and enlarged by Chandler B. Grannis (New York: R. R. Bowker, 1978), 55.

19. Mrs. Gaskell was troubled by the reaction to *Ruth,* one of the first sympathetic depictions of the fallen woman. In one of her letters she notes: "in several instances I have *forbidden* people to write, for their expressions of disapproval (although I have known that the feeling would exist in them,) would be very painful and stinging at the time, 'An unfit subject or fiction' is

the thing to say about it . . . 'Deep regret' is what my friends here . . . feel and express." See Elizabeth Gaskell to Anne Robson, before January 27, 1853, *The Letters of Mrs. Gaskell,* ed. J. A. V. Chapple and Arthur Pollard (Manchester: Manchester University Press, 1966), 220, quoted in Mitchell, *Fallen Angel* 40. Like *Ruth,* Frances Trollope's novel *Jessie Phillips* provoked a great deal of complaint, leading the author to complain of receiving "such a multitude of communications urging various and contradictory modes of treating the subject." See Frances Trollope, *Jessie Phillips: A Tale of the Present Day* (London: Colburn, 1844), chap. 56, quoted in Mitchell, *Fallen Angel* 25.

20. Haight, *Banned Books* 40, 45, 51. Sally Mitchell notes that in order to be published in book form, several magazine serials dealing with the fallen woman had to be revised to meet the requirements of publishers and circulating libraries (*Fallen Angel* 88–89).

21. Dominick LaCapra, *Madame Bovary on Trial* (Ithaca: Cornell University Press, 1982).

22. Ernest Boyd, Introduction to the Modern Library Edition of *Nana* (New York: Random House, 1928), v–vi.

23. On the question of sexual practices outside the dictates of the ideology of purity see Michel Foucault, *The History of Sexuality,* vol. 1: *An Introduction,* trans. Robert Hurley (New York: Vintage Books, 1978); Peter Gay, *Education of the Senses,* vol. 1 of *The Bourgeois Experience: Victoria to Freud* (Oxford: Oxford University Press, 1984). On the feminine ideal see Barbara Welter, "The Cult of True Womanhood: 1820–1860," *American Quarterly* 18 (Summer 1966): 151–74; Mitchell, *Fallen Angel* x–xvi; and Nancy F. Cott, "Passionlessness: An Interpretation of Victorian Sexual Ideology, 1790–1850" *Signs* 4, no. 2 (Winter 1978): 219–36.

24. Haight, *Banned Books* 53.

25. George Bernard Shaw, Preface to *Mrs. Warren's Profession,* in *Bernard Shaw: Collected Plays with Their Prefaces,* vol. 1 (New York: Dodd, Mead, 1975), 231–32.

26. Dreiser's difficulties with his publisher, Doubleday, Page and Company, are discussed by John C. Berkey and Alice M. Winters in the "Historical Commentary" to *Sister Carrie* (Philadelphia: University of Pennsylvania Press, 1981).

27. Elizabeth Janeway, Afterword, *Susan Lenox: Her Fall and Rise* (Carbondale: Southern Illinois University Press, 1977), xviii.

28. David Graham Phillips, *Susan Lenox: Her Fall and Rise* 150.

29. John S. Sumner, Anthony Comstock's successor as head of the New York Society for the Suppression of Vice, attempted to dissuade D. Appleton from publishing the book. See Haight, *Banned Books* 59; Janeway, Afterword xi–xii:

30. Haight, *Banned Books* 27.

31. The Formula is reprinted in Garth Jowett, *Film: The Democratic Art* (Boston: Little, Brown, 1976), 466–67.

32. The Code is reprinted in Raymond Moley, *The Hays Office* (New York: Bobbs Merrill, 1945), 241–48, and a somewhat shorter version appears in Jowett, *Film* 468–72.

33. While I discuss only American fallen woman films, there are also many European variants of the story. For example, in the Italian diva film *Lydia* (tentatively dated 1910 by the Cineteca Italiana), the heroine runs off with a wealthy nobleman, an act which precipitates her ailing mother's death and leads to public disgrace, and eventually death, for her lover and herself. Many Asta Nielsen films of the same period deal with the fallen woman, including *Afgrunden* (1910), *Heisses Blut* (1911), *Im grossen Augenblick* (1911), *Die arme Jenny* (1912), and *Die Sünden der Väter* (1913). Nielsen's films are described in *Asta Nielsen: Ihr Leben in Fotodokumenten, Selbstzeugnissen und zeitgenössischen Betrachtungen,* ed. Renate Seydel and Allan Hagedorff (Munich: Universitas Verlag, 1981). The German "street" films of the twenties are also a prime example of the genre, most notably *Die freudlose Gasse.* Patrice Petro discusses the German variants of the genre in *"Dirnentragödie:* Sexual Mobility, Social Mobility, and

Melodramas of the Street," in her *Joyless Streets: Women and Melodramatic Representation in Weimar Germany* (Princeton: Princeton University Press, 1989), 160–74.
34. For examples, see the review of *It* in *Variety* (February 9, 1927) and Harry Edington, Letter to George J. Schaefer, August 15, 1940, *Kitty Foyle*, RKO Production Files, RKO Archive, Los Angeles.
35. Griffith, "Cycles and Genres," 438–39; and see McLane, "Hollywood's Fallen Women Features," 206–7.
36. Viviani, "Who Is without Sin?"
37. William Troy, "Virtue in 1933," in a weekly column "Films," *Nation*, March 29, 1933, 354–55.
38. Edgar Dale, *The Content of Motion Pictures* (New York: Macmillan, 1935), 108.
39. Ibid., 107.
40. Alice Ames Winter to Will Hays, July 10, 1933, Hays Collection, Indiana State Library.
41. *Photoplay*, September 1931, cited in Campbell, "RKO's Fallen Women."
42. Mildred Martin, of the *Philadelphia Inquirer*, July 23, 1933, as quoted in a public relations report to Will Hays from K. L. Russell, July 26, 1933, Hays Collection, Indiana State Library.
43. Blumer and Hauser, *Movies, Delinquency, and Crime* 96.
44. Ibid., 42.
45. Jason Joy to William A. Orr, June 14, 1932, *Red Headed Woman*, MPPDA Case Files, Academy Library.
46. James Wingate to Will Hays, n.d., *Jennie Gerhardt*, MPPDA Case Files, Academy Library.
47. Moley, *Hays Office* 77–82.
48. Not surprisingly, Moley, in what amounts to a celebration of Hays and the wonders of industry self-regulation, does not emphasize the majors' oligopolistic control of the first-run exhibition outlets. For a discussion of the significance of theater ownership see Mae D. Huettig, *Economic Control of the Motion Picture Industry: A Study in Industrial Organization* (Philadelphia: University of Pennsylvania Press, 1944).
49. Jack Vizzard, *See No Evil: Life inside a Hollywood Censor* (New York: Simon & Schuster, Pocket Book Edition, 1971); James M. Wall, "Oral History with Geoffrey Shurlock," Louis B. Mayer Library, American Film Institute, Los Angeles (A.F.I., 1975).
50. Wall, "Oral History with Geoffrey Shurlock," 254–300.
51. I have run across one case in which the MPPDA sought to block the exhibition of a film, the 1929 version of *White Cargo*. The film was produced in Britain by an independent, J. B. Williams, who was not a member of the association. Significantly, the 1942 version, made by 20th Century-Fox, was released with MPPDA approval.
52. Vizzard, *See No Evil* 63. Shurlock also mentions the importance of reviewing scripts prior to production in Wall, "Oral History with Geoffrey Shurlock," 126: "As usual in those days they had to take it [problematic material] out of the script before anything lurid could be even conceived. It was our policy to question everything, to be sure we had a basis to raise questions later on; we didn't want him [the producer?] asking us afterward: 'Why didn't you tell me at the script level?' "
53. Discussing the MPPDA's pledge to "enforce" the Code in 1934, Sklar writes: "The movie producers already possessed a code of moral standards, the Production Code of 1930, which went about as far as it could toward expressing the Catholic bishops' viewpoint without converting the movies from entertainment to popular theology" (*Movie-Made America*, 173). Garth Jowett writes: "by 1935 the motion picture industry was essentially under the control of a Catholic hegemony" (*Film*, 256).
54. The Legion printed ratings of current releases and circulated these among its members. "C" (Condemned) films were "considered to be those which, because of theme or treatment, have

been described by the Holy Father as 'positively bad' " ("Explanation of Film Classifications," National Catholic Office for Motion Pictures, undated pamphlet held by the Library of Performing Arts, New York Public Library, New York). Shurlock discusses the case of Cukor's *Two-Faced Woman* which was condemned by the Legion; see Wall, "Oral History with Geoffrey Shurlock," 249–50. A listing of films classified by the Legion shows a somewhat larger number of films given a "B" (Objectionable in part, for all) rather than an outright "C" rating. Examples are *Kitty Foyle, Forever Amber, The Gay Sisters,* and *Dance, Girls, Dance.* See the fascinating "Motion Pictures Classified by the National Legion of Decency, February 1936–November 1948," undated pamphlet held in the Library of Performing Arts, New York Public Library.

55. Annette Kuhn has also analyzed film censorship as a constructive force in the elaboration of meaning. See the essay on the Production Code and Howard Hawks's *The Big Sleep* in *The Power of the Image: Essays on Representation and Sexuality* (London: Routledge & Kegan Paul, 1985),74–95, and, on British cinema, *Cinema, Censorship, and Sexuality 1909–1925* (London: Routledge, 1988).

56. This approach toward the relationship between film and ideology is proposed by Jean-Louis Comolli and Jean Narboni, "Cinema/Ideology/Criticism," *Cahiers du Cinéma* (Oct/Nov 1969), translated in *Screen* 12, no. 1 (Spring 1971): 27–36. The *Cahiers* produced two collective texts on film which, they argued, revealed the contradictions within ideology. See "John Ford's *Young Mr. Lincoln*" (July/Aug 1970), translated in *Screen* 13, no. 3 (Autumn 1972), reprinted in *Movies and Methods,* vol. I, ed. Bill Nichols (Berkeley: University of California Press, 1976), and *"Morocco"* (Nov/Dec 1970), translated in *Sternberg,* ed. Peter Baxter (London: BFI Publishing, 1980).

57. See, for example, Claire Johnston, "Woman's Cinema as Counter-Cinema," in *Notes on Women's Cinema,* BFI pamphlet (London: 1973), reprinted in *Movies and Methods,* vol. 1, ed. Bill Nichols (Berkeley: University of California Press, 1976). For a critique of Johnston's methods of analysis see Janet Bergstrom, "Rereading the Work of Claire Johnston," *Camera Obscura* 3/4 (1979): 21–32.

58. Richard Maltby, " 'Baby Face' or How Joe Breen Made Barbara Stanwyck Atone for Causing the Wall Street Crash," *Screen* 27, no. 2 (March/April 1986): 24. Barbara Klinger also finds the category of the subversive text problematic, suggesting that it is necessary to take account of the multiplicity of discourses which determine the consumption of the supposedly subversive or progressive text, see "Cinema/Ideology/Criticism Revisited: The Progressive Text," *Screen* 25, no. 1 (Jan/Feb 1984): 44.

59. On April 4, 1928, Jason Joy writes to Will Hays from the West Coast, announcing that he has secured furniture for the establishment of an office, Letter, Hays Collection, Indiana State Library. I suspect that the establishment of censorship on the West Coast was in response to the coming of sound. The relationship between the Bureau of Motion Pictures and the MPPDA in the forties is discussed in Clayton R. Koppes and Gregory D. Black, *Hollywood Goes to War: How Politics, Profits, and Propaganda Shaped World War II Movies* (New York: Macmillan, 1987), 82–112.

LESSON FIVE

The Studios

Columbia Pictures: The Making of a Motion Picture Major, 1930–1943

Tino Balio

Starting out in Poverty Row, Columbia Pictures survived the battle for the theaters, the conversion to sound, and the Great Depression to emerge as a full-fledged member of the Hollywood establishment by 1934. In that year, giant film companies such as Paramount, Fox, and RKO had been dragged down by their theater chains into receivership or bankruptcy, but little Columbia won the respect of Wall Street by earning over $1 million in profits. In 1934, Columbia also won accolades from the critics by releasing two surprise hits, Victor Schertzinger's *One Night of Love,* a modern-dress operetta starring soprano Grace Moore, and Frank Capra's *It Happened One Night,* a screwball comedy starring Claudette Colbert and Clark Gable. *It Happened One Night* had the distinction of sweeping the top five Academy Awards—an achievement that has occurred only one other time in the history of the Oscars.[1]

The economic arena Columbia operated in was a virtual oligopoly dominated by the so-called Big Five—Loew's Inc. (MGM), Paramount Pictures, Warner Bros., Twentieth Century-Fox, and RKO. These companies were fully integrated—that is, they produced practically all the top-quality pictures, operated worldwide distribution networks, and owned large affiliated theater chains. Columbia, Universal Pictures, and United Artists were the Little Three. Columbia and Universal produced and distributed mostly low-budget pictures that played on the bottom half of double bills; United Artists functioned solely as a distributor for a small group of elite independent producers. These eight companies constituted the majors.

Although Columbia's role in the business during the studio system era is well established, the company's entrée into the Hollywood establishment has never been fully explored.[2] A definitive account of Columbia's escape from Poverty Row must wait until the studio opens its corporate records to researchers, but even without the benefit of primary sources much can be inferred about Columbia's development from articles in the trade press, movie reviews, and the occasional piece in business magazines. Using these sources, I have isolated the goals that Columbia met in becoming a major motion picture company, which were: volume production, national distribution, first-run exhibition, a roster of one or two stars, and a few hits.

These goals were consonant with the business practices of the American film industry as it entered the era of big business in the twenties,[3] And as Columbia's entrée into the majors will demonstrate, these goals were mutually dependent. In practice, they had to be targeted pretty much in succession. As a result, this case study has certain implications for understanding the history of the film industry. First, the major studios had no preordained right to succeed. Each company had to acquire the pragmatic skills to carve a niche for itself in the market, to stabilize its operations, and to generate profits. Second, production had to be tailored first and foremost to the paying public. Producing films to suit the personal tastes of studio moguls, boards of directors, or financiers would have ruined a company. Third, the market presented companies with an array of options. All motion picture companies had the goal of profit maximization, but they chose different means to achieve that end.

To place some perspective on Columbia's maneuverings, I have compared its strategies to those of United Artists and Eagle-Lion Pictures. At first glance, such comparisons might seem odd; after all, UA was founded in 1919 by Mary Pickford, Charles Chaplin, Douglas Fairbanks, and D. W. Griffith exclusively as a distributor of high-quality independent productions, while Eagle-Lion didn't get started until after World War II and functioned partly as a distributor of British films. But a closer look will reveal that Columbia, United Artists, and Eagle-Lion confronted similar problems but solved them in different ways.

Poverty Row Beginnings

Columbia Pictures got its start as CBC Film Sales Company, which was founded by Jack Cohn, Joe Brandt, and Harry Cohn in 1919 to produce and market novelty shorts.[4] Jack Cohn and Joe Brandt handled sales and managed the business affairs of the company in New York, while Harry Cohn handled the production end in Hollywood where he operated out of a rented studio in Poverty Row. The American film industry had entered the era of big business during the twenties and CBC had to expand or perish. Gradually branching out into Westerns, comedies, and even a few inexpensive features, CBC signaled its growing aspirations by incorporating as Columbia Pictures on January 10, 1924.[5] The immediate objective was to take control of its own distribution. Severing its ties to states'-rights operators, Columbia acquired its first exchange in 1925; by 1929 it had established a national distribution network and by 1931 it had branched out into foreign markets. Meanwhile, Columbia shored up its feature film production by purchasing a small studio on Gower Street in Hollywood in 1926 and by signing new directors, most notably Frank Capra, soon after.

Despite such moves, Columbia found itself in a bind. The quality of its features was not good enough to secure regular bookings in the affiliated theater chains, and the quantity of its output could not meet the needs of smaller independent theaters. That Columbia overcame these barriers to entry was largely the handiwork of Harry Cohn. Columbia underwent a management shakeup in 1931 when Jack Cohn and Joe Brandt attempted to oust Harry Cohn from the company. The details of the attempted coup are unclear, but when Columbia financier A. H. Giannini of the Bank of America threw his support to Harry Cohn, Brandt retired from the company and sold his interest to Harry Cohn. Harry Cohn took over the presidency of the company while retaining his job as chief of production, which made him the only executive in the business to hold the two posts; Jack Cohn moved up to executive vice-president in charge of distribution and remained in New York. Harry and Jack Cohn retained most of the equity and voting stock in the company and operated Columbia as a family-run business throughout the studio system era.[6]

Reorganizing Production

Columbia, with its limited financial resources, could not compete with the Big Five in important first-run situations, but it could hope to tap the low end of the market by servicing unaffiliated theaters that changed bills up to three times a week. In contrast, United Artists targeted the high end of the market by distributing high-quality independent productions. During the thirties, UA released the films of Charles Chaplin, Samuel Goldwyn, Alexander Korda, Howard Hughes, and Twentieth Century Pictures, a production company operated by Joseph Schenck and Darryl Zanuck. All specialized in "prestige pictures," although not exclusively. Prestige pictures, by far the most popular production trend of the decade, did not constitute a genre. The term implied production values and treatment—a big-budget special based on a presold property, often as not a literary "classic," and tailored for top stars.[7] For Goldwyn, prestige meant adaptations of Pulitzer Prize winners (*Street Scene* [1931]) or novels written by Nobel laureates (*Arrowsmith* [1932]); for Korda, it meant historical biopics (*The Private Life of Henry VIII* [1933] and *Catherine the Great* [1934]); for Howard Hughes, it meant spectacular action films (*Hell's Angels* [1930]). United Artists released relatively few pictures each year, from fifteen to twenty, but the pictures earned the company a reputation as the Tiffany's of the industry.

To service the low end of the market, Columbia continued its policy of marketing shorts and Westerns. Columbia's roster of shorts was immense and consisted of Walt Disney's Mickey Mouse cartoons and Silly Symphonies, Krazy Cat cartoons, Eddie Buzzell's Bedtime Stories, Scrappy cartoons, Screen Snapshots, and Sunrise Comedies, among others; its roster of Westerns included the Buck Jones and Tim McCoy series. Since the demand for these types of pictures was seemingly limitless, they provided a stable financial base for the company.

On this base, Columbia expanded feature film production. Harry Cohn modified studio operations in 1931 by converting from the central producer system to the producer-unit system and by delegating the day-to-day details of production to a group of associate producers.[8] Columbia released around thirty features a year from 1930 to 1934, when output rose to forty-three. The cause of this jump is not known exactly, but double features no doubt played a role.

Showing two pictures for the price of one was an old business practice. The shortage of talking pictures during the conversion to sound and the higher rentals they commanded stemmed the practice for a while, but the Depression gave double-featuring a boost. Independent theaters adopted the practice to break down the barriers of booking protection, which is to say, excessive clearances enjoyed by first-run theaters. Indies reasoned that if they could not present hit pictures in a timely manner to their patrons, they would offer quantity instead. Although the affiliated theater chains initially fought the practice, they too soon fell into line and by 1934, nearly every theater in competitive situations—the markets that generated the bulk of the box-office gross—showed double features. Double features essentially doubled the demand for product. Since the production facilities and talent of the Big Five limited the number of pictures they could produce, a gap existed that was soon filled by Columbia, Universal, and Poverty Row studios.

Surveying Columbia's releases from 1930 to 1934 reveals that the studio specialized in low-budget pictures having ordinary contemporary settings. Of the more than 150 features produced in this period, approximately 50 were dramas, 20 were crime/gangster pictures, 18 were mysteries, 10 were comedies, 9 were women's films, and 8 were action/adventures. In addition, the studio produced 15 Buck Jones and 7 Tim McCoy series Westerns. It is significant that the studio's roster included only 3 musicals and 2 horror films—genres that are expensive to produce because of their technical demands and special effects.

In its quest for profits, Columbia's policy was to produce economy models of class-A pictures. This meant following trends closely and relying heavily on remakes. Concerning the quality of a typical Columbia release, *Variety* had this to say: "Nothing new in a familiar story" (*Fugitive Lady* [1934]); "Makes no pretense of being above the split-week grade" (*The Sky Raiders* [1931]); and "Just a western with airplanes instead of horses" (*Air Hostess* [1933]). Concerning Columbia's cost-cutting techniques, *Variety* said of *Murder on the Roof* (1930): "The obvious inexpensive manner in which Columbia produced this all-talker won't be noticed by lay audiences. When a producing company can turn one out like this on this kind of dough, that company is bound to make money with it. So are the theatres playing it—certain theatres." Occasionally, a Columbia picture generated special appeal. *Variety* described *By Whose Hand?* (1932) as follows: "This Columbia [picture] is the answer to the grind house exhib's prayer. It is a vigorous melodrama, loaded with climaxes and speed, trimly played and expertly produced for the lesser grade house."[9] Occasionally, pictures like *By Whose Hand?* might qualify as programmers, which meant they could fill either the top or bottom half of a bill, depending on the genre, location of the theater, and audience.[10]

Expanding Distribution

Expanding feature film production required an efficient distribution system, since the two areas were interdependent. Branching out into distribution after incorporating had been expensive, but Columbia no longer had to pay commissions to states'-rights exchanges. A national distribution system also meant that Columbia could coordinate domestic release patterns, control advertising and publicity at every level of the market, and set prices for its pictures—requirements if the company ever expected to release class-A pictures.

Columbia's B production operated on tight margins and it was crucial for the company to wring every possible dollar in film rentals from the market. Columbia's B features cost from $50,000 to $100,000 to produce; in contrast, the majors spent as much as $300,000 on B films and Poverty Row as little as $10,000. Regardless of cost, Columbia's routine films were sold in blocks on a flat-fee basis following industry custom.

Although block booking had been harshly attacked by federal agencies, independent theaters, and citizen's groups, the trade practice persisted throughout the thirties as a form of wholesaling which permitted studios to peddle their entire season's output to exhibitors on an all-or-nothing basis. Block booking offered distributors several advantages, among them the scale economies of selling in bulk and the guarantee that every picture released by the company would find a market regardless of quality.[11] Unlike percentage terms used for class-A pictures, flat fees prevented a distributor from capturing the extraordinary profits of an unexpected hit; on the other hand, flat fees had the advantage of generating predictable returns, so that if a studio kept costs within limits, its pictures could earn a profit. Since Harry Cohn was a notorious penny-pincher, we can assume that Columbia's conservative spending habits and its control over distribution helped secure a steady flow of financing from its principal backer, the Bank of America.

The Case of United Artists

To get some perspective on Columbia's operations thus far, we can take a closer look at the way United Artists structured its operations.[12] United Artists was founded by Mary Pickford, Douglas Fairbanks, Charles Chaplin, and D. W. Griffith in 1919 as a distribution company to be owned and operated by stars. The founders had risen through the ranks of the business to become prominent independent producers. They had obtained financing and had released their pictures through leading firms such as Famous Players-Lasky and First National, but the founders decided to team up in response to the merger movement in the film industry which promised, among other things, to contain the skyrocketing salaries of big-name talent like themselves.

The founders of UA gained control of a key element of the film business. As independent producers, the founders controlled the making of their pictures. By forming UA, they could oversee the sales, promotion, and advertising of their pictures as well. Under this plan, UA's founders had to secure their own financing, but UA would reduce the risks of production financing by selling pictures individually on a percentage basis rather than in blocks and by charging producers a modest distribution fee for its services. United Artists was supposed to operate at just above breakeven and to funnel most of the distribution gross to its independent producers, thereby permitting them to pay off the production loans on their pictures promptly and to reach profits sooner. In other words, the founders decided to forgo the profits of the middleman—that is, the profits from owning a distribution company—in the hope of maximizing profits as independent producers.

To function efficiently—that is, to meet the overhead expenses of maintaining a sales staff in the principal markets of the world—United Artists required a larger volume of quality pictures than the founders as a group could provide. UA hoped to attract other stars and big-name directors to the fold; however, the thought of leaving the paternalistic care of the studio system appealed to few Hollywood luminaries and UA faced a chronic product shortage from the start.[13]

UA found a way out of its dilemma by aligning itself with a different type of independent—the creative producer. Unlike Chaplin, Fairbanks, and Pickford, who were actor-producers, the creative producer, typified by Joseph Schenck and Samuel Goldwyn, was an entrepreneur who operated in much the same way as the head of a studio, only on a much smaller scale. Schenck and Goldwyn chose suitable properties for the stars they had under contract, oversaw the development of their scripts, secured the financing, and supervised production. Every prominent producer who released through United Artists from 1930 to 1950 functioned in this manner. And only this type of independent could be relied on to deliver enough pictures on a regular basis to keep UA's distribution pipeline full. However, because UA did not have the financial resources to provide production financing, it remained the smallest of the eight majors.

What lessons could Columbia have learned from United Artists? None really, since during the early thirties Columbia had precious little money to devote to any class-A production. And besides, Harry Cohn was not about to entrust the studio's most important projects to outside producers. Columbia eventually opened its doors to independent producers, but not until the breakdown of the studio system after World War II.

Strengthening Exhibition

Having acquired a studio and exchanges, Columbia's next objective was to gain access to first-run theaters. Unlike the Big Five companies, which were completely integrated, the Little Three did not own theater chains. (Universal owned a small chain for a while but was forced to sell it during the Depression.) An analysis of Columbia Pictures by *Barron's* magazine, a national financial weekly, noted that the studio's financial health in 1935 resulted partly from its steadfast refusal to own theaters.[14] The magazine made this observation during the depths of the Depression when Paramount, Fox, and RKO seemed hopelessly mired in red ink as a result of their investments in real estate. With the return of prosperity, however, the assessment of *Barron's* would no longer be valid. Ownership of theaters, first-run houses in particular, would become the tool that enabled the Big Five to maintain control of the market. Columbia, Universal, and United Artists remained in a subservient position vis-à-vis the Big Five precisely because they did not own important theater chains.

Columbia released its pictures primarily to two types of theaters. Most were subsequent-run houses, typically small independent operations; less numerous were first-run houses, typically affiliates of the majors. Since the studio had meager financial resources, it could only occasionally produce a contender and only then did the studio want access to first-run houses. (As I will discuss later, Columbia would be relegated to subsequent-run venues until it had big-name stars on its roster.) First-run playing time meant longer runs—usually a week—in large, prestigious theaters and the opportunity of renting a picture on a percentage-of-the-gross basis. Thus if a release struck the public's fancy, the studio could enjoy a substantial share of the box-office take.

United Artists had gained access to first-run houses not only because it handled quality pictures, but also because the company had indirectly gone into exhibition. Alarmed by the battle for theaters, UA's owners, with the exception of Chaplin, invested $1 million to form United Artists Theatre Circuit in 1926. With an additional $4 million from a public stock issue, the Theatre Circuit constructed and/or purchased first-run theaters in key cities. What linked United Artists to United Artists Theatre Circuit was a ten-year franchise that granted the theater chain the preferential right to exhibit UA's pictures. The maneuver worked, with the result that affiliated theater chains recognized United Artists as a forceful competitor and booked its pictures.

How did Columbia gain access to first-run theaters? Reviews in *Variety* reveal that Columbia signed a franchise agreement with RKO in 1930 granting the theater chain first call on Columbia's releases. Unlike the other members of the Big Five, RKO was a relative newcomer to the business. Founded by RCA in 1928 to complete head on with AT&T in the sound recording and playback field, RKO merged Joseph P. Kennedy's Film Booking Office, the Keith-Albee-Orpheum circuit of vaudeville houses, and RCA's Photophone sound system into a vertically integrated firm containing three hundred theaters, four studios, and $80 million in working capital.

Despite RKO's impressive pedigree, the company faced the same challenges breaking into the market that Columbia did, plus one more—choice attractions to fill the playing time of its theaters. Since the Big Five had their own interests to protect, RKO turned to independent producers and the Little Three for help. The terms of RKO's franchise agreement with Columbia are not known, but if they are similar to the terms of RKO's franchise agreements with United Artists, the deal probably went something like this. RKO agreed to exhibit a specific number of better-quality pictures each year in selected theaters and to pay a film rental for each engagement based on the production cost of the picture and on the overhead expense of the respective theater.[15] In practice, RKO made a down payment based on a sliding scale that measured the relative production cost of the picture (the higher the production cost, the higher the down payment) and then split the box-office gross fifty-fifty after deducting the overhead expenses of the theater. These terms constituted a variation of the percentage of the gross form of rental and enabled Columbia to receive remuneration in relation to the box-office performance of its pictures.

The RKO franchise agreement may have been a turning point for Columbia. It provided both an incentive to produce higher quality pictures and a venue for their exhibition. If this assumption holds good, having a Frank Capra on the lot gains significance. A talented director, a star or two, and a few acceptable literary properties provided the leverage to lift Columbia into the majors.

After joining the studio in 1927, Capra quickly earned Harry Cohn's confidence and was awarded the task of handling the studio's occasional class-A picture. Capra responded by directing a series of inexpensive but well-received comedies. Going into the thirties, Capra's stature as a director grew with each successive release. By the time he made *American Madness* in 1932, critics were referring to him as "one of Hollywood's best."[16] Capra's *The Bitter Tea of General Yen* (1932) was chosen as the first feature presentation of RKO's new Radio City Music Hall in New York. After *It Happened One Night* swept the Academy Awards in 1934, Capra literally became a star and received top billing in Columbia's ads. Beginning with *The Bitter Tea of General Yen*, all the pictures Capra made for Columbia received a Music Hall send-off. Since his pictures received royal handling in New York, we can assume that a similar treatment awaited them in first-run situations around the country.

The fate of Columbia's other class-A products in this period is more difficult to assess. What is clear, however, is that simply having one Frank Capra was not enough to maintain Columbia's status as a member of the Little three. All of Columbia's competitors relied not only upon masterful directors but also upon stars. Star vehicles typically enjoyed a ready-made market, reduced the risk of production financing, and commanded the best rental terms.[17] Could a substitute be found for stars in the making of class-A pictures?

The Case of Eagle-Lion

A glance at Eagle-Lion Films suggests how one studio pursued such a strategy.[18] Eagle-Lion was a short-lived venture founded in 1946 by American industrialist Robert R. Young. The owner of Producers Releasing Corporation (PRC), a Poverty Row studio that specialized in cheap Westerns starring Buster Crabbe, Tim McCoy, Al "Lash" LaRue, and others, Young wanted nothing less than to create a new motion picture company. An alliance with British film magnate J. Arthur Rank, who was trying to break into the U.S. exhibition market, seemed an excellent way to begin.

At the end of World War II, Rank dominated all branches of the film business in Great Britain. Outside Great Britain, Rank owned or controlled theaters in France, Canada, and Australia and had close ties with exhibitors throughout the British Commonwealth. Although Britain was the most important overseas market for American films, it was not large enough to support indigenous production. Rank therefore had to export to survive, but getting playing time in the affiliated theater chains of the Big Five proved daunting. Rank had no other choice but to deal with the second tier of the American film industry. Universal agreed to distribute part of the Rank line in return for a reciprocal favor from Rank in Great Britain and in other markets. Since Rank produced more pictures than Universal could comfortably handle alone, he also agreed to collaborate along similar lines with Robert Young.

The alliance with Rank provided Young with instant prestige and access to important theaters overseas—a passport out of Poverty Row, or so it was thought. To comply with the agreement, Young spent over $12 million of his own money to form a vertically integrated operation, Eagle-Lion Films, a distribution company, and Eagle-Lion Studios, a production company. The former had offices in New York and had as its goal doing business with a higher grade exhibitor; the latter operated out of the PRC studio in Hollywood, which was upgraded at a cost of $1 million, and had as its goal the making of class-A pictures.

But Eagle-Lion faced formidable barriers to entry in the American market, not the least of which was an industrywide recession. All the optimistic predictions about the postwar prosperity for the movies soon began to ring hollow. Although the domestic box office rose steadily to peak in 1946, late in 1947 it began a steady decline that would last ten years. Producing a roster of lackluster pictures its first year, Eagle-Lion found itself shut out of first-run theaters. Much had to do with Eagle-Lion's stars. Unlike Columbia, Eagle-Lion could not borrow stars from the majors for the simple reason that majors would never entrust one of their valuable properties to a Poverty Row studio, or in this case a studio without an established track record. Because Eagle-Lion did not have the resources to develop stars, the studio limped along for a while using aging leading men on their way down (that is, George Brent and Louis Hayward) and a few young people working their way up (that is, Richard Basehart, June Lockhart, and Scott Brady).

Neither strategy succeeded and to stay afloat Eagle-Lion developed a radical production policy that substituted action, color, natural locations, and authenticity for the usual combination of stars and pre-sold stories. The result was a form of product differentiation—a string of film noir pictures that put Eagle-Lion, albeit temporarily, in the limelight. Produced on low budgets, these pictures included Anthony Mann's *T-Men* (1947), a semidocumentary based on Treasury Department cases; Crane Wilbur's *Canon City* (1948), a reenactment of a jailbreak at the Canon City, Colorado, state penitentiary that was shot on the site; and Alfred Werker's *He Walked by Night* (1948), a thriller depicting a brilliant psychotic killer. All made money and all received favorable press. For example, *Canon City*, which introduced Scott Brady as one of the prison busters, grossed $1.2 million on a budget of $424,000 and was cited by *Life* and *Look* as one of the top pictures of the year.

The postwar recession at the box office proved fatal to Eagle-Lion. Since the market for B films had declined, the company could not use this type of picture to create a firm financial base. With audiences becoming selective in their moviegoing tastes, even class-A features found the going rough. Had conditions been better, Eagle Lion's product differentiation strategy might have saved the company. Regardless, the studio demonstrated that an alternative existed to expensive star-studded pictures. But this option was not a viable one for Columbia. For one thing, location shooting just was not practical until new technology was introduced after World War II. For another, censorship forces during the early thirties were up in arms over the depiction of violence and crime in the movies.

Acquiring Stars

Columbia therefore had no choice but to adopt the star system if it wanted to produce class-A pictures. Commenting on Columbia's star power in the period from 1930 to 1934, *Barron's* said, "Another factor in [Columbia's] success has been the avoidance of onerous long-term contracts with stars, the long-term appeal of which is bound to be uncertain. It has followed a policy of signing artists and directors for a few pictures a year or of borrowing actors and actresses from other companies, a program that makes for economy and flexibility of production cost."[19] This assessment needs qualification; Columbia would have been fortunate indeed to have had real stars under long-term contract. Because *Barron's* assessment was likely based in part on interviews with company executives, it has the ring of a rationalization for the studio's lackluster roster.

Concerning star development, a studio had three options: (1) It could develop stars by casting players in different roles and testing audience reaction; (2) it could borrow stars from other studios; or (3) it could pretend it had stars and hope that exhibitors and the public would play along. The first option obviously consumed the most time and money; the second was feasible only for studios that had already achieved major status; the third required the most chutzpah.

During the early thirties, Columbia had the chutzpah to "star" veteran actor Jack Holt in over a dozen pictures. A typical Holt picture was an action story containing "love interest, melodramatics, outdoors and he-man stuff," said *Variety*. In its review of *The Woman I Stole* (1933), *Variety* said, "Jack Holt has been making pictures like this for years and has prospered. There's nothing especially distinguished in the output, but it is all eminently saleable material. Factory product, but factory product of a successful kind, with a ready market and satisfactory returns."[20] Columbia's supporting male players were Ralph Graves and Ralph Bellamy. That was it. Columbia had one true female star under contract—Barbara Stanwyck—but Columbia saw her name in lights only briefly. Stanwyck got her big break as the leading lady in Frank Capra's *Ladies of Leisure* (1930). *Variety* said that Stanwyck saved the picture "with her ability to convince in heavy emotional scenes," but that she had "small gifts for graceful comedy."[21] After testing her in several roles, Columbia gave her star billing in Frank Capra's *The Miracle Woman* (1931). Her biggest hit and final Columbia release was Capra's *The Bitter Tea of General Yen* (1933). Afterward, Stanwyck departed for Warner Bros., leaving Columbia temporarily with only one female personality of any magnitude on its roster—opera singer Grace Moore.

To bolster class-A production, Columbia had to exploit the second star based tactic: reliance on loan-outs from other studios. The majors loaned talent to one another on a regular basis. Try as they might, studios found it impossible to keep high-priced players busy all the time. Since an idle star was a heavy overhead expense, loan-outs could spread the costs. Studios devised various formulas to determine loan-out fees: the most common one was to charge a minimum fee of four weeks salary plus a surcharge of three weeks; another was to charge the basic salary for however long the star was needed plus a surcharge of 25 percent.[22]

The Big Five, having large stables of stars, would consider loan-outs to the Little Three, including the top-ranked independent producers associated with United Artists. Myth has it that the majors used loan-outs to discipline stars and to keep difficult people in line. But this argument does not make much sense, because it implies that a studio would risk its investment in a star by allowing him or her to appear in an inferior picture produced by a second-rate company. Actually, most stars were on the lookout for challenging parts and wanted the opportunity to play them anywhere. Given Columbia's lowly status in the early thirties, most of the loan-outs to the studio were on their way down. Claudette Colbert and Clark Gable were in lulls when Columbia borrowed them from Paramount and MGM, respectively, to star in *It Happened One Night;* the picture revitalized both their careers, but their home studios, not Columbia, enjoyed most of the benefits.

Producing Hits

By demonstrating the ability to produce the occasional hit, Columbia met its final goal. Columbia could have existed as a Poverty Row studio without hits, but the company needed a winner or two each year as a major to strengthen its financial reserves, to retire its debt, and to retain the interest of Wall Street. Yet producing a box-office winner has always been a difficult task. As *Barron's* pointed out, "Gauging the box-office appeal of a play or motion picture before production has, in the long run, proved to be . . . as hazardous as guessing the results of a horse race. Public taste is fickle, and the mere success of a single 'movie' offers no assurance that its type—gangster, biography, musical comedy, etc.—will maintain its appeal. 'Will they buy it?' is the nightmare of the producer of every theatrical production, and the answer can never be accurately foretold."[23] Therefore, producing hits not only generated profits, but also established a studio's credibility in the marketplace.

At Columbia, the task of producing winners fell mainly to Frank Capra. Columbia produced only three big hits from 1930 to 1934: Frank Capra's *Lady for a Day* in 1933 (Columbia's first release to make it to *Film Daily's* Ten Best pictures list), Victor Schertzinger's *One Night of Love,* and Capra's *It Happened One Night* (both in 1934). The latter two pictures enabled Columbia to generate profits of $1,009,000 in 1934, nearly equaling the company's peak pre-Depression earnings of $1,030,000 in 1929.

The question is: what strategy did the studio use to produce hits? Let's examine *It Happened One Night*. This picture and two other 1934 comedy hits—Howard Hawks's *Twentieth Century* (Columbia) and W. S. Van Dyke's *The Thin Man* (MGM)—have traditionally been regarded as initiating the screwball cycle in the thirties. However, contemporaneous sources saw *It Happened One Night* as a continuation of ongoing trends. Noting that Robert Riskin's screenplay about a runaway heiress who falls in love with a tough reporter was based on a short story in *Cosmopolitan* by Samuel Hopkins Adams entitled "Night Bus," *Variety,* saw the picture as "another long distance bus story," a variation on MGM's *Fugitive Lovers* and Universal's *Cross Country Cruise,* which had been released a month earlier.[24] Others considered the picture a "traveling hostelry" film similar to *Grand Hotel* and such spin-offs as Fox's *Transatlantic* (1931), Paramount's *Shanghai Express* (1932), and Columbia's own *American Madness* (1932).[25] Seen from this perspective, *It Happened One Night* did not materialize out of nowhere, but from Columbia's strategy of following trends.

Capitalizing on the success of *It Happened One Night,* Columbia decided to specialize in screwball comedies. Again, Capra carried most of the burden and produced three hits, *Mr. Deeds Goes to Town* (1936), *You Can't Take It with You* (1938), and *Mr. Smith Goes to Washington* (1939). If one line of screwball comedy featured the madcap adventures of wealthy heroines in comedies of remarriage, the Capra pictures, which were written in collaboration with either Robert Riskin or with Sidney Buchman, followed another line by depicting "utopian fantasies" where the little guy always comes out on top.[26] To play the heroes of these pictures, Columbia borrowed Gary Cooper from Paramount for *Mr. Deeds* and James Stewart from MGM for the other two. Jean Arthur, Columbia's only contract star, costarred in all three.

Capra's stature as a director had grown enormously after *It Happened One Night* and, beginning with *Mr. Deeds,* Columbia placed Capra's name above the title of his pictures. The three Capra comedies were named to *Film Daily's* Top Ten and won numerous awards, including special honors for Capra. *You Can't Take It with You,* the most acclaimed of the group, was hailed by *Time* as "the Number 1 cinema comedy of 1938" and received Academy Awards for best picture and best direction.

The returns on these pictures was another matter. Columbia budgeted $500,000 for *Mr. Deeds,* double the amount it spent on *It Happened One Night* and made a prudent investment. But Columbia permitted the budgets for Capra's subsequent productions, including his prestige picture *Lost Horizon* (1937), to escalate well beyond $1.5 million. The pictures did well at the box office, but as a group they barely recouped their production costs. Few pictures in the thirties could support such investments, with the result that Capra's pictures enhanced the reputation of the studio but earned modest profits.[27]

Columbia's other attempts at exploiting the screwball cycle fared less well. The studio borrowed Claudette Colbert from Paramount a second time to produce Gregory La Cava's *She Married Her Boss* (1935), a comic variation of the traditional "sob-and-hanky" melodrama. The picture did only so-so business. Columbia then designed two vehicles for Irene Dunne. Dunne had previously made a name for herself at other studios performing in melodramas and musicals but Columbia offcast her in Richard Boleslawski's *Theodora Goes Wild* (1936) and Leo McCarey's *The Awful Truth* (1937). In the former, Dunne played a "female Mr. Deeds" opposite Melvyn Douglas in a "distaff version" of Capra's *Mr. Deeds Goes to Town,* noted a review. In the latter, she played opposite Cary Grant in a comedy of remarriage. Neither picture made it to *Variety's* annual list of box-office champions, although *The Awful Truth* won considerable acclaim by being named to *Film Daily's* Ten Best pictures list and by winning the best direction Oscar for McCarey.

Lacking a roster of stars and a large financial cushion, Columbia was forced to concentrate mainly on one production trend as a source of its class-A pictures during the second half of the thirties. The Big Five, on the other hand, had the resources to spread risks by focusing on a range of production cycles and by producing pictures with trend-setting possibilities. And as owners of first-run theaters, the Big Five profited from any picture that struck the public's fancy regardless of which studio released it. Members of the Little Three would not secure an equal footing with the Big Five until the *Paramount* decrees went into effect beginning in 1948.

This case study has plotted a "bottom-up" course of development for Columbia Pictures as it struggled to become a member of the motion picture establishment. I have thereby rejected the conventional portrait of the studio era as a mature oligopoly in which Columbia, along with the other members of the Little Three, were somehow consigned by the Big Five to the second tier of the majors. In its place, this case study has offered a more dynamic account of industrial behavior depicting how one company successfully pursued a series of mutually dependent goals and objectives. Comparing Columbia to United Artists and Eagle-Lion adds perspective to the account by revealing how other small studios attempted to solve similar problems. Each choice affected the fortunes of the respective companies and as a consequence the ways in which they made their pictures.

Notes

1. *One Flew Over the Cuckoo's Nest,* a United Artists release, swept the top Academy Awards in 1975. Producers Saul Zaentz and Michael Douglas received the Best Picture Oscar; the other winners were director Miloš Forman, actor Jack Nicholson, actress Louise Fletcher, and screenwriters Laurence Hauben and Bo Goldman.
2. Douglas Gomery's concise overview of Columbia Pictures in *The Hollywood Studio System* ([New York: St. Martin's Press, 1986], esp. pp. 161–72) is the most authoritative account of the studio currently available; Edward Buscombe's essay, "Notes on Columbia Pictures Corporation, 1926–1941" (*Screen* 15 [Autumn 1975]: 65–82) suggests a relationship between the financing of Columbia's pictures and the ideology of Capra's films; and Joel Finler's chapter on the studio in his *The Hollywood Story* ([New York: Crown, 1988], pp. 68–87) contains a wealth of data on the studio's releases and personnel.
3. See, for example, Halsey, Stuart & Co's prospectus, "The Motion Picture Industry as a Basis for Bond Financing" (27 May 1927) in *The American Film Industry,* rev. ed., ed. Tino Balio, (Madison: University of Wisconsin Press, 1985), pp. 195–217.
4. Gomery, *The Hollywood Studio System,* p. 162. Anthony Slide's *The American Film Industry: An Historical Dictionary* ([New York: Greenwood Press, 1986], p. 70) states that CBC was founded in 1922; David Bordwell, Janet Staiger, and Kristein Thompson's *The Classical Hollywood Cinema: Film Style and Mode of Production to 1960* ([New York: Columbia University Press, 1985], p. 403) gives 1918 as the founding date.
5. Temporary National Economic Committee, *The Motion Picture Industry—A Pattern of Control* (Washington, D.C.: U.S. Government Printing Office, 1941), p. 62.
6. Warner Bros. was the only other major that continued to be run by its founders, the others having passed into the hands of professional managers during the twenties.
7. For a discussion of the importance of the prestige film as a production trend, see Tino Balio, *Grand Design: Hollywood as a Modern Business Enterprise, 1930–1939* (New York: Charles Scribner's Sons, 1993), pp. 179–211.
8. Bordwell, Staiger, and Thompson, *The Classical Hollywood Cinema,* p. 321.
9. *Variety Film Reviews* (New York: Garland, 1983–). See the entries for the following dates: 11 December 1934; 2 June 1931; 24 January 1933; 29 January 1930; 16 August 1932.
10. Brian Taves, "The B Film: Hollywood's Other Half," in *Grand Design: Hollywood as a Modern Business Enterprise, 1930–1939:* pp. 317–18.
11. For a contemporaneous discussion of block booking, see Howard T. Lewis, *The Motion Picture Industry* (New York: D. Van Nostrand, 1933), pp. 142–80, and TNEC, *The Motion Picture Industry,* pp. 21–33.
12. Tino Balio, *United Artists: The Company Built by the Stars* (Madison: University of Wisconsin Press, 1975).
13. Gloria Swanson was the only other big star to join United Artists during the twenties. Unfortunately, Miss Swanson's decision proved disastrous to her career since she failed to learn the skills to oversee both the business and artistic sides of independent production. See Balio, *United Artists,* pp. 82–84.
14. "Unique Motion Picture Enterprise," *Barron's* 15 (25 March 1935): 14.
15. Balio, *United Artists,* pp. 65–66.
16. Charles Wolfe, *Frank Capra: A Guide to References and Resources* (Boston: G.K. Hall, 1987), p. 11.

17. A fuller discussion of the economics of the star system is found in Cathy Klaprat, "The Star as Market Strategy: Bette Davis in Another Light," in *The American Film Industry*, pp. 351–76.
18. Tino Balio, *United Artists: The Company That Changed the Film Industry* (Madison: University of Wisconsin Press, 1987), pp. 11–39.
19. "Unique Motion Picture Enterprise," *Barron's*, p. 14.
20. *Variety Film Reviews*, 4 July 1933.
21. *Variety Film Reviews*, 28 May 1930.
22. "Less Than 2,000 Players Work," *Variety*, 7 September 1938, p. 2.
23. "Unique Motion Picture Enterprise," *Barron's*, p. 14.
24. *Variety Film Reviews*, 27 February 1934.
25. Heidi Kenaga, "Studio Differentiation of 'Screwball' Comedy" (unpublished paper, University of Wisconsin, Department of Communication Arts, 1990).
26. Wolfe, *Frank Capra: A Guide*, p. 22.
27. Finler, *The Hollywood Story*, p. 75.

LESSON SIX

Genres

Authorship and Genre: Notes on the Western

Jim Kitses

First of all, the western is American history. Needless to say, this does not mean that the films are historically accurate or that they cannot be made by Italians. More simply, the statement means that American frontier life provides the milieu and mores of the western, its wild bunch of cowboys, its straggling towns and mountain scenery. Of course westward expansion was to continue for over a century, the frontier throughout that period a constantly shifting belt of settlement. However, Hollywood's West has typically been, from about 1865 to 1890 or so, a brief final instant in the process. This twilight era was a momentous one: within just its span we can count a number of frontiers in the sudden rash of mining camps, the building of the railways, the Indian Wars, the cattle drives, the coming of the farmer. Together with the last days of the Civil War and the exploits of the badmen, here is the raw material of the western.

At the heart of this material, and crucial to an understanding of the gifts the form holds out to its practitioners, is an ambiguous, mercurial concept: the idea of the West. From time immemorial the West had beckoned to statesmen and poets, existing as both a direction and a place, an imperialist theme and a pastoral Utopia. Great empires developed ever westward: from Greece to Rome, from Rome to Britain, from Britain to America. It was in the West as well that the fabled lands lay, the Elysian fields, Atlantis, El Dorado. As every American schoolboy knows, it was in sailing on his passage to India, moving ever westward to realize the riches of the East, that Columbus chanced on the New World. Hand in hand with the hope of fragrant spices and marvelous tapestries went the ever-beckoning dream of life eternal: surely somewhere, there where the sun slept, was the fountain of youth.

As America began to be settled and moved into its expansionist phases, this apocalyptic and materialist vision found new expression. In his seminal study *Virgin Land,* Henry Nash Smith has traced how the West as symbol has functioned in America's history and consciousness. Is the West a Garden of natural dignity and innocence offering refuge from the decadence of civilization? Or is it a treacherous Desert stubbornly resisting the gradual sweep of agrarian progress and community values? Dominating America's intellectual life in the nineteenth century, these warring ideas were most clearly at work in attitudes surrounding figures like Daniel Boone, Kit Carson and Buffalo Bill Cody, who were variously seen as rough innocents ever in flight from society's artifice, and as enlightened pathfinders for the new nation. A folk-hero manufactured in his own time, Cody himself succumbed towards the end of his life to the play of these concepts that so gripped the imagination of his countrymen: "I stood between savagery and civilization most all my early days."

Refracted through and pervading the genre, this ideological tension has meant that a wide range of variation is possible in the basic elements of the form. The plains and mountains of western landscape can be an inspiring and civilizing environment, a moral universe productive of the western hero, a man with a code. But this view, popularized by Robert Warshow in his famous essay, "The Westerner", is one-sided. Equally the terrain can be barren and savage, surroundings so demanding that men are rendered morally ambiguous, or wholly brutalized. In the same way, the community in the western can be seen as a positive force, a movement of refinement, order and local democracy into the wilds, or as a harbinger of corruption in the form of Eastern values which threaten frontier ways. This analysis over-simplifies in isolating the attitudes: a conceptually complex structure that draws on both images is the typical one. If Eastern figures such as bankers, lawyers and journalists are often either drunkards or corrupt, their female counterparts generally carry virtues and graces which the West clearly lacks. And if Nature's harmonies produce the upright hero, they also harbour the animalistic Indian. Thus central to the form we have a philosophical dialectic, an ambiguous cluster of meanings and attitudes that provide the traditional thematic structure of the genre. This shifting ideological play can be described through a series of antinomies, so:

The Wilderness	**Civilization**
The Individual	**The Community**
freedom	restriction
honor	institutions
self-knowledge	illusion
integrity	compromise
self-interest	social responsibility
solipsism	democracy
Nature	**Culture**
purity	corruption
experience	knowledge
empiricism	legalism
pragmatism	idealism
brutalization	refinement
savagery	humanity
The West	**The East**
America	Europe
the frontier	America
equality	class
agrarianism	industrialism
tradition	change
the past	the future

In scanning this grid, if we compare the tops and tails of each sub-section, we can see the ambivalence at work at its outer limits: the West, for example, rapidly moves from being the spearhead of manifest destiny to the retreat of ritual. What we are dealing with here, of course, is no less than a national world-view: underlying the whole complex is the grave problem of identity that has special meaning for Americans. The isolation of a vast unexplored continent, the slow growth of social forms, the impact of an unremitting New England Puritanism obsessed with the cosmic struggle of good and evil, of the elect and the damned, the clash of allegiances to Mother Country and New World, these factors are the crucible in which American consciousness was formed. The thrust of contradictions, everywhere apparent in American life and culture, is clearest in the great literary heritage of the romantic novel that springs from Fenimore Cooper and moves through Hawthorne and Melville, Mark Twain and Henry James, Fitzgerald and Faulkner, Hemingway and Mailer. As Richard Chase has underlined in his *The American Novel and Its Tradition,* this form in American hands has always tended to explore rather than to order, to reflect on rather than to moralize about, the irreconcilables that it confronts; and where contradictions are resolved the mode is often that of melodrama or the pastoral. For failing to find a moral tone and a style of close social observation—in short, for failing to be *English*—the American novel has often had its knuckles rapped. As with literature, so with the film: the prejudice that even now persists in many quarters of criticism and education with reference to the Hollywood cinema (paramountly in America itself) flows from a similar lack of understanding.

The ideology that I have been discussing inevitably filters through many of Hollywood's genres: the western has no monopoly here. But what gives the form a particular thrust and centrality is its historical setting; its being placed at exactly that moment when options are still open, the dream of a primitivistic individualism, the ambivalence of at once beneficent and threatening horizons, still tenable. For the film-maker who is preoccupied with these motifs, the western has offered a remarkably expressive canvas. Nowhere, of course, is the freedom that it bestows for personal expression more evident than in the cinema of John Ford.

It would be presumptuous to do more than refer here to this distinguished body of work, the crucial silent period of which remains almost wholly inaccessible. Yet Ford's career, a full-scale scrutiny of which must be a priority, stands as unassailable proof of how the historical dimensions of the form can be orchestrated to produce the most personal kind of art. As Andrew Sarris has pointed out, "no American director has ranged so far across the landscape of the American past." But the journey has been a long and deeply private one through green valleys of hope on to bitter sands of despair. The peak comes in the forties where Ford's works are bright monuments to his vision of the trek of the faithful to the Promised Land, the populist hope of an ideal community, a dream affectionately etched in *The Grapes of Wrath, My Darling Clementine, Wagonmaster.* But as the years slip by the darker side of Ford's romanticism comes to the foreground, and twenty years after the war—in *The Man Who Shot Liberty Valance, Two Rode Together, Cheyenne Autumn*—we find a regret for the past, a bitterness at the larger role of Washington, and a desolation over the neglect of older values. The trooping of the colors has a different meaning now. As Peter Wollen has described in his chapter on *auteur* theory in *Signs and Meaning in the Cinema*, the progression can be traced in the transposition of civilized and savage elements. The Indians of *Drums Along the Mohawk* and *Stagecoach*, devilish marauders that threaten the hardy pioneers, suffer a sea-change as Ford's hopes wane, until with *Cheyenne Autumn* they are a civilized, tragic people at the mercy of a savage community. The ringing of the changes is discernible in the choice of star as well, the movement from the quiet idealism of the early Fonda through the rough pragmatism of the Wayne *persona* to the cynical self-interest of James Stewart. As Ford grows older the American dream sours, and we are left with nostalgia for the Desert.

Imperious as he is, Ford is not the western; nor is the western history. For if we stand back from the western, we are less aware of historical (or representational) elements than of form and *archetype*. This may sound platitudinous: for years critics have spoken confidently of the balletic movement of the genre, of pattern and variation, of myth. This last, ever in the air when the form is discussed, clouds the issues completely. We can speak of the genre's celebration of America, of the contrasting images of Garden and Desert, as national myth. We can speak of the parade of mythology that is mass culture, of which the western is clearly a part. We can invoke Greek and medieval myth, referring to the western hero as a latter-day knight, a contemporary Achilles. Or we can simply speak of the myth of the western, a journalistic usage which evidently implies that life is not like that. However, in strict classical terms of definition myth has to do with the activity of gods, and as such the western has no myth. Rather, it incorporates elements of *displaced* (or corrupted) myth on a scale that can render them considerably more prominent than in most art. It is not surprising that little advance is made upon the clichés, no analysis undertaken that interprets how these elements are at work within a particular film or director's career. What are the archetypal elements we sense within the genre and how do they function? As Northrop Frye has shown in his monumental *The Anatomy of Criticism,* for centuries this immensely tangled ground has remained almost wholly unexplored in literature itself. The primitive state of film criticism inevitably reveals a yawning abyss in this direction.

Certain facts are clear. Ultimately the western derives from the long and fertile tradition of Wild West literature that had dominated the mass taste of nineteenth-century America. Fenimore Cooper is again the germinal figure here: Nash Smith has traced how the roots of the formula, the adventures of an isolated, aged trapper/hunter (reminiscent of Daniel Boone) who rescues genteel heroines from the Indians, were in the *Leatherstocking Tales* which began to emerge in the 1820s. These works, fundamentally in the tradition of the sentimental novel, soon gave way to a rush of pulp literature in succeeding decades culminating in the famous series edited by Erastus Beadle which had astonishing sales for its time. Specialists in the adventure tale, the romance, the sea story, turned to the West for their setting to cash in on the huge market. As the appetite for violence and spectacle grew, variations followed, the younger hunter that had succeeded Cooper's hero losing his pristine nature and giving way to a morally ambiguous figure with a dark past, a Deadwood Dick who is finally redeemed by a woman's love. The genre, much of it sub-literary, became increasingly hungry for innovation as the century wore on, its Amazon heroines perhaps only the most spectacular sign of a desperation at its declining hold on the imagination. As the actual drama of the frontier finally came to a close, marked by Frederick J. Turner's historic address before the American Historical Association in 1893 where he advanced his thesis on free land and its continual recession westward as the key factor in America's development, the vogue for the dime novel waned, its hero now frozen in the figure of the American cowboy.

In 1900 the Wild Bunch held up and robbed a Union Pacific railway train in Wyoming; in 1903 Edwin S. Porter made *The Great Train Robbery* in New Jersey. The chronology of these events, often commented on, seems less important than their geography: it had been the East as well from which Beadle westerns such as *Seth Jones; or, The Captives of the Frontier* had flowed. The cinema was born, its novel visual apparatus at the ready, the heir to a venerable tradition of reworking history (the immediate past) in tune with ancient classical rhythms. In general, of course, the early silent cinema everywhere drew on and experimented with traditional and folkloric patterns for the forms it required. What seems remarkable about the western, however, is that the core of a formulaic lineage already existed. The heart of this legacy was romantic narrative, tales which insisted on the idealization of characters who wielded near-magical powers. Recurrent confrontations between the personified forces of good and evil, testimony to the grip of the New England Calvinist ethic, had soon focused the tales in the direction of morality play. However, in any case, the structure was an impure one which had interpolated melodramatic patterns of corruption and redemption, the revenge motif borrowed from the stage towards the end of the century, and humour in the Davy Crockett and Eastern cracker-barrel traditions. The physical action and spectacle of the Wild West shows, an offshoot of the penny-dreadful vogue, was to be another factor.

This complex inheritance meant that from the outset the western could be many things. In their anecdotal *The Western* George N. Fenin and William K. Everson have chronicled the proliferating, overlapping growth of early days: Bronco Billy Anderson's robust action melodramas, Thomas H. Ince's darker tales, W. S. Hart's more "authentic" romances, the antics of the virtuous Tom Mix, the Cruze and Ford epics of the twenties, the stunts and flamboyance of Ken Maynard and Hoot Gibson, the flood of "B" movies, revenge sagas, serials, and so on. Experiment seems always to have been varied and development dynamic, the pendulum swinging back and forth between opposing poles of emphasis on drama and history, plots and spectacle, romance and "realism," seriousness and comedy. At any point where audience response was felt the action could freeze, the industrial machine moving into high gear to produce a cycle and, in effect, establish a minor tradition within the form. Whatever "worked" was produced, the singing westerns of the thirties perhaps only the most prominent example of this policy of eclectic enterprise.

For many students of the western Gene Autry and Roy Rogers have seemed an embarrassing aberration. However, such a view presupposes that there is such an animal as *the* western, a precise model rather than a loose, shifting and variegated genre with many roots and branches. The word "genre" itself, although a helpful one, is a mixed blessing: for many the term carries literary overtones of technical *rules*. Nor is "form" any better; the western is many *forms*. Only a pluralist vision makes sense of our experience of the genre and begins to explain its amazing vigour and adaptability, the way it moves closer and further from our own world, brightening or darkening with each succeeding decade. Yet over the years critics have ever tried to freeze the genre once and for all in a definitive model of the "classical" western. Certainly it must be admitted that works such as *Shane* and *My Darling Clementine* weld together in remarkable balance historical reconstruction and national themes with personal drama and archetypal elements. In his essay, "The Evolution of the Western," Bazin declared *Stagecoach* the summit of the form, an example of "classic maturity," before going on to see in Anthony Mann's early small westerns the path of further progress. Although there is a certain logic in searching for films at the center of the spectrum, I suspect it is a false one and can see little value in it. Wherever definitions of *the* genre movie have been advanced they have become the weapons of generalization. Insisting on the purity of his classical elements, Bazin dismisses "superwesterns" (*Shane, High Noon, Duel in the Sun*) because of their introduction of interests "not endemic." Warshow's position is similar, although his conception of the form is narrower, a particular kind of moral and physical texture embodied in his famous but inadequate view of the hero as "the last gentleman." Elsewhere Mann's films have been faulted for their neurotic qualities, strange and powerful works such as *Rancho Notorious* have been refused entry because they are somehow "not westerns." This impulse may well be informed by a fear that unless the form is defined precisely (which inevitably excludes) it will disappear, wraith-like, from under our eyes. The call has echoed out over the lonely landscape of critical endeavour: what is the western?

The model we must hold before us is of a varied and flexible structure, a thematically fertile and ambiguous world of historical material shot through with archetypal elements which are themselves ever in flux. In defining the five basic modes of literary fiction Northrop Frye has described myth as stories about gods; romance as a world in which men are superior both to other men and to their environment; high mimetic where the hero is a leader but subject to social criticism and natural law; low mimetic where the hero is one of us; and ironic where the hero is inferior to ourselves and we look down on the absurdity of his plight. If we borrow this scale, it quickly becomes apparent that if the western was originally rooted between romance and high mimetic (characteristic forms of which are epic and tragedy), it rapidly became open to inflection in any direction. Surely the only definition we can advance of the western hero, for example, is that he is both complete and incomplete, serene and growing, vulnerable and invulnerable, a man and a god. If at juvenile levels the action approaches the near-divine, for serious artists who understand the tensions within the genre the focus can be anywhere along the scale . . . For example, in Anthony Mann there is a constant drive towards mythic quality in the hero; in Sam Peckinpah there is a rich creative play with the romantic potential; with Budd Boetticher it is the ironic mode that dominates.

The romantic mainstream that the western took on from pulp literature provided it with the stately ritual of displaced myth, the movement of a god-like figure into the demonic wasteland, the death and resurrection, the return to a paradisal garden. Within the form were to be found seminal archetypes common to all myth, the journey and the quest, the ceremonies of love and marriage, food and drink, the rhythms of waking and sleeping, life and death. But the incursions of melodrama and revenge had turned the form on its axis, the structure torn in the directions of both morality play and tragedy. Overlaying and interpenetrating the historical thematic there was an archetypal and metaphysical ideology as well. Manifest destiny was answered by divine providence, a Classical conception of fate brooding over the sins of man. Where history was localizing and authenticating archetype, archetype was stiffening and universalizing history.

The western thus was—and is—a complex variable, its peculiar alchemy allowing a wide range of intervention, choice and experiment by script-writer and director. History provides a source of epics, spectacle and action films, pictures sympathetic to the Indian, "realistic" films, even anti-westerns (Delmer Daves' *Cowboy*). From the archetypal base flow revenge films, fables, tragedies, pastorals, and a juvenile stream of product. But of course the dialectic is always at work and the elements are never pure. Much that is produced, the great bulk of it inevitably undistinguished, occupies a blurred middle ground. But for the artist of vision in *rapport* with the genre, it offers a great freedom for local concentration and imaginative play.

"My name is John Ford. I make westerns." Few film-makers can have been so serene about accepting such a label. After all, the industry must have ambivalent attitudes about the "horse-opera" which has been their bread and butter for so long. And of course the western has been at the heart of mass culture, the staple of television, its motifs decorating advertisements and politicians, the pulp fiction and comic books flowing endlessly as do the films themselves. But in fact its greatest strength has been this very pervasiveness and repetition. In this context, the western appears a huge iceberg the small tip of which has been the province of criticism, the great undifferentiated and submerged body below principally agitating the social critic, the student of mass media, the educationalist. This sharp division has been unfortunate: sociology and education have often taken up crude positions in their obliviousness to the highest achievements; criticism has failed to explore the dialectic that keeps the form vigorous. For if mass production at the base exploits the peak, the existence of that base allows refinement and reinvigoration. It is only because the western has been everywhere before us for so long that it "works." For over the years a highly sophisticated sub-language of the cinema has been created that is intuitively understood by the audience, a firm basis for art.

It is not just that in approaching the western a director has a structure that is saturated with conceptual significance: the core of meanings is in the imagery itself. Through usage and time, recurring elements anchored in the admixture of history and archetype and so central as to be termed *structural*—the hero, the antagonist, the community, landscape—have taken on an everpresent cluster of possible significances. To see a church in a movie—any film but a western—is to see a church; the camera records. By working carefully for it a film-maker can give that church meaning, through visual emphasis, context, repetitions, dialogue. But a church in a western has *a priori* a potential expressiveness rooted in the accretions of the past. In Ford's *My Darling Clementine* a half-built church appears in one brief scene: yet it embodies the spirit of pioneer America. Settlers dance vigorously on the rough planks in the open air, the flag fluttering above the frame of the church perched precariously on the edge of the desert. Marching ceremoniously up the incline towards them, the camera receding with an audacious stateliness, come Tombstone's knight and his "lady fair," Wyatt Earp and Clementine. The community are ordered aside by the elder as the couple move on to the floor, their robust dance marking the marriage ceremony that unites the best qualities of East and West. It is one of Ford's great moments.

However, the scene is not magic, but flows from an exact understanding (or intuition) of how time-honored elements can have the resonance of an *icon*. This term, which I borrow from art history, should connote an image that both records and carries a conceptual and emotional weight drawn from a *defined* symbolic field, a tradition. Like Scripture, the western offers a world of metaphor, a range of latent content that can be made manifest depending on the film-maker's awareness and preoccupations. Thus in Boetticher's *Decision at Sundown* a marriage ceremony is completely violated by the hero who promises to kill the bridegroom by nightfall. Here the meaning flows completely from the players, in particular Randolph Scott's irrational behavior; the church itself is devoid of meaning. In Anthony Mann churches rarely appear. In Peckinpah churches have been a saloon and a brothel, and religion in characters has masked a damaging repressiveness. If we turn to the Indian we find that, apart from the early *Seminole,* he functions in Boetticher as part of a hostile universe, no more and no less. In Mann, however, the Indian is part of the natural order and as such his slaughter stains the landscape; it is not surprising that at times he comes, like an avenging spirit, to redress the balance. In Peckinpah the Indian, ushering in the theme of savagery, brings us to the very center of the director's world.

Central to much that I have been saying is the principle of convention. I have refrained from using the term only because it is often loosely used and might have confused the issues. At times the term is used pejoratively, implying cliché; at others it is employed to invoke a set of mystical rules that the master of the form can juggle. In this light, a western is a western is a western. If we see the term more neutrally, as an area of agreement between audience and artist with reference to the form which his art will take, it might prove useful at this stage to recapitulate the argument by summarizing the interrelated aspects of the genre that I have tried to isolate, all of which are in some measure conventional.

> *(a) History:* The basic convention of the genre is that films in western guise are about America's past. This constant tension with history and the freedom it extends to script-writer and film-maker to choose their distance is a great strength.
> *(b) Themes:* The precise chronology of the genre and its inheritance of contradictions fundamental to the American mind dictate a rich range of themes expressed through a series of familiar character types and conflicts (e.g. law ver-

sus the gun, sheep versus cattle). These motifs, situations and characters can be the focus for a director's interests or can supply the ground from which he will quarry what concerns him.

(c) Archetype: The inherent complexity and structural confusion (or the *decadence*) of the pulp literature tradition that the western drew on from the beginning meant that westerns could incorporate elements of romance, tragedy, comedy, morality play. By a process of natural commercial selection cycles emerged and began to establish a range of forms.

(d) Icons: As a result of mass production, the accretions of time, and the dialect of history and archetype, characters, situations and actions can have an emblematic power. Movement on the horizon, the erection of a community, the pursuit of Indians, these have a range of possible associations. Scenes such as passing on gun-lore, bathing or being barbered, playing poker, have a latent ritualistic meaning which can be brought to the surface and inflected. The quest, the journey, the confrontation, these can take on moral or allegorical overtones.

What holds all of these elements together (and in that sense provides the basic convention) is narrative and dramatic structure. It is only through mastery of these that a film-maker can both engage his audience and order the form in a personally meaningful way. At a general level this means the understanding and control necessary for any expression of emotion in terms of film—the creating of fear, suspense, amusement, awe. However, with an art as popular as the western this must also mean a precise awareness of audience expectation with reference to a range of characters—preeminently hero and antagonist—and testing situations, conflicts, spectacle, landscape, physical action and violence. Fundamental to success would seem to be the understanding that the world created must be essentially fabulous. While treating situations that have their relevance for us, the form must not impinge too directly on our experience. The world that the film creates is self-contained and its own; it comments not on our life but on the actions and relationships it reveals to us. So long as the world evoked is *other,* few limitations exist. A commonplace about the form, that it is handy for exploring simple moral issues, does not survive the experience of attending to any number of works: the maturity of relationships in Robert Parrish's *Wonderful Country,* the complex moral and metaphysical rhetoric of *Johnny Guitar,* the work, certainly, of Mann, Boetticher and Peckinpah, these could hardly be called simple. Nor are social and psychological elements impossible so long as they are held in a fruitful tension with the romantic thrust of the genre. *Showdown at Boot Hill,* where Charles Bronson has become a bounty hunter because he feels he is too *short,* is an unsuccessful Freudian tale. *The Left-Handed Gun,* where the murder of a father-figure turns Billy the Kid antisocial and self-destructive, is a distinguished psychological tragedy. *3:10 to Yuma* and *Shane,* both maligned because of their success where the genre proper fails (i.e. with most film journalists), are honorable works. Rather than dogma, the grounds must be quality. And the challenge always is to find the dramatic structure that best serves both film-maker and audience.

The western is not just the men who have worked within it. Rather than an empty vessel breathed into by the film-maker, the genre is a vital structure through which flow a myriad of themes and concepts. As such the form can provide a director with a range of possible connections and the space in which to experiment, to shape and refine the kind of effects and meanings he is working towards. We must be prepared to entertain the idea that *auteurs* grow, and that genre can help to crystallize preoccupations and contribute actively to development. Moreover, we must be clear about directors who return to the western time and again. To work with "stark reality" (Boetticher's phrase) may be the dream of many a Hollywood film-maker; yet it does not follow that the closer he comes to articulating private worlds directly, the higher the achievement. Certainly the western compels distance if the result is to be both personal and commercially viable. Bazin came to praise both Mann and Boetticher for returning to what he felt was the essence of the genre in their small revenge movies. But in my view the reverse is true: these two men, together with Sam Peckinpah, can be said to have found *their* essence within the western.

The White Man's Indian: An Institutional Approach

John E. O'Connor

The most obvious explanation for the Native American's Hollywood image is that the producers, directors, screenwriters, and everyone else associated with the movie industry have inherited a long intellectual and artistic tradition. The perceptions that Europeans and Americans have had of the Native American were both emotional and contradictory. Either an enemy or a friend, he was never an ordinary human being accepted on his own terms. As Robert Berkhofer explains in his book *The White Man's Indian: Images of the American Indian from Columbus to the Present* (1977), the dominant view of the Indians has reflected primarily what the white man thought of himself.

As the positive concept of the "Noble Savage" took shape, especially in eighteenth-century France, it was conceived as evidence to support the arguments of Enlightenment philosophers like Rousseau. Paris-bound thinkers believed that people would be better off as children of nature, free of the prejudices and conventions imposed by such established European institutions as the monarchy and the church. The negative view of many of the captivity narratives common in the literature of the New England Puritans proved to the faithful that the forces of the Devil were alive and at work in the dark forests of America. Berkhofer argues that from the first contacts of the European explorers, white men tended to generalize about Indians rather than discriminate among individual tribes, to describe Indians primarily in terms of how they differed from whites, and to incorporate strict moral judgments in their descriptions of Indian life. This judgmental approach has proved true in prose, painting, and documentary photography—in every art form that chose the Indian as its subject, including film. Consider, for example, the characteristic view of the Indians' relationship to the land. The view that the Indian impeded progress because he lacked the ambition and "good sense" the whites used in developing the American landscape has prevailed throughout our history. Movies and television, the popular art forms of today, continue to present images of Native Americans that speak more about the current interests of the dominant culture than they do about the Indians.

As war clouds rose overseas in the late 1930s and early 1940s and the dominant American culture sought to reaffirm its traditional patriotic values, the negative stereotype of the Indian (a traditional enemy) served a broader purpose in films such as *Drums Along the Mohawk* (1939) and *They Died With Their Boots On* (1941). Thirty years later, with America embroiled in a different kind of war—and millions of its citizens challenging the government's policies—the movies reflected its divided consciousness. In films of the 1960s and 1970s like *Tell Them Willie Boy Is Here* (1969) and *Little Big Man* (1970), Berkhofer perceives that "the Indian became a mere substitute for the oppressed black or hippie white youth alienated from the modern mainstream of American society".

One must take care, however, in drawing generalizations. Even with the gradual shift in public interests and values, certain plot formulas have persisted. The Indian raids, for example, on the stagecoach *(Orphans of the Plains* [1912], *Stagecoach* [1939], *Dakota Incident* [1956]), on the wagon train *(Covered Wagon* [1923], *Wagon Wheels* [1934], *Wagonmaster* [1950]), on the heralds of technological progress *(Iron Horse* [1924], *Union Pacific* [1939], *Western Union* [1941]), and on the peaceful frontier homestead *(The Heritage of the Desert* [1924], *The Searchers* [1956], *Ulzana's Raid*

[1972]) have changed little. There have been cycles of Indian pictures such as the string of sympathetic films that followed *Broken Arrow* (1950), but at times a romanticized, even glorified, image could coexist with the vicious one. In 1936, for example, when most screen Indians were the essence of cruelest savagery, Twentieth Century-Fox made the fourth screen version of the idyllic Indian drama *Ramona,* starring Loretta Young.

Even in the very early days, when small production companies churned out two-reel westerns weekly for the nickelodeon trade, a patron might leave one movie house where he had just seen a sympathetic—though not necessarily accurate—Indian drama and walk into another theatre where the natives on the screen were totally inhuman. Thomas Ince's *Heart of an Indian* (1912), for example, allowed that some Indians might be sensitive people; but D.W. Griffith's *The Battle at Elderbush Gulch* (1914), though it showed the provocation for battle, presented the Indians as absolute savages—they even wanted to steal Mae Marsh's puppy dogs to kill and eat in a ritual sacrifice. Another common Indian image was the comic one in Western spoofs like Charlie Chase's *Uncovered Wagon* (1920), the Marx Brothers' *Go West!* (1940) and Mel Brooks's *Blazing Saddles* (1974). Over the last ten years a series of film documentaries and docudramas, especially those made for television, have taken strides toward presenting the Indians more on their own terms, but by and large the Hollywood product continues to present the white man's Indian.

The serious scholarship of historians, anthropologists, and other professionals should have helped to dispel the assumptions that tainted the popular concepts of Native Americans. But the conclusions of Helen Hunt Jackson's landmark history *Century of Dishonor* (1881) and such detailed studies of tribal life as those by Steward (1938) and Eggan (1955) were painfully slow in finding their way into school textbooks and into the broader culture.

Filmmakers who perceive the Indians through the distorted lens of the broader culture will invariably produce movies filled with twisted images. However, in spite of a more or less subtle racial bias, Hollywood is presumably not filled with Indian-haters intent on using their power to put down the natives. One need only observe how quickly a director or a studio might switch from portraying a "bloodthirsty" to a "noble savage" if the market seems to call for it. Far from purposeful distortion, significant elements of the Indian image can be explained best through analyzing various technical and business-related production decisions that may never have been considered in terms of their affect on the screen image.

Film is a collaborative art. It requires the creative contributions of dozens of people, who will subtly—sometimes unconsciously—alter the movie's message or the way it is presented. Moreover, although almost any artist would be happy to sell work—to that extent commercial concerns may influence all art—the huge monetary investments necessary to produce a feature film make art and commerce inseparable. If producers, set designers, script writers, cinematographers, directors, and actors want to practice their craft, the films they make must earn a profit. Therefore, the creative process involved in producing a Hollywood movie demands the artistic judgment of a team of professionals and its utmost effort to make the film appeal to the broadest possible audience. The poet, the painter, and (to some extent) the novelist may escape these pressures. In some ways, they complicate the analysis of film art more than the other forms, but they are indispensable to understanding a film's point of view.

To simplify analysis I have grouped some of these production factors into three general areas: dramatic considerations, commercial considerations, and political considerations. These designations are imprecise. Certain elements of filmmaking may fit as well into two or three of the categories, whereas others may not fit easily into any. Such divisions, however, may make the artistic, financial, political and other forces that influence the artistic process easier to understand.

The influence of such production factors is not unique to movies about Native Americans. The three types of considerations figure in the production of every Hollywood film. A similar analysis would be fruitful in studying gangster movies or science fiction films. Of significance in analyzing films about Native Americans is the way in which seemingly unrelated production decisions may have superseded interest in historical accuracy or cultural integrity and how they may have dictated the image of the Indian in particular films.

In many ways, film is a literary form. Like a novel, a play, or any other narrative structure, its purpose is to tell a story. The filmmaker (a composite of all the collaborators), like the novelist and the playwright, must resolve questions of format, structure, and the relationships of characters so that they are comprehensible to the audience. A good filmmaker, like any other artist, will try to solve these problems so that they illuminate some aspect of the human condition. Rather than use words on a page or paints on a palette, the filmmaker works with a complex combination of images projected on a screen, and the demands of this medium influence the dramatic language used to tell the story. This is especially evident in films that have been adapted from another form. *Massacre* (1934) began as a book-length journalistic exposé of the state of Indian affairs in the early 1930s. A well-organized and effective book, it dealt with reservation life, unemployment, inadequate medical care, and other problems. The filmmakers had to create a different structure using fictional characters with whom the audience might identify. Walter Edmunds's novel *Drums Along the Mohawk* was a bestseller in the 1930s. Though some regard it as a classic of historical fiction, the structure did not lend itself to the movies. The story of how the Iroquois "destructives" had terrorized the farmers of the Mohawk Valley year after year was long and episodic. In some ways its drawn-out descriptions of successive attacks must have given the reader a sense of desperation similar to what the colonists must have felt. Moguls at the studio decreed that the film script needed tightening and careful pacing to allow a series of lesser climaxes to lead up to a single major climax that would end the film on a positive note.

Whether told in a book or on film, every story has a point of view. Establishing any point of view, especially a complex one, may be more difficult in film than in print. One reason for this difficulty is that filmmaking conventions discourage the use of a narrator, preferring that characters develop the plot and point of view through dialog. Only two of the films discussed here use narration. They use it sparingly, and, as the study of the manuscripts at Twentieth Century-Fox indicates, the narration by Tom Jeffords that begins and ends *Broken Arrow* was a device decided on at the last minute. The visual medium lends itself well to describing the landscape or the ambience, but communicating the personality of a character becomes difficult. Without a narrator, the audience's perception of what the characters say and do (and what other characters say about them) is all there is to delineate their personalities. This restriction helps to explain why, even with some narration, Arthur Penn's *Little Big Man* fails to capture the subtle characterization of Old Lodge Skins that Thomas Berger achieves in his novel.

Communicating with images can be more difficult than with words. Images are more open to misinterpretation by the viewer taking in the message on a sensual and emotional level, and at a predetermined rate, in contrast to the basically intellectual, self-paced process of reading a book. Camera angles, composition, lighting, editing, and a host of other factors can influence the viewer's unconscious perception. Imagine how difficult it was to develop characterizations before the innovation of sound. For example, the makers of *The Vanishing American* (1926) had to try to match Zane Grey's skillfully written characterizations working only with pictures and a few subtitles. Of course, even in the silent era the filmmaker may have provided a musical score for the theater pianist to play along with the film, or he might have tinted the images on the screen to suggest a mood, as D.W. Griffith did for *America* (1924). But the development of synchronized sound and Technicolor further complicated the process of producing and decoding movies. For example, might the funeral scene in *Massacre* have had a different tone if Hal Wallis had allowed it to be screened with the sounds of weeping and sobbing Indians in the background? In *Drums Along the Mohawk,* would the Indians have seemed so menacing if their painted faces and the farmhouses they set on fire had been filmed in black and white instead of color?

With few exceptions, Indians have come to the screen most often in films about the American West. As Will Wright points out in his *Sixguns and Society: A Structural Study of the Western* (1975), Western films have a mythology and a method all their own. Wright makes it clear that although the Western has several standard plot variations, its popularity with filmmakers (and other artists) over the years depends mainly on the human conflicts involved in life on the critical edge between wilderness and civilization. Whenever this drama allows the full development of an Indian character so that the viewer gets to know him, the film almost always induces some empathy. But little time has been spent in developing the screen personalities of Indians. They become flat characters, relatively nondescript evil forces that help establish an atmosphere of tension within which the cattle ranchers, the townspeople, the stagecoach riders, the outlaws, the sheepherders, the cavalry officers, the schoolmarms, and the barmaids can relate to one another. As another scholar of the Western, John Cawelti, puts it: "The western formula seems to prescribe that the Indian be a part of the setting to a greater extent than he is ever a character in his own right. The reason for this is twofold: to give the Indian a more complex role would increase the moral ambiguity of the story and thereby blur the sharp dramatic conflicts; and, second, if the Indian represented a significant way of life rather than a declining savagery, it would be far more difficult to resolve the story with a reaffirmation of the values of modern society" (p. 38)

Therefore, the demands of dramatic structure and visual communication may have shaped the Indian image in Western movies as much as the traditional myths about which Robert Berkhofer has written. In fact, it seems clear that translation into a visual medium, where characters with complex personalities and subtle motivations are harder to portray than simple good guys and bad guys, accentuated the dichotomy between the bloodthirsty and the noble savage that Berkhofer traced back to the beginnings of the white man's experience in America.

Let us move on to commercial considerations. For the longest time, Hollywood businessmen reasoned that films had to appeal to the broadest possible audience. In some ways this exaggerated the impact of such dramatic considerations as narrative structure and point of view. For a mass audience, for example, the dramatic situations should be straightforward and unconfused. Typically, the audience could easily decide which characters were good and which were evil (white hats or black?). In the studio tradition, "moral ambiguities" were kept to a minimum. (*Devil's Doorway* [1949], a film that played up complex moral questions related to race and prejudice, is a rare exception to an almost ironclad Hollywood rule.)

The same was true for stereotypes of all kinds, particularly for Native Americans. Moviegoers came to expect Indians to be presented in a characteristic way. The designers of Indian movie costumes have generally given little attention to the actual dress of the tribes. Language elements, cultural beliefs, and religious rituals of one tribe have been attributed to others—or, more often, invented on the set. Frequently, Native American actors have been denied roles as Indians in favor of non-Indian actors whom the producers thought "looked better." Not many Americans noticed: where the finer points of Indian culture and history are concerned, moviegoers have never been particularly discriminating.

Especially in Western films, the bloodthirsty, war-crazed Indian has been Hollywood's stock in trade. Something different on the screen might distract the audience from the theme of the film. Distract it too often, and it will not be entertained—and selling entertainment is the name of the game. From time to time the stereotype even had to be reinforced. For *Geronimo* (1939), for example, it was thought that Native American actor Chief Thundercloud would not live up to the public's expectations of a menacing savage. Not only did the makeup artists take on the project of making him look the part, the publicity department prepared a series of photos for the press that showed the transformation.

It is interesting that the attempt to satisfy the total public usually led to a Hollywood film including some element, however small, of explanation for the Indian's brutal behavior. Therefore any viewer of *America* or *Drums Along the Mohawk* who might find it hard to believe in such bloodthirsty Indians could rationalize that the Tory leaders (played by Lionel Barrymore and John Carradine) had whipped the "ignorant natives" into their frenzy. No one could doubt that the Indian was the enemy in *They Died With Their Boots On,* but the film allowed a grudging respect for Crazy Horse (Anthony Quinn) and stressed the fact that white men had broken their treaty and provoked the Indians' final resort to the warpath.

One reason that westerns have enjoyed such long-term popularity is that they include lots of action, and the Indians have always served such scenes well. On the other hand, peace-loving Indians make for little excitement. Even in a sympathetic movie, such as *The Vanishing American,* the obligatory battle serves as a climax. The coming of sound further emphasized the excitement of the Indian attack. The war whoops screeched by the Indians in *Massacre* allowed the studio's sound engineers sensational use of their relatively new medium. The publicity material for *Geronimo* suggested that exhibitors play an Indian sound-effects record in their theater lobbies, with tom-toms and war cries to reinforce the impression that the movie being shown inside was action-packed and replete with exotic sounds of a primitive West.

The publicity efforts the studios mounted deserve special attention. Although it may be impossible to determine how much impact such "exploitation campaigns" had on the success or failure of any picture, the studios certainly viewed them as a necessary part of the business. Ironically, in suggesting ways that exhibitors might get public attention for their shows, sometimes the publicity "press books" presented ideas at odds with the theme of the movie itself.

Commercial considerations also help to explain the evolving Indian image. Over time the American movie audience has changed. Since the movies began a financial comeback in the early 1960s, producers have decided that the typical American moviegoer is younger and better educated than his counterpart of the 1930s or 1940s. As a result, audiences want movies to do more than merely entertain. The old stereotypes are less likely to convince today though new clichés seem to have taken their place. And, although pressure groups have always tried to control the presentation of particular images in the movies, Indian activists have only achieved any real clout in the last decade or two.

The bottom line of a successful movie, as in any other commercial venture, can be found on the profit-and-loss statement. Low production and distribution costs will make the breakeven point easier to reach, and the cost of producing Western movies with Indians can be minimal. For example, sets could be put together inexpensively and extras found on the reservation for far less than union scale. The unavailability of most studio financial records makes it impossible to speak with any precision about the actual costs or profits. It is clear, however, that major productions shot on location with large casts of well-known actors become costly. Cost overruns for location shooting on *Cheyenne Autumn* (1964) necessitated the elimination of many scenes, and they may have contributed to the film's artistic and commercial failure.

Finally, a significant percentage of the Hollywood film industry's income since the 1930s has come from foreign sales. A film such as *Tell Them Willie Boy Is Here* could make up for some of its disappointing domestic sales by becoming a hit for European and Third World audiences.

Many would argue that every Hollywood film is a political document. As Soviet films have characteristically excoriated the czarist regime and extolled the Communist Revolution, the Hollywood movie industry—imbued as it is with the capitalist ethic—has supported the political and economic systems on which it relies. Although the process of filmmaking and the role of government may differ considerably, the product is much the same. Apart from this general orientation, however, political factors have influenced the shape of what reaches the screen in more specific ways.

At times political and commercial factors could coincide. When Warner Brothers' early 1930s films of social consciousness, such as *Massacre,* supported the National Recovery Administration and the New Deal that Franklin D. Roosevelt offered the American public, they expressed in part the liberal political point of view that prevailed in Hollywood. But the moviemakers also hoped that their films would ride on the wave of positive popular opinion that accompanied the new president's efforts to kickstart a stalled economy. As the American people began to renew their hope in the future, Hollywood movies helped to feed their growing confidence in the new administration.

In another era, when a studio reasoned that assistance from the U.S. War Department could be a crucial element in keeping down production costs, the military's production suggestions could be a great influence. Nothing could be more political than the way in which Warner Brothers tried to convince the U.S. army that it should help make *They Died With Their Boots On*. The movie's producers heard suggestions from many quarters about various elements of their project on the portrayal of the Indians, for example. But the only recommendations that seem to have received close attention were the War Department's ideas on how to portray the U.S. military.

A different type of a political influence may have shaped D.W. Griffith's work on *America,* especially the Indians' role in that film. Griffith's papers suggest that he and others on his production staff were sensitive to the demands of various patriotic organizations concerned about the images that got to the screen. The Indians were the only group they could portray as "heavies" without inviting the political wrath of the cultural establishment. In an interview for the recent images of Indians television series, director King Vidor noted that although many minorities and ethnic groups had "lobbies" in Hollywood to protect their movie image, no one spoke for the Indians. Perhaps the ultimate irony is that in Western films, where Indians most often appear, producers have always had to consider the demands of the American Humane Society about the treatment of the horses—yet the Native Americans are not treated with nearly as much politesse.

International politics could play a part too. As Twentieth Century-Fox prepared *Drums Along the Mohawk* for release in 1939, decision-makers tried to weigh the impact such a film could have on current tensions in Europe. Might Germany read a popular film that played up the long-forgotten hatred and resentments associated with the American Revolution as a sign that the alliance between the United States and Great Britain was perhaps not so secure? This conclusion would be less likely if, as in the film, Indians and American Tories were the enemy portrayed and no British officers were shown.

Most recently, political influence found its way into movies of the late 1960s and early 1970s in the form of Indian allegories of the American experience in Southeast Asia. The Indian movies made then, such as *Little Big Man* and *Soldier Blue* (both 1970), films that indicted the American Army for practicing genocide on the Native American, were partly the expressions of the producers' and directors' feelings about Vietnam. Even more important, however, they were commercial products aimed at the moviegoing public of young adults who, by profitable coincidence, also represented the age group most deeply involved in the antiwar movement.

Some of the films discussed here offer striking contrasts and similarities. *The Vanishing American* and *Broken Arrow* present a "noble savage" stereotype, while *Drums along the Mohawk* deals with the era of the American Revolution, and its production was fraught with worries about how to portray the British as an enemy. Interesting similarities exist in the ways that *The Vanishing American*, *Massacre*, and *Tell Them Willie Boy Is Here* address the pressures of reservation life, even though the contemporary styles of filmmaking (in the silent era, the early sound era, and the era of the independent producer, respectively) differ considerably. *They Died with Their Boots On* and *Little Big Man*, made almost thirty years apart, sharply contrast in their views of the United States military and their Indian enemies at times (1941 and 1970) when war was much on the mind of the American public. The producers of other films, such as *Devil's Doorway* and *Cheyenne Autumn*, bent over backward to sympathize with the Indians' plight, but they did nothing to correct Hollywood's characteristic carelessness in portraying historical events and the complexity of Native American cultures. In spite of the forces that changed the shape of the movie business over the past three-quarters of a century and transformed the precise nature of the stereotypes, Hollywood Indians are still far from real.

Works Cited

1. Berger, Thomas. *Little Big Man.* New York: Dial Press, 1964.
2. Berkhofer, Robert F. Th*e White Man's Indian: Images of the American Indian from Columbus to the Present.* New York: Random House, 1977.
3. Cawelti, John. *The Six-gun Mystique.* Bowling Green, Ohio: Popular Culture Press, 1978.
4. Edmunds, Walter. *Drums Along the Mohawk.* Boston: Little, Brown, 1936.
5. Eggan, Fred. *Social Anthropology of North American Tribes.* Chicago: University of Chicago Press, 1955.
6. Gessner, Robert. *Massacre.* New York: Jonathan Cope and Harrison Smith, 1931.
7. Grey, Zane. *The Vanishing American.* New York: Harper, 1925.
8. Jackson, Helen Hunt. *A Century of Dishonor.* New York: Little, Brown, 1881.
9. Steward, Julian Haynes. *Basin-Plateau Aboriginal Socio-Political Groups.* Washington, D.C.: U.S. Government Printing Office, 1938.
10. Wright, Will. *Sixguns and Society: A Structural Study of the Western.* Berkeley: University of California Press, 1975.

John Ford Talks to Philip Jenkinson about Not Being Interested in Movies

Philip Jenkinson

Philip Jenkinson: *Were you interested in movies way back?*
John Ford: Not really—not interested in them now actually. It's a way of making a living.
J: *Was filmmaking in 1917 as primitive as everyone suggests?*
F: I hardly think that "primitive" is the right word. We had no lights and we had a big stage—just a board and over that we stretched cambric cotton to hold the light off—and there'd be five or six companies working side by side. We thought it was rather nice. We all knew one another and visited back and forth. We'd go over to the actors and say, "Do you mind coming over and playing a butler for us?" Well, not a butler—we didn't have butlers in those days: they were mostly Westerns.
J: *When did you become interested in Westerns?*
F: When I left school I went to college and didn't like it. So I left and worked in Arizona as a cowboy, and eventually ended up in Hollywood. I like to make Western pictures because I like to get out and live in the open: you get up early, you work late, you eat dinner with an appetite, you sleep well, and I do like the people you meet and work with. That is really my only interest in Westerns. As story material I am not particularly fascinated by them. It's not my metier by any means. None of my so-called better pictures are Westerns.
J: *What do you remember of* The Lost Patrol, *made in 1934?*
F: We had one of the first of the so-called "producers" on this picture. We had a shot where the British cavalry were supposed to come to the rescue and it was very hard. When it was time to come on, this airplane flew over their heads and of course the horses scattered. The plane finally landed in a little satellite airfield they had, and this idiot producer got out with a big cigar. Of course it spoiled the shot for that day and we had to wait until the next day. He said to me: "Jack, I've been looking over your schedule. You start working at seven, then you quit at eleven, and start working at 2:30 or three. Look at those hours you're losing. If you worked right on through, you'd finish five or six days ahead."

I said: "Cliff, you can't work in this heat."

He said: "It's wonderful, I love it, It's great."

I said: "I'm sorry, I've got to line this shot up," and he wandered away. We finally got the shot and I said, "Where's Mr. So-and-So? Yes, the so-called producer who flew in last night."

"We've just taken him to the hospital with sunstroke."

J: *There's a story that on the film* Wee Willie Winkie, *after the death of Victor McLaglen, you spontaneously suggested that they include a funeral scene.*
F: Well, we were out there and I said: "It's a mistake in the story to kill McLaglen off, because he's one of the leading characters, but at least if we're going to kill him off, let's give him a funeral." It was in the rain, so I said, "Let's shoot it in the rain." Which we did. That's all there is to it. Just enough to fill in a day's work.

J: *It looks like a sequence that would have taken a week to shoot, and instead you tell me you did it all in a day.*
F: Oh no, we didn't do it in a day. Nothing of the sort. We did it in about an hour and a quarter.
J: Stagecoach *was the first time you filmed in Monument Valley. Why did you decide to shoot there?*
F: I used to stay occasionally with the chap who ran the trading post, and he said, "You know, the Navajos are starving. I understand you're going to do a Western. If you come up there and do it, you'd probably save a lot of lives." I think we left about $500,000 there. A man that rode a horse, if he provided his own horse, got ten dollars a day, the women got five dollars, and the children got three dollars a day. It put them on their feet and they appreciated it. If anybody else tries to come in there, they object. They don't want anybody in there but me.
J: *Do you see the systematic destruction of the Red Indian as something inevitable, or a blot on American history?*
F: That's a political question. I don't think it has anything to do with pictures. All I could say is "No comment." I wasn't alive then, I had nothing to do with it. My sympathy is all with the Indians. Do you consider the invasion of the Black and Tans in Ireland a blot on English history? Being Irish, it's my prerogative to answer a question with a question. Do you consider that a blot on English history?
J: *I don't know enough about it.*
F: It's the same thing.
J: *Can you tell me about the incredible story of your filming of the* Battle of Midway?
F: What was incredible about it?
J: *You running out there with a camera under direct attack.*
F: I did what?
J: *You were making shots and directing shots while the place was literally being blasted to bits.*
F: That was what I was getting paid for. There's nothing extraordinary about that. I was on this turret to report the position and the numbers of Japanese planes to the officers who were fifty feet under the ground, and meanwhile I had a little 16mm camera. I just reported the different things and took the pictures. That was what the Navy was for. What else could you do?
J: *In between making "A" pictures, you turned out scores and scores of "B" films.*
F: One of the troubles with directors is that they make a big picture—which might be a hit—and then they try to top it. And they usually fall flat on their faces. So I try to make it as a rule: if I make a big picture which is a hit I do a cheap picture next. Relax for three or four weeks while preparing another story. Usually, of course, to my mind the little picture is better. My favorite picture, for example, is one you've never heard of called *The Sun Shines Bright*.
J: *What aspects of American society at this moment dismay you the most?*
F: I'm worried about these riots, these students. I'm worried about this antiracism (sic). It doesn't mean the Negroes are doing it. They're being influenced by outside. Some other country. They are agents, the people who are doing things, that are being arrested . . . and the poor Negroes are getting the blame. That's why I think our ancestors would be . . . bloody ashamed of us if they saw us now. But things will get better.
J: *Your films often depict bloodshed, yet I get the feeling you hate violence.*
F: I do, and my pictures do not always show violence. Very, very few of them do. And if they show violence, it's over quickly. I suggest it more than anything else. I hate violence in pictures just as I do all this sex and incest and all the things that are going on now.

LESSON SEVEN

Stars

Introduction to Heavenly Bodies

Richard Dyer

Eve Arnold's portrait of Joan Crawford gathers into one image three dimensions of stardom. Crawford is before two mirrors, a large one on the wall, the other a small one in her hand. In the former we see the Crawford image at its most finished; she is reduced to a set of defining features: the strong jaw, the gash of a mouth, the heavy arched eyebrows, the large eyes. From just such a few features, an impressionist, caricaturist or female impersonator can summon up Joan Crawford' for us. Meanwhile, in the small mirror we can see the texture of the powder over foundation, the gloss of the lipstick, the penciling of the eyebrows—we can see something of the means by which the smaller image has been manufactured.

Neatly, we have two Crawford reflections. The placing of the smaller one, central and in sharpest focus, might suggest that this is the one to be taken as the 'real' Crawford. Eve Arnold is known as a photographer committed to showing women 'as they really are', not in men's fantasies of them. This photo appears in her collection *The Unretouched Woman* (1976), the title proclaiming Arnold's aim; it is accompanied by the information that Crawford wanted Arnold to do the series of photos of her to show what hard work being a star was. The style and context of the photo encourage us to treat the smaller image as the real one, as do our habits of thought. The processes of manufacturing an appearance are often thought to be more real than the appearance itself—appearance is mere illusion, is surface.

There is a third Crawford in the photograph, a back view slightly less sharply in focus than the mirror images. Both the large and the small facial images are framed, made into pictures. The fact that the different mirrors throw back different pictures suggests the complex relationship between a picture and that of which it is a picture, something reinforced by the fact that both mirrors reflect presentation: making-up and decorating the face. Both mirrors return a version of the front of the vague, shadowy figure before them. Is this third Crawford the real one, the real person who was the occasion of the images? This back view of Crawford establishes her as very much there, yet she is beyond our grasp except through the partial mirror images of her. Is perhaps the smaller mirror image the true reflection of what the actual person of Crawford was really like, or can we know only that there was a real person inside the images but never really know her? Which is Joan Crawford, really?

We can carry on looking at the Arnold photo like this, and our mind can constantly shift between the three aspects of Crawford; but it is the three of them taken together that make up the phenomenon Joan Crawford, and it is the insistent question of 'really' that draws us in, keeping us on the go from one aspect to another.

Logically, no one aspect is more real than another. How we appear is no less real than how we have manufactured that appearance, or than the 'we' that is doing the manufacturing. Appearances are a kind of reality, just as manufacture and individual persons are. However, manufacture and the person (a certain notion of the person; as I'll discuss) are generally thought to be more real than appearance in this culture. Stars are obviously a case of appearance—all we know of them is what we see and hear before us. Yet the whole media construction of stars encourages us to think in terms of 'really'—what is Crawford really like? which biography, which word-of-mouth story, which moment in which film discloses her as she really was? The star phenomenon gathers these aspects of contemporary human existence together, laced up with the question of 'really'.

The rest of this chapter looks at this complex phenomenon from two angles—first, the constitutive elements of stars, what they consist of, their production; secondly, the notions of personhood and social reality that they relate to. These are not separate aspects of stardom, but different ways of looking at the same overall phenomenon. How anything in society is made, how making is organised and understood, is inseparable from how we think people are, how they function, what their relation to making is. The complex way in which we produce and reproduce the world in technologically developed societies involves the ways in which we separate ourselves into public and private persons, producing and consuming persons and so on, and the ways in which we as people negotiate and cope with those divisions. Stars are about all of that, and are one of the most significant ways we have for making sense of it all. That is why they matter to us, and why they are worth thinking about.

Making Stars

The star phenomenon consists of everything that is publicly available about stars. A film star's image is not just his or her films, but the promotion of those films and of the star through pin-ups, public appearances, studio hand-outs and so on, as well as interviews, biographies and coverage in the press of the star's doings and 'private' life. Further, a star's image is also what people say or write about him or her, as critics or commentators, the way the image is used in other contexts such as advertisements, novels, pop songs, and finally the way the star can become part of the coinage of everyday speech. Jean-Paul Belmondo imitating Humphrey Bogart in *A bout de souffle* is part of Bogart's image, just as anyone saying, in a mid-European accent, 'I want to be alone' reproduces, extends and inflects Greta Garbo's image.

Star images are always extensive, multimedia, intertextual. Not all these manifestations are necessarily equal. A film star's films are likely to have a privileged place in her or his image, and I have certainly paid detailed attention to the films in the analyses that follow. However, even this is complicated. In the case of Robeson, his theatre, recording and concert work were undoubtedly more highly acclaimed than his film work—he was probably better known as a singer, yet more people would have seen him in films than in the theatre or concert hall. Later, in the period not covered here, he became equally important as a political activist. Garland became more important in her later years as a music hall, cabaret and recording star, although, as I argue in the *Garland chapter,* that later reputation then sent people back to her old films with a different kind of interest. Again, Monroe may now have become before everything else an emblematic figure, her symbolic meaning far outrunning what actually happens in her films.

As these examples suggest, not only do different elements predominate in different star images, but they do so at different periods in the star's career. Star images have histories, and histories that outlive the star's own lifetime. In the chapters that follow I have tried to reconstruct something of the meanings of Robeson and Monroe in the period in which they were themselves still making films—I've tried to situate them in relation to the immediate contexts of those periods. Robeson and Monroe have continued to be ethnic and sexual emblems as they were in their lifetime, but I have wanted to situate them in relation to the specific ways of understanding and feeling ethnic and sexual questions which were available in the thirties and fifties respectively, rather than in relation to what they mean in those terms now, although this would be an equally proper enquiry. (I did not, by the way, put ethnic and sexual in relation to Robeson and Monroe 'respectively', because Robeson is importantly situated in relation to ideas of sexuality just as Monroe is a profoundly ethnic image.) With Garland I have done the opposite—I have tried to look at her through a particular world-view, that of the white urban male gay subculture that developed in relation to her after her major period of film stardom and as she was becoming better known as a cabaret, recording and television star (and subject of scandal). The studies of Monroe, Robeson and Garland that follow are partial and limited, not only in the usual sense that all analyses are, but in being deliberately confined to particular aspects of their images, at particular periods and with a particular interest in seeing how this is produced and registered in the films.

Images have to be made. Stars are produced by the media industries, film stars by Hollywood (or its equivalent in other countries) in the first instance, but then also by other agencies with which Hollywood is connected in varying ways and with varying degrees of influence. Hollywood controlled not only the stars' films but their promotion, the pin-ups and glamour portraits, press releases and to a large extent the fan clubs. In turn, Hollywood's connections with other media industries meant that what got into the press, who got to interview a star, what clips were released to television was to a large extent decided by Hollywood. But this is to present the process of star making as uniform and oneway. Hollywood, even within its own boundaries, was much more complex and contradictory than this. If there have always been certain key individuals in controlling positions (usually studio bosses and major producers, but also some directors, stars and other figures) and if they all share a general professional ideology, clustering especially around notions of entertainment, still Hollywood is also characterized by internecine warfare between departments, by those departments getting on with their own thing in their own ways and by a recognition that it is important to leave spaces for individuals and groups to develop their own ideas (if only because innovation is part of the way that capitalist industries renew themselves). If broadly everyone in Hollywood had a sense of what the Monroe, Robeson and Garland images were, still different departments and different people would understand and inflect the image differently. This already complex image-making system looks even more complex when one brings in the other media agencies involved, since there are elements of rivalry and competition between them and Hollywood, as well as co-operation and mutual influence. If the drift of the image emanates from Hollywood, and with some consistency within Hollywood, still the whole image-making process within and without Hollywood allows for variation, inflection, and contradiction.

What the audience makes of all this is something else again—and, as I've already suggested, the audience is also part of the making of the image. Audiences cannot make media images mean anything they want to, but they can select from the complexity of the image the meanings and feelings, the variations, inflections and contradictions, that work for them. Moreover, the agencies of fan magazines and clubs, as well as box office receipts and audience research, mean that the audience's ideas about a star can act back on the media producers of the star's image. This is not an equal to-and-fro–the audience is more disparate and fragmented, and does not itself produce centralised, massively available media images; but the audience is not wholly controlled by Hollywood and the media, either. In the case, for example, of feminist readings of Monroe (or of John Wayne) or gay male readings of Garland (or Montgomery Clift), what those particular audiences are making of those stars is tantamount to sabotage of what the media industries thought they were doing.

Stars are made for profit. In terms of the market, stars are part of the way films are sold. The star's presence in a film is a promise of a certain kind of thing that you would see if you went to see the film. Equally, stars sell newspapers and magazines, and are used to sell toiletries, fashions, cars and almost anything else.

This market function of stars is only one aspect of their economic importance. They are also a property on the strength of whose name money can be raised for a film; they are an asset to the person (the star him/herself), studio and agent who controls them; they are a major part of the cost of a film. Above all, they are part of the labour that produces film as a commodity that can be sold for profit in the market place.

Stars are involved in making themselves into commodities; they are both labour and the thing that labour produces. They do not produce themselves alone. We can distinguish two logically separate stages. First, the person is a body, a psychology, a set of skills that have to be mined and worked up into a star image. This work, of fashioning the star out of the raw material of the person, varies in the degree to which it respects what artists sometimes refer to as the inherent qualities of the material; make-up, coiffure, clothing, dieting and body-building can all make more or less of the body features they start with, and personality is no less malleable, skills no less learnable. The people who do this labour include the star him/herself as well as make-up artistes, hairdressers, dress designers, dieticians, body-building coaches, acting, dancing and other teachers, publicists, pin-up photographers, gossip columnists, and so on. Part of this manufacture of the star image takes place in the films the star makes, with all the personnel involved in that, but one can think of the films as a second stage. The star image is then a given, like machinery, an example of what Karl Marx calls 'congealed labour', something that is used with further labour (scripting, acting, directing, managing, filming, editing) to produce another commodity, a film.

How much of a determining role the person has in the manufacture of her or his image and films varies enormously from case to case and this is part of the interest. Stars are examples of the way people live their relation to production in capitalist society. The three stars examined in subsequent chapters all in some measure revolted against the lack of control they felt they had—Robeson by giving up feature film-making altogether, Monroe by trying to fight for better parts and treatment, Garland by speaking of her experiences at MGM and by the way in which her later problems were credited to the Hollywood system. These battles are each central parts of the star's image and they enact some of the ways the individual is felt to be placed in relation to business and industry in contemporary society. At one level, they articulate a dominant experience of work itself under capitalism—not only the sense of being a cog in an industrial machine, but also the fact that one's labour and what it produces seem so divorced from each other—one labours to produce goods (and profits) in which one either does not share at all or only in the most meagre, back-handed fashion. Robeson's, Monroe's, Garland's sense that they had been used, turned into something they didn't control is particularly acute because the commodity they produced is fashioned in and out of their own bodies and psychologies.

Other stars deliver different stories, of course. June Allyson, in interviews and in her biography 'with Frances Spatz-Leighton', sings the praises of the job security provided by the studio system, of big capital, just as in her movies she perfected the role of the happy stay-at-home housewife who saw it as her role to support her man in his productive life, whether he produced music (as in *The Glenn Miller Story*) or profits (as in *Executive Suite*). There is a consistency between her 'contented housewife' screen image, her satisfaction with her working conditions, the easygoing niceness in the tone of the biography and interviews. She thus represents the possibility of integrated, mutually supporting spheres of life, not the tension between screen image, manufacture and real person that Monroe, Garland and Robeson suggest.

Many male stars—Clark Gable, Humphrey Bogart, Paul Newman, Steve McQueen—suggest something else again. In each, sporting activity is a major—perhaps the major—element in their image; they are defined above all as people for whom having uncomplicated fun is paramount, and this is implicitly carried over into their reported attitude to their work. But equally work isn't important, it's just something you do so as to have the wherewithal to play polo, sail yachts, race cars. This is, then, an instrumental attitude towards manufacture, not the antagonistic one of Garland, Robeson and Monroe, nor the integrated one of Allyson, nor yet again the committed one of, for example, Fred Astaire, Joan Crawford or Barbra Streisand. These last three suggest different relations of commitment to work—Astaire to technical mastery, in the endless stories of his perfectionist attitude towards rehearsal and the evidence of it on the screen; Crawford in her total slogging away at all aspects of her image and her embodiment of the ethic of hard work in so many of her films; Streisand in her control over the films and records she makes, a reported shopfloor control that also shows in the extremely controlled and detailed nature of her performance style. Whatever the particular inflection, stars play out some of the ways that work is lived in capitalist society. My selection of Monroe, Robeson and Garland is different only in that there is in them an element of protest about labour under capitalism which you do not find in Allyson, Gable, Astaire, Streisand and the rest.

The protests of Robeson, Monroe and Garland are individual protests. Robeson and Monroe could be taken as protests emblematic of the situation of black people and women respectively, and have been properly used as such. But they remain individualised, partly because the star system is about the promotion of the individual. Protest about the lack of control over the outcome of one's labour can remain within the logic of individualism. The protests of Robeson, Monroe and Garland are of the individual versus the anomic corporation; they are protests against capitalism that do not recognise themselves as such, protests with deep resonances within the ideologies of entrepreneurial capitalism. They speak in the name of the individual and of the notion of success, not in the name of the individual as part of a collective organisation of labour and production. (Robeson alone began to move in that direction in his ensemble theatre work, and in his deliberately emblematic role in political activity in later years.)

A star image consists both of what we normally refer to as his or her 'image', made up of screen roles and obviously stage-managed public appearances, and also of images of the manufacture of that 'image' and of the real person who is the site or occasion of it. Each element is complex and contradictory, and the star is all of it taken together. Much of what makes them interesting is how they articulate aspects of living in contemporary society, one of which, the nature of work in capitalist society, I've already touched on. In the chapters that follow I want to look at the ways in which three particular stars relate to three aspects of social life—sexuality, ethnicity and sexual identity. Even being that specific, it is still complicated, I'm still wanting to keep some sense of the multiplicity of readings even of those stars in those terms. In the rest of this chapter, however, I want to risk even wider generalisations. Work, sexuality, ethnicity and sexual identity themselves depend on more general ideas in society about what a person is, and stars are major definers of these ideas.

Living Stars

Stars articulate what it is to be a human being in contemporary society; that is, they express the particular notion we hold of the person, of the 'individual'. They do so complexly, variously—they are not straightforward affirmations of individualism. On the contrary, they articulate both the promise and the difficulty that the notion of individuality presents for all of us who live by it.

'The individual' is a way of thinking and feeling about the discrete human person, including oneself, as a separate and coherent entity. The individual is thought of as separate in the sense that she or he has an existence apart from anything else—the individual is not just the sum of his or her social roles or actions. He or she may only be perceived through these things, may even be thought to be formed by them, yet there is, in this concept of the person, an irreducible core of being, the entity that is perceived within the roles and actions, the entity upon which social forces act. This irreducible core is coherent in that it is supposed to consist of certain peculiar, unique qualities that remain constant and give sense to the person's actions and reactions. However much the person's circumstances and behaviour may change, 'inside' they are still the same individual; even if 'inside' she or he has changed, it is through an evolution that has not altered the fundamental reality of that irreducible core that makes her or him a unique individual.

At its most optimistic, the social world is seen in this conception to emanate from the individual, and each person is seen to 'make' his or her own life. However, this is not necessary to the concept. What is central is the idea of the separable, coherent quality, located 'inside' in consciousness and variously termed 'the self', 'the soul', 'the subject' and so on. This is counterposed to 'society', something seen as logically distinct from the individuals who compose it, and very often as inimical to them. If in ideas of 'triumphant individualism' individuals are seen to determine society, in ideas of 'alienation' individuals are seen as cut adrift from and dominated, battered by the anonymity of society. Both views retain the notion of the individual as separate, irreducible, unique.

It is probably true to say that there has never been a period in which this concept of the individual was held unproblematically throughout society. The notion of the individual has always been accompanied by the gravest doubts as to its tenability. It is common, for instance, to characterize Enlightenment philosophy as one of the most shiningly optimistic assertions of individuality; yet two of its most sparkling works, Hume's *An Essay on Human Understanding* and Diderot's *Rameau's Nephew*, fundamentally undercut any straightforward belief in the existence of the coherent, stable, inner individual; Hume by arguing that all we can know as our self is a series of sensations and experiences with no necessary unity or connection, Diderot by focusing on the vital, theatrical, disjointed character of Rameau's nephew, so much more 'real' than Diderot, the narrator's stodgily maintained coherent self.

If the major trend of thought since the Renaissance, from philosophical rumination to common sense, has affirmed the concept of the individual, there has been an almost equally strong counter-tradition of ideas that have severely dented our confidence in ourselves: Marxism, with its insistence that social being determines consciousness and not vice versa, and, in its economist variant, with its vision of economic forces propelling human events forward; psychoanalysis, with its radical splitting of consciousness into fragmentary, contradictory parts; behaviourism, with its view of human beings controlled by instinctual appetites beyond consciousness; linguistics and models of communication in which it is not we who speak language, but language which speaks us. Major social and political developments have been understood in terms of the threat they pose to the individual: industrialisation can be seen to have set the pace for a whole society in which people are reduced to being cogs in a machine; totalitarianism would seem to be the triumph, easily achieved, of society over the individual; the development of mass communications, and especially the concomitant notion of mass society, sees the individual swallowed up in the sameness produced by centralised, manipulative media which reduce everything to the lowest common denominator. A major trajectory of twentieth-century high literature has examined the disintegration of the person as stable ego, from the fluid, shifting self of Woolf and Proust to the minimal self of Beckett and Sarraute. 'Common sense' is no less full of tags acknowledging this bruised sense of self: the sense of forces shaping our lives beyond our control, of our doing things for reasons that we don't understand, of our not recognising ourself in actions we took yesterday (to say nothing of years ago), of not seeing ourselves in photographs of ourselves, of feeling strange when we recognise the routinised nature of our lives—none of this is uncommon.

Yet the idea of the individual continues to be a major moving force in our culture. Capitalism justifies itself on the basis of the freedom (separateness) of anyone to make money, sell their labour how they will, to be able to express opinions and get them heard (regardless of wealth or social position). The openness of society is assumed by the way that we are addressed as individuals—as consumers (each freely choosing to buy, or watch, what we want), as legal subjects (free and responsible before the law), as political subjects (able to make up our mind who is to run society). Thus even while the notion of the individual is assailed on all sides, it is a necessary fiction for the reproduction of the kind of society we live in.

Stars articulate these ideas of personhood, in large measure shoring up the notion of the individual but also at times registering the doubts and anxieties attendant on it. In part, the fact that the star is not just a screen image but a flesh and blood person is liable to work to express the notion of the individual. A series of shots of a star whose image has changed—say, Elizabeth Taylor—at various points in her career could work to fragment her, to present her as nothing but a series of disconnected looks; but in practice it works to confirm that beneath all these different looks there is an irreducible core that gives all those looks a unity, namely Elizabeth Taylor. Despite the elaboration of roles, social types, attitudes and values suggested by any one of these looks, one flesh and blood person is embodying them all. We know that Elizabeth Taylor exists apart from all these looks, and this knowledge alone is sufficient to suggest that there is a coherence behind them all.

It can be enough just to know that there was one such person, but generally our sense of that one person is more vivid and important than all the roles and looks s/he assumes. People often say that they do not rate such and such a star because he or she is always the same. In this view, the trouble with, say, Gary Cooper or Doris Day, is that they are always Gary Cooper and Doris Day. But if you like Cooper or Day, then precisely what you value about them is that they are always 'themselves'—no matter how different their roles, they bear witness to the continuousness of their own selves.

This coherent continuousness within becomes what the star 'really is'. Much of the construction of the star encourages us to think this. Key moments in films are close-ups, separated out from the action and interaction of a scene, and not seen by other characters but only by us, thus disclosing for us the star's face, the intimate, transparent window to the soul. Star biographies are devoted to the notion of showing us the star as he or she really is. Blurbs, introductions, every page assures us that we are being taken 'behind the scenes', 'beneath the surface', 'beyond the image', there where the truth resides. Or again, there is a rhetoric of sincerity or authenticity, two qualities greatly prized in stars because they guarantee, respectively, that the star really means what he or she says, and that the star really is what she or he appears to be. Whether caught in the unmediated moment of the close-up, uncovered by the biographer's display of ruthless uncovering, or present in the star's indubitable sincerity and authenticity, we have a privileged reality to hang on to, the reality of the star's private self.

The private self is further represented through a set of oppositions that stem from the division of the world into private and public spaces, a way of organising space that in turn relates to the idea of the separability of the individual and society:

private	public
individual	society
sincere	insincere
country	city
small town	large town
folk	urban
community	mass
physical	mental
body	brain
naturalness	artifice
sexual intercourse	social intercourse
racial	ethnic

When stars function in terms of their assertion of the irreducible core of inner individual reality, it is generally through their associations with the values of the left-hand column. Stars like Clark Gable, Gary Cooper, John Wayne, Paul Newman, Robert Redford, Steve McQueen, James Caan establish their male action-hero image either through appearing in Westerns, a genre importantly concerned with nature and the small town as centres of authentic human behaviour, and/or through vivid action sequences, in war films, jungle adventures, chase films, that pit the man directly, physically against material forces. It is interesting that with more recent examples of this type—Clint Eastwood, Harrison Ford—there has been a tendency either to give their films a send-up or tongue-in-cheek flavour (Eastwood's chimp films, Ford as Indiana Jones) or else a hard, desolate, alienated quality (Eastwood in *Joe Kidd*, Ford in *Blade Runner*), as if the values of masculine physicality are harder to maintain straightfacedly and unproblematically in an age of microchips and a large scale growth (in the USA) of women in traditionally male occupations.

The private self is not always represented as good, safe or positive. There is an alternative tradition of representing the inner reality of men, especially, which stretches back at least as far as the romantic movement. Here the dark, turbulent forces of nature are used as metaphors for the man's inner self: Valentino in *The Son of the Sheik*, the young Laurence Olivier as Heathcliff in *Wuthering Heights* and as Maxim de Winter in *Rebecca*. In the forties and fifties the popularisation of psychoanalysis added new terms to the private:public opposition. Thus:

private	public
subconscious	conscious
Id	Ego

and in the still more recent Lacan inflection:

Imaginary	Symbolic

These have been particularly important in the subsequent development of male stars, where the romantic styles of brooding, introspective, mean-but-vulnerable masculinity have been given Oedipal, psychosexual, paranoid or other crypto-psychoanalytical inflections with stars like Montgomery Clift, James Dean, Marlon Brando, Anthony Perkins, Jack Nicholson, Richard Gere. Recent black male stars such as Jim Brown, Richard Roundtree and Billy Dee Williams are interesting in that their fiercely attractive intensity seems closer to the 'dangerous' romantic tradition proper; at the same time they also draw on the old stereotype of the black man as brute, only now portraying this as attractive rather than terrifying; and they are almost entirely untouched by the psychoanalytical project of rationalising and systematising and naming the life of the emotions and sensations. All these male stars work variations on the male inner self as negative, dangerous, neurotic, violent, but always upholding that as the reality of the man, what he is really like.

The stars analysed in the rest of this book also have strong links with the left-hand, 'private' column. Monroe was understood above all through her sexuality—it was her embodiment of current ideas of sexuality that made her seem real, alive, vital. Robeson was understood primarily through his racial identity, through attempts to see and, especially, hear him as the very essence of the Negro folk. Both were represented insistently through their bodies—Monroe's body was sexuality, Robeson's was the nobility of the black race. Garland too belongs with the left-hand column, initially through her roles as country or small-town girl, later through the way her body registered both her problems and her defiance of them. All the descriptions of her from her later period begin by describing the state of her body and speculating from that on what drugs, drink, work and temperament have done to it, and yet how it continues to be animated and vital. Not only are Monroe, Robeson, Garland stars who are thought to be genuine, who reveal their inner selves, but the final touchstone of that genuineness is the human body itself. Stars not only bespeak our society's investment in the private as the real, but also often tell us how the private is understood to be the recovery of the natural 'given' of human life, our bodies. Yet as the chapters that follow argue, what we actually come up against at this point is far from straightforwardly natural; it is particular, and even rather peculiar, ways of making sense of the body. The very notions of sexuality and race, so apparently rooted in the body, are historically and culturally specific ideas about the body, and it is these that Monroe and Robeson, especially, enact, thereby further endowing them with authenticity.

What is at stake in most of the examples discussed so far is the degree to which, and manner in which, what the star really is can be located in some inner, private, essential core. This is how the star phenomenon reproduces the overriding ideology of the person in contemporary society. But the star phenomenon cannot help being also about the person in public. Stars, after all, are always inescapably people in public. If the magic, with many stars, is that they seem to be their private selves in public, still they can also be about the business of being in public, the way in which the public self is endlessly produced and remade in presentation. Those stars that seem to emphasise this are often considered 'mannered', and the term is right, for they bring to the fore manners, the stuff of public life. When such stars are affirmative of manners and public life they are often, significantly enough, European or with strong European connections—stars to whom terms like suave, gracious, debonair, sophisticated, charming accrue, such as Fred Astaire, Margaret Sullavan, Cary Grant, David Niven, Deborah Kerr, Grace Kelly, Audrey Hepburn, Rex Harrison, Roger Moore. These are people who have mastered the public world, in the sense not so much of being authentically themselves in it nor even of being sincere, as of performing in the world precisely, with poise and correctness. They get the manners right. An additional example might be Sidney Poitier, only with him the consummate ease of his public manners comes up against the backlog of images of black men as raging authenticities, with the result that in his films of the fifties and sixties he is not really able to be active in public, he is a good performer who doesn't perform anything. It is only with *In the Heat of the Night* that something else emerges, a sense of the tension attendant on being good in public, a quality that brings Poitier here into line with a number of other stars who suggest something of the difficulty and anxiety attendant upon public performance.

Many of the women stars of screwball comedy—Katharine Hepburn, Carole Lombard, Rosalind Russell, and more recently Barbra Streisand—have the uncomfortable, sharp quality of people who do survive and succeed in the public world, do keep up appearances, but edgily, always seem to be in the difficult process of doing so. Bette Davis's career has played variations on this representation of public performance. Many of her films of the thirties and forties exploit her mannered style to suggest how much her success or survival depends upon an ability to manipulate manners, her own and those of people around her, to get her own way (*Jezebel*, *The Little Foxes*), to cover her tracks out of courage (*Dark Victory*) or guilt (*The Letter*), to maintain a public presence at all costs for a greater good than her own (*The Private Life of Elizabeth and Essex*), to achieve femininity (*Now Voyager*) and so on. If being in public for Davis in these films is hypertense, registered in her rapid pupil movements, clenching and unclenching fists, still in the thirties and forties she is enacting the excitement, the buzz of public life, of being a person in public. Later films become something like the tragedy of it. *All About Eve* details the cost of keeping up appearances, maintaining an image. *Whatever Happened to Baby Jane?* evokes the impossibility of achieving again the public role that made her character feel good. Yet the end of *Baby Jane* affirms the public self as a greater reality than the private self cooped up in the dark Gothic mansion—we learn that it is Crawford not Davis who is the baddie; away from the house, on the beach, surrounded by people, the ageing Jane can become the public self she really is, Baby Jane. Davis's career thus runs the gamut of the possibilities of the private individual up against public society; from, in the earlier films, triumphant individualism, the person who makes their social world, albeit agitatedly, albeit at times malignantly, to, in the later films, something like alienation, the person who is all but defeated by the demands of public life, who only hangs on by the skin of their teeth—until the up-tempo happy ending.

The private/public, individual/society dichotomy can be embodied by stars in various ways; the emphasis can fall at either end of the spectrum, although it more usually falls at the private, authentic, sincere end. Mostly too there is a sense of 'really' in play—people/stars are really themselves in private or perhaps in public but at any rate somewhere. However, it is one of the ironies of the whole star phenomenon that all these assertions of the reality of the inner self or of public life take place in one of the aspects of modern life that is most associated with the invasion and destruction of the inner self and corruptibility of public life, namely the mass media. Stars might even seem to be the ultimate example of media hype, foisted on us by the media's constant need to manipulate our attention. We all know how the studios build up star images, how stars happen to turn up on chat shows just when their latest picture is released, how many of the stories printed about stars are but titillating fictions; we all know we are being sold stars. And yet those privileged moments, those biographies, those qualities of sincerity and authenticity, those images of the private and the natural can work for us. We may go either way. As an example, consider the reactions at the time to John Travolta in *Saturday Night Fever*. I haven't done an audience survey, but people seemed to be fairly evenly divided. For those not taken with him, the incredible build-up to the film, the way you knew what his image was before you saw the film, the coy but blatant emphasis on his sex appeal in the film, the gaudy artifice of the disco scene, all merely confirmed him as one great phoney put-on on the mass public. But for those for whom he and the film did work, there were the close-ups revealing the troubled pain behind the macho image, the intriguing off-screen stories about his relationship with an older woman, the spontaneity (= sincerity) of his smile, the setting of the film in a naturalistically portrayed ethnic subculture. A star's image can work either way, and in part we make it work according to how much it speaks to us in terms we can understand about things that are important to us.

Nonetheless, the fact that we know that hype and the hard sell do characterize the media, that they are supreme instances of manipulation, insincerity, inauthenticity, mass public life, means that the whole star phenomenon is profoundly unstable. Stars cannot be *made* to work as affirmations of private or public life. In some cases, the sheer multiplicity of the images, the amount of hype, the different stories told become overwhelmingly contradictory. Is it possible still to have any sense of Valentino or Monroe, their persons, apart from all the things they have been made to mean? Perhaps, but at best isn't it a sense of the extraordinary fragility of their inner selves, endlessly fragmented into what everyone else, including us, wanted them to be? Or it may be that what interests us is the public face, accepting the artifice and fantasy for what it is—do we ask for sincerity and authenticity from Jayne Mansfield or Diana Ross, Groucho, Harpo or Chico Marx?

Or we may read stars in a camp way, enjoying them not for any supposed inner essence revealed but for the way they jump through the hoops of social convention. The undulating contours of Mae West, the lumbering gait and drawling voice of John Wayne, the thin, spiky smile of Joan Fontaine—each can be taken as an emblem of social mores: the ploys of female seduction, the certainty of male American power, the brittle niceness of upper class manners. Seeing them that way is seeing them as appearance, as image, in no way asking for them to be what they are, really.

On rare occasions a star image may promote a sense of the social constructedness of the apparently natural. The image of Lena Horne in her MGM films does this in relation to ideas of black and female sexuality. Her whole act in these films—and often it is no more than a turn inserted into the narrative flow of the film—promotes the idea of natural, vital sexuality, with her flashing eyes, sinuous arm movements and suggestive vocal delivery. That people saw this as the ultimate in unfettered feminine libido is widely attested, yet as an act it has an extraordinary quality, a kind of metallic sheen and intricate precision that suggests the opposite of animal vitality. In an interview with Michiko Kakutani in the *New York Times* (Sunday, 3 May 1981, section D, pp1,24), Lena Horne discussed her image in this period in relation to her strategy of survival in the period as a black women:

> *Afraid of being hurt, afraid of letting her anger show, she says she cultivated an image that distanced her from her employers, her colleagues, and from her audiences as well. If audience members were going to regard her as no more than an exotic performer—'Baby, you sure can sing, but don't move next door'—well, then, that's all they'd get. By focusing intently on the notes and lyrics of a song, she was able to shut out the people who were staring at her, and over the years, she refined a pose of sophisticated aloofness, a pose that said, 'You're getting the singer, but not the woman.' I used to think, "I'm black and I'm going to isolate myself because you don't understand me,' ", she says. 'All the things people said—sure, they hurt, and it made me retreat even further. The only thing between me and them was jive protection.'*

It is rare for a performer to understand and state so clearly both how they worked and the effect of it, but this catches exactly Horne's image in the forties and fifties, its peerless surface, its presentation of itself *as* surface, its refusal to corroborate, by any hint of the person giving her self, the image of black sexuality that was being wished on her. This could not, did not stop audiences reading her as transparently authentic sexuality; but it was some sort of strategy of survival that could also be seen for what it was, a denaturalising of the ideas of black sexuality.

I have been trying to describe in this chapter some of the ways in which being interested in stars is being interested in how we are human now. We're fascinated by stars because they enact ways of making sense of the experience of being a person in a particular kind of social production (capitalism), with its particular organisation of life into public and private spheres. We love them because they represent how we think that experience is or how it would be lovely to feel that it is. Stars represent typical ways of behaving, feeling and thinking in contemporary society, ways that have been socially, culturally, historically constructed. Much of the ideological investment of the star phenomenon is in the stars seen as individuals, their qualities seen as natural. I do not wish to deny that there are individuals, nor that they are grounded in the given facts of the human body. But I do wish to say that what makes them interesting is the way in which they articulate the business of being an individual, something that is, paradoxically, typical, common, since we all in Western society have to cope with that particular idea of what we are. Stars are also embodiments of the social categories in which people are placed and through which they have to make sense of their lives, and indeed through which we make our lives—categories of class, gender, ethnicity, religion, sexual orientation, and so on. And all of these typical, common ideas, that have the feeling of being the air that you breathe, just the way things are, have their own histories, their own peculiarities of social construction.

Because they go against the grain of the individualising, naturalising emphasis of the phenomenon itself, these insistences on the typical and social may seem to be entirely imported from theoretical reflection. Yet ideas never come entirely from outside the things they are ideas about, and this seems particularly so of the star phenomenon. It constantly jogs these questions of the individual and society, the natural and artificial, precisely because it is promoting ideas of the individual and the natural in media that are mass, technologically elaborated, aesthetically sophisticated. That central paradox means that the whole phenomenon is unstable, never at a point of rest or equilibrium, constantly lurching from one formulation of what being human is to another. This book is an attempt to tease out some of those formulations in particular cases, to see how they work, to get at something of the contradictions of what stars are, really.

References

1. Allyson, June with Spatz-Leighton, Frances (1982) *June Allyson* (New York: G.P. Putnam).
2. Arnold, Eve (1976) *The Unretouched Woman* (New York: Knopf).

Ingrid From Lorraine to Stromboli: Analyzing the Public's Perception of a Film Star

James Damico

As a symbol of the height of glamour and artifice—plucked eyebrows, dyed hair, phony "exotic" name—and the victim of numerous scandals, Lana Turner may well epitomize our image of the classical era's Movie Star. But we should remember that the species of stardom to which she belongs is just one within the genus stardom. As James Damico's comments on Ingrid Bergman illustrate, not all stars are perceived as glamorous and artificial. The star image may be constructed as "natural" rather than artificially glamorous—although it must be stressed that even such "naturalness" is an ideologically delimited construct. Indeed, in the paradox that defines Hollywood, naturalness can become part of star fabrication. Bergman was extolled for her natural purity, her lack of makeup, her unplucked eyebrows. These were the terms that David O. Selznick's promotional team used to construct a vocabulary—a "lexicon" in Damico's words—for the public to know and idolize Bergman, for them to read Bergman. As always in the mainstream cinema, the viewers choose their stars and select their salient characteristics, but the studios determine the limits of the selection—until "real-life" events overwhelm even the manipulative efforts of the studios' public-relations departments, as they did with Ingrid Bergman.

Damico's analysis chronicles Bergman's promotional buildup by Selznick and her early association with the role of Joan of Arc, but his central interest is the impact—on her fans, her career, and her image—of her extramarital liaison with director Roberto Rossellini. Damico argues that the publicity attending that situation brought to the surface elements of Bergman's persona that had previously been misapprehended, ignored, or repressed. Suddenly, Bergman's sexual, "earthly love"—now publicly available—seemed to besmirch the transcendent, natural, Joan-of-Arc spirituality that Selznick had constructed for her. Damico traces these contrasting themes through Bergman's screen roles, the criticism of those roles, and the publicity material surrounding the Rossellini affair.

Although Damico provides interesting speculations on Bergman's image, he actually stops short of analyzing the "public's perception" of Bergman (and ignores the issue of the subject-viewer's, positioning by the text). He cites general evidence of the furor surrounding her, but the specifics of her affront are presented mostly through the comments of critics and gossip columnists—neither of which is an accurate barometer of public opinion. This essay includes no empirical audience research and no attempt to analyze the discourse of actual viewers (which could begin, perhaps, with the letters fans sent to the studios). As is often the problem with film historical research, scholars are forced to extrapolate meanings from secondary sources that may or may not accurately represent the primary object of study. In this case, the writings of critics and columnists are presumed to express the views of Ingrid Bergman's viewers and fans.

> Oh, sing me a saga of Joan
> Whose actions we cannot condone.
> From Boudoir to Altar
> Her steps never falter.
> She quips 'Get me God on the phone.'
> Who is this pure maid of Lorraine?
> Whose voices she cannot explain?
> From a life so licentious
> She is turned so repentious,
> It's driven her simply insane....[1]

Today when adultery and a panoply of what were once held to be sexual sins are not only publicly admitted by film stars, but often committed and filmed as part of their work, and when actresses openly form liaisons specifically to have children whom they intend to rear outside marriage, all without fear of adverse public reaction, it is intriguing to recall that there was a recent time when one film star's adultery with and illegitimate child by a film director was headline news for more than a year; caused the entire motion picture industry a long moment of apprehension; prompted local, state and national lawmaking bodies to indignant tirades and to the preparation of restrictive legislation; mobilized professional, religious and civic groups to vociferous protest; and moved a legion of everyday moviegoers to towering outrage.

Exactly what caused the extensive and spontaneous national reaction that attended Ingrid Bergman's affair-cum-marriage with Roberto Rossellini is not easy to identify, but it is important to speculate on in the context of determining the function that films and film stars have in society and especially informative in tracing the process by which the public arrives at a perception of a star's personality.

Ingrid Bergman was born in Sweden in 1915, married Dr. Peter Lindstrom in 1937, had a daughter in 1938, was brought to America in 1939 by David O. Selznick, and very soon thereafter became an important Hollywood star. Though not generally known, by at least 1946 her marriage had begun to sour, and it has been suggested that she had at a minimum a pair of extramarital affairs at this time (with Robert Capa, the photographer, and Victor Fleming, the director). But, in critical contrast to her subsequent involvement with Rossellini, these were discreetly managed and the public remained totally ignorant of them.

In 1948, struck by the power of *Open City* and *Paisan,* she wrote worshipfully to Rossellini, in effect pleading to work with him;[3] he responded enthusiastically; and during the shooting of *Under Capricorn* in England, she and her husband (who also acted as her business manager) met with the Italian in Paris on numerous occasions to plan the production of what was finally called *Stromboli* (named after the film's locale specifically to capitalize on the international tide of notoriety that identified the volcanic island as the place where Ingrid and Roberto had carried on their romance). Subsequently, they all repaired to Hollywood, ostensibly to find a way to shoot their film there, but it seems Rossellini had the further intention, as he announced to a reporter, of putting "the horns on Mr. Bergman."[4] Soon though, finding that he couldn't work in Hollywood, he returned to Italy where it was decided the film would be done.

What initially directed all the curiosity towards Bergman's arrival in Rome on March 20, 1949, was the much-ballyhooed meeting of two diametrically opposed cinematic worlds—the Hollywood glossy and the Italian neorealistic. But what inflated worldwide interest to extraordinary proportions and created the bedlam that never really afterwards subsided, was the openly conducted, apparently flaunted romance between the married actress and director begun in full view of the assembled international press from the moment she stepped off the plane. Front-page articles and photos documented the affair, Ingrid and Roberto strolled hand-in-hand across full pages in *Life,* and gossip column items became superfluous.

In the temper of the times, it was, to be sure, tactless, brazen and almost calculated to create a scandal. But totally unexpected was the breadth of the attack on Bergman, which reached epic scale when the news broke that she was pregnant and when eventually she had Rossellini's child out of wedlock.

Ministerial groups, women's organizations and private citizens bombarded Hollywood with resolutions and letters. Legislatures the country over spent hours discussing the scandal. A Sioux City Catholic bishop declared that it was about time Hollywood did something about "persons whose dirty, lousy, filthy conditions are ruining the industry."[5]

Editorials were written by newspapers of all sizes and persuasions, most condemning Bergman but some championing the artist's right to individual freedom. Her death scene from *Joan of Arc*, which had been included as part of an educational film, *History Brought to Life*, was hurriedly excised from final prints.[6] Louella Parsons, in announcing her pregnancy, compared what she called Bergman's "sacrifice for love" to those of Mary, Queen of Scots, and Lady Hamilton, and to the abdication of Edward VII[7].

Senator Edwin Johnson of Colorado, a leader in the Swedish-American community, felt particularly aggrieved, having previously held up Bergman as a perfect model of Nordic womanhood. For more than an hour on the floor of the U.S. Senate, he fulminated against the actress, calling her "a free-love cultist," "a powerful influence for evil," and "Hollywood's apostle of degradation"; and he urged passage of a resolution barring her forever from returning to the United States for "moral turpitude," predicting that "from the ashes of Ingrid Bergman a better Hollywood will rise."[8]

Attempts were made to get the then very active local and state censor boards to ban *Stromboli* as immoral, not because of any salacious content in the film, but by virtue of the extracinematic conduct of its principals. A Memphis censor tried unsuccessfully to ban all Bergman pictures, present and past, stating that "Miss Bergman's conduct is a disgrace, not only to her profession, but to all American women. I'm glad she's a foreigner." This was balanced by the police captain and head of Chicago's censor board, who said, "If we're going to delve into the past of every Hollywood actor, we'd be eliminating about two-thirds of all films."[9]

Not satisfied with oratory, Senator Johnson presented to the Senate a bill which would have made it mandatory for all entertainment industry members to be licensed before being permitted to work. This would have given those responsible complete control over all film artists simply by investing in them the power to revoke licenses for whatever they deemed reprehensible public behavior. It failed to gain acceptance.[10]

The extent of the furor this affair aroused, however, is evident, and it indicates the wide social implications of what amounted in reality to little more than a sexual peccadillo in an element of society well known for and indulged in its promiscuities. The question therefore arises: Why did this particular film star's affair generate such a momentous reaction when many another's hardly caused a ripple? And why was this adulterous act so condemned when, for instance, at approximately the same time, Robert Mitchum's apparent transgression of an even stronger societal taboo was revealed with his arrest for drug possession, and it, though widely reported, barely affected his career and raised nothing like the storm of disapproval that Bergman's actions did?

Essentially, the answer lies in the way in which the public perceives film stars and in the peculiarities of the Bergman image. The public images of a majority of stars are constructed out of a mixture of the off-screen characters of the actors, their on-screen personas, how publicity defines both of these, and how the general public interprets and fuses all the foregoing elements into assimilable phenomena which it then labels with, and thereafter identifies by, the stars' names. Although audiences and professional observers, such as critics and reviewers, are often perceptive in recognizing authentic artistic temperament, they are by no means infallible in correctly interpreting the nature of and defining that temperament. Arbitrarily, or out of their own psychological needs, or from suggestions made by publicity, they will often ascribe to film personalities characteristics, attitudes, beliefs, virtues and vices for which they think they see validation on the screen in the stars' behavior and expression. Such judgments, however, may in fact be essential misunderstandings of these indicators of authentic temperament and consequently of the personality components of which they are expressive (as has been the case, for example, in such popular and basic misconceptions as of Wallace Reid's "wholesomeness," Will Rogers' "lack of sophistication," Jayne Mansfield's "dumbness," etc.). It is this kind of critical misinterpretation that seems to have been made of Bergman's personality.

From her initial appearance in Swedish films, through her Hollywood years, which included many public and stage appearances, Bergman provoked reactions whose language verged on the monotonous. "Beautiful," "natural," "clean," "fresh," "glowing," and "spiritual" turned up again and again in articles and reviews. Her performance in *Intermezzo: A Love Story*, her first American film, brought from Frank S. Nugent, the not normally effusive critic of *The New York Times*, an analysis of the actress and her acting that might be thought of as cutting the pattern to be followed by most subsequent reviewers:

> *She is beautiful, and not at all pretty. Her acting is surprisingly mature, yet singularly free from the stylistic traits—the mannerisms, postures, precise intonations—that become the stock in trade of the matured actress. Our impression of her Anita, who is pallid one moment, vivacious the next, yet always consistent, is that of a lamp whose wick burns bright or dull, but always burns. There is that incandescence about Miss Bergman, that spiritual spark which makes us believe that Selznick has found another great lady of the screen.*[11]

Six months later, in appraising her first English-speaking stage performance in *Liliom*, Brooks Atkinson matched his colleague's enthusiasm:

> *Ingrid Bergman acts with incomparable loveliness . . . is personally beautiful and endows Julie with an awakened, pulsing grace of spirit. One is timidly reluctant to praise an actress too highly on her first appearance, but the time will come when it will be hard to praise Miss Bergman enough. There is something wonderfully enkindling about the way she illuminates Julie's character.*[12]

These are, of course, exceptional notices from different observers of her work in entirely different media, and they testify to a common recognition of authentic and essential qualities in the Bergman acting persona.

It was precisely these qualities that Selznick had seen in the original Swedish *Intermezzo* and that he took great care to ensure Bergman projected in his remake. In a memo to Gregory Ratoff, the director of the American *Intermezzo*, the producer issued methodical instructions about photographing her:

> *The [Gregg] Toland tests of Miss Bergman prove indubitably . . . the difference between a great photographic beauty and an ordinary girl with Miss Bergman lies in proper photography of her—and that this in turn depends not simply on avoiding the bad side of her face; keeping her head down as much as possible; giving her the proper hairdress, giving her the proper mouth make-up, avoiding long shots so as not to make her look too big [she was nearly 5'10"], and, even more importantly, but for the same reason, avoiding low cameras on her, as well as being careful to build people who work with her . . . but most important of all, on shading her face and in invariably going for effect lighting on her.*[13]

Selznick's painstaking attention to the actress' physical appearance extended not only to her make-up, but made a rather large issue out of her eyebrows—as it turned out, a matter of some significance.

> *Thanks to clubbing everybody on the head about avoiding make-up on Miss Bergman, it looks as though we have a new star in her, with the public and the press all commenting widely on the fact that her eyebrows look natural, and that she isn't smeared with Hollywood make-up.*[14]

> *Ann Rutherford [a young film actress] told me . . . that all the girls she knows are letting their eyebrows grow in as a result of Bergman's unplucked eyebrows. . . . So apparently our decision about Miss Bergman's eyebrows, based upon this studio's feeling that the public was sick and tired of the monstrosities that had been*

> *inflicted on the public by most of Hollywood's glamour girls is going to have a national reaction.*[15]

The studio's internecine battles over seeming inconsequentialities, such as the retention of the actress' eyebrows, her unmade-up look, and her name (which raged hotly for a time), were all settled in favor of her "naturalness," and had the desired effect not only upon audiences, but also on critics, as Graham Greene's review of *Intermezzo* testifies:

> *The film is most worth seeing for the new star, Miss Ingrid Bergman, who is as natural as her name . . . a performance that doesn't give the effect of acting at all, but of living—without make-up.*[16]

But beyond being methodically built, the image of the actress was just as precisely disseminated. Long before her first picture was released, the producer assiduously labored at shaping the public's concept of his star-to-be:

> *I think Miss Bergman's interview in the [Los Angeles] Examiner was awfully bad publicity . . . our being quoted as thinking she is sexy . . . is not the way we should publicize her. . . . Please don't have her interviewed unless somebody you can rely on . . . can be present.*[17]

In a subsequent memo to his publicity department, he set out the correct "angle" on the actress. It involved stressing for public consumption her conscientiousness as an artist, her devotion to her work, her thrift and her unaffectedness (manifested, for example, in her acceptance of less than a star's dressing room and her desire not to have a stand-in).

> *All of this is completely unaffected and completely unique and I should think would make a grand angle of approach to her publicity, spreading these stories all around, and adding to them as they occur, so that her natural sweetness and consideration and conscientiousness become something of a legend. Certainly there could be nothing more popular, and nothing could win for her the affection of fans more than this. . . . It is completely in keeping with the character she plays in the picture and completely in keeping with the fresh and pure personality and appearance which caused me to sign her. . . .*[18]

Through his campaign, Selznick was in effect offering filmgoers a ready-made lexicon with which to label all the startling qualities of the Bergman personality, in the expectation that the provided labels would be synthesized into a sympathetic interpretation of both the actress' personal character and her screen performances. The process, of course, was a Hollywood tradition, and had been tried before with great and, more often, utterly no success. Its obvious risk was that the public would not agree that the lexicon provided for it was appropriate to what it saw on the screen. But a more essential risk underlay the first: even if the public did accept them, the proffered labels and consequent directed interpretation of the star's qualities might eventually turn out to be misleading and false, and that out of a sense of having been duped, the general audience might turn on and reject the star.

Almost unanimously, however, the public did accept Selznick's campaign on Bergman. Not only did descriptions and judgments of the actress in reviews match the producer's scenario, but countless interviews and articles reemphasized the same points. *The Richmond* (Va.) *News-Leader*, for example, said she looked like an American college girl and made other stars look phoney because she "buys her own groceries and even wears her own eyelashes."[19] *The Milwaukee Journal* praised her for having her family "form the background of her life away from the studio," and for never posing for cheesecake art.[20] But this *Baltimore Sun* summation of August 20, 1944, can serve as the essence of the public conception of Bergman:

> *A big star who is satisfied with her roles, her salary and her life in general. . . . There isn't a superlative left which hasn't been used about her person and her acting. She is probably the only woman here [Hollywood] who hasn't an enemy. She has never in the five years she's lived here, been mentioned unfavorably in a gossip column.*

> *... There is nothing star-ish about her, except her personality, smile and charm ... she doesn't dear and darling everybody. She never wears make-up, except a little lipstick occasionally, and she lives quietly with her husband ... and daughter. ... She has no conceit, except about her ability as an actress ....*

These quotations make evident how much the supposed stability of her family life had entered into the publicity picture, when, in reality, her domestic situation at the time was rapidly deteriorating.

Equally a part of the Bergman "legend" from its beginnings was her identification with Joan of Arc. She had had a fixation on the French saint from girlhood and got Selznick to announce, as her second American film, a dramatization of Joan's life. The film was not made because the approaching war rendered it inappropriate to portray the British burning France's woman saint. But a publicity barrage at the time implanted the historical figure in the public consciousness as a kind of alter-ego for the actress. The alter-ego was finally given palpable form shortly before the Rossellini affair when Bergman appeared on Broadway as *Joan of Lorraine* in Maxwell Anderson's play. Not only did she triumph, but she was also "immortalized" in the role for the nation at large on the cover of *Life*. This was immediately followed by the culmination of her personal and career aspirations with the filming of *Joan of Arc*, which, though a financial and artistic failure, was critical in solidifying the connection between the actress and the saint.

But entirely hidden from the public during this time, besides her romantic involvements, were what has been called "the Bergman temper,"[21] her obstinancy, her chronic restlessness, her compulsive eating, and the fact that as a girl her next most cherished personage after Saint Joan was Isolde, because she "was a symbol of earthly love."[23] There appeared no public hint of the woman Robert Capa described as

> *all tied up in a million knots ... so naive it hurts ... afraid to let go ... a damn sight more woman than actress. And people should stop treating her like an adolescent schoolgirl—or like a saint.*

Or of the person that a Hollywood producer saw as "a very selfish, self-centered woman ... only interested in herself."[25] Or of what Bergman said of herself to her press agent:

> *We Swedes are not supposed to show our emotions in front of strangers. That's the way we're brought up. On the set, when I'm working, they think I'm so placid, and the fan magazines keep saying I'm so normal and simple. But you know me better.*
>
> *I wish I could rage and throw things, but if I did I'd feel foolish and wonder how I looked. So when I get angry I think to myself, will I lose my dignity? And I hold it inside and wait until I'm alone in my bedroom, then I throw myself on the bed and scream and cry.*[26]

And after Rossellini:

> *I was regarded as the wholesome, well-mannered girl, the actress without make-up, the Hollywood exception. People didn't expect me to have emotions like other women.*[27]

Selznick has also testified to the importance of his publicity campaign and the image of the actress it attempted to present to the public.

> *I'm afraid I'm responsible for the public's image of her as Saint Ingrid. I hired a press agent who was an expert at shielding stars from the press, and we released only stories that emphasized her sterling character. We deliberately built her up as the normal, healthy, unneurotic career woman, devoid of scandal and with an idyllic home life. I guess that backfired later.*[28]

One thing the promulgated image of Bergman did do was to cause the general public to ignore or rationalize away the specifically sexual character of the largest proportion of her roles and, even more essentially, the almost totally sexual nature of her screen persona.

In her twelve American films prior to *Joan of Arc,* Bergman is a whore or promiscuous in four (*Dr. Jekyll and Mr. Hyde, Saratoga Trunk, Notorious, Arch of Triumph*); is having or has had an affair in four (*Intermezzo, Casablanca, For Whom the Bell Tolls* [in which she has also been gang-raped], *Spellbound*); and is a virtual slave of sexual dependency in one (*Gaslight*). Of the three remaining films, she is accused of infidelity in *Rage in Heaven*; self-sacrificingly admits to someone else's infidelity in *Adam Had Four Sons*; and even in *The Bells of St. Mary,* as James Agee observed, uses;

> sex appeal . . . to play a Mother Superior . . . and in general, I grieve to say, justifies a recent piece of radio promotion which rather startlingly describes a nun: "Ingrid Bergman has never been lovelier, hubba hubba hubba."[29]

Most critics, however, ambivalently sought to reconcile the Bergman "legend" with those of her roles containing sexual specifics too obvious to ignore by simply accepting the validity of her acting while denying the character it portrayed. Of her Clio Dulane in *Saratoga Trunk,* for example, Bosley Crowther said:

> *Miss Bergman gives ample surface evidence of a coquettish, impulsive miss and looks quite fetching with dark hair and eyebrows, but there is no genuine spirit in her act. It is hard to accept this proper lady as the willful courtesan she's supposed to be.*[30]

And of her "unemployed courtesan" and "tramp" in *Arch of Triumph*

> *. . . we watch love as it is made by two of the movies' most able craftsmen [Bergman and Charles Boyer, but] she with her clean-cut, graceful style [is] quite hard to reconcile with her characterization.*[31]

Even her co-workers saw this "able craftsman's" love-playing as spiritual. As her press agent put it after *The Bells of St. Mary* was released:

> *Forgotten were the "bad girls" she had previously played, which had never fooled anyone anyway. Through all the painted women of her former films had shone the artless, virginal look, which her adherents now insisted was the true Bergman.*[32]

The difficulty in reconciling the actress' publicity image with her screen persona lay in the fact that the two were not identical but complementary. In contradiction of the "legend," the constituents of Bergman's film persona arise from a central motivating concept of an "earthly love" that is total, orgasmic, all-consuming and the only essential experience in life. It is a love desperately to be hoped for, anxiously anticipated, struggled with, but then surrendered to entirely—mind, heart, soul and body; a surrender in its complementary concept of "unearthly" love no less applicable to the Maid Joan than to Isolde.

Surrender, as Selznick realized in recognizing "how superbly" Bergman played "scenes of surrender,"[33] is possibly the prime element of her screen personality. It is the action to which *Casablanca* builds, and which is capped by her line, "You'll have to do the thinking for both of us." It is the emotional impetus behind the celebrated kissing scene in *Notorious* that makes it more than just a technical exercise—the sense of her natural giving in contrast to Cary Grant's rather removed acceptance of her.

Of the many physical manifestations of the passionate intensity of her portrayals (misunderstood not only by audiences but by old Hollywood hands as well, who are as susceptible to the processes of legend making as the general public), one was singled out by Sam Wood, director of both *For Whom the Bell Tolls* and *Saratoga Trunk*. He attempted to explain it, however, in terms of the Bergman publicity image.

> *Bergman's loveliness is more than external. It comes from in here (he patted his abdomen). When she plays a love scene she blushes—real blushes. And when her cheeks get pink you can see it on the screen because there's no make-up to hide it. It's a beautiful sight to see.*

The distinction between blush and flush is more than alphabetical. Bergman's coloring in such circumstances is less an indication of her virginal tendencies than an expression of the restraint she is exercising before the overwhelming character of her understanding of love—her tremulous anxiety at the prospect of a surrender that will mark the commitment to an all-encompassing passion.

It was a characteristic of the actress that another director, Anatole Litvak, recognized and defined:

> *Her great quality is that the moment she understands a part, her intellect gives way to emotion. When her emotion takes over, it comes out all right.*[35]

Ben Hecht recounts that Bergman did not want to do *Spellbound* because, as she said:

> *I don't believe the love story. The heroine is an intellectual woman, and an intellectual woman simply can't fall in love so deeply.*[36]

The author wryly remarks that she played the part convincingly. What he doesn't note is that she played it as she did all her successful roles—with an underlying emotional rationale—and that the woman in the film consequently came out far more emotional than intellectual. According to the producer, Walter Wanger, this approach extended beyond the confines of the part. "She always imagined herself in love with the leading man or director in every picture she did."[37] In other words, the entire filmmaking process was an extension of the total and emotional nature of the love experience at the center of her films.

The close relationship that an all-encompassing and finally transcendental romantic sexual love bears to a spiritual love of an equal intensity is critical to the misapprehension of Bergman's film persona; for those physical and emotional attributes that constitute her screen personality could just as easily be read as expressive of the spiritual torment of a soul reaching for communion with and salvation from God. Her nearly metaphysical agony at the prospect of a total personal surrender could as well delineate the agony of a surrender to the will of a heavenly power; and her fear and trembling before the commitment to an overwhelming romantic love might as well express a deep anxiety at the possibility of loss of one's identity in the acceptance of God.

It would appear, therefore, that filmgoers accepted the readymade interpretation provided by the actress' publicity image of those qualities comprising the phenomenon they knew as Ingrid Bergman and which they recognized as authentically artistic, because they assumed that the judgments already devised for them were accurate, and that the view which saw Bergman as essentially representative of spiritual concerns had been validated by the persona itself as it appeared and performed on the screen.

As it turned out, however, those judgments were neither accurate nor complete, and in their errors of omission and commission they provided, at least partially, the basis for the broad social disappointment, anger and resentment that attended Bergman's affair with Rossellini. For it is possible to speculate that in accepting the publicity image of the actress, a segment of the moviegoing public came to regard her as a totem figure (as it often seems to do other celebrities, out of other needs and to fulfill other functions) because her apparent film persona could conveniently serve as a focus, reflector and symbolic rehearser of the audience's indefinite spiritual longings and aspirations. But when it was dramatically shown that the central passion of the Bergman personality was not exclusively spiritual, but also quite specifically sexual, when the totem had in effect despoiled itself, the now wrathful public rose up in an effort to pull down what it saw as a self-proclaimed false idol.

Such a speculation, at any rate, offers a partial explanation of how a film star's inconsequential act of adultery could be aggrandized into an international incident and become a matter of legislative, professional and deep personal concern. It also provides a further sounding of the profound depths of the public's psychic investment in films and film stars.

Notes

1. Doggerel by Lewis Milestone, David Lewis, Charles Boyer, Russell Metty and Norman Lloyd, sent to Bergman during the first week of October 1946, on the occasion of the start of rehearsals for *Joan of Lorraine;* quoted in Joseph Steele, *Ingrid Bergman: An Intimate Portrait*

(New York: David McKay Company, Inc., 1959), pp. 111–12. The "life so licentious" is that portrayed by the actress in *Arch of Triumph,* which she had just completed filming in collaboration with the writers of the verse, and in which she played another Joan (Madou), a prostitute. The sudden change from this Joan to Joan of Arc is what has "driven her simply insane."

2. Steele, pp. 63–66, 91–92, 138–39.
3. The letter may be found in Bill Davidson, "Anatomy of a Scandal," in *The Real and the Unreal* (New York: Harper & Brothers, Publishers, 1961), p. 161.
4. Steele, p. 168.
5. *The New York Herald Tribune,* February 7, 1950.
6. *Variety,* February 15, 1950.
7. Steele, p. 261.
8. Ibid., p. 142.
9. *Variety,* February 8, 1950.
10. Jack Vizzard, *Speak No Evil* (New York: Simon and Schuster, Inc., 1970), p. 148.
11. October 6, 1939.
12. *The New York Times,* March 31, 1940.
13. David O. Selznick, *Memo From David O. Selznick,* ed. Rudy Behlmer (New York: The Viking Press, 1972), p. 130.
14. Ibid., p. 280.
15. Ibid., pp. 133–34.
16. *The Spectator,* January 26, 1940.
17. Selznick, p. 130.
18. Ibid., pp. 131–32.
19. February 15, 1940.
20. October 26, 1943.
21. Steele, p. 52.
22. Davidson, p. 144.
23. Steele, p. 17.
24. Ibid., p. 92.
25. Davidson, p. 148.
26. Steele, p. 75.
27. Davidson, pp. 157–58.
28. Ibid.
29. *The Nation,* January 5, 1946.
30. *The New York Times,* November 22, 1945.
31. Ibid., April 21, 1948.
32. Steele, p. 76.
33. Selznick, pp. 338–39.
34. Steele, p. 39.
35. Davidson, pp. 149–50.
36. *A Child of the Century* (New York: The New American Library, 1954), p. 449.
37. Davidson, p. 145.

Are Stars Necessary?

Alfred Hitchcock

Ever since the birth of films, I suppose, producers have been asking themselves this question, and with ever-growing insistence the public have answered "yes."

There are idealists who consider films as an art pure and simple, and who say that all actors should be subordinate to the film.

As a film producer, I *know* that art must first of all be commercially popular to be successful, and that one of the greatest factors which make a film commercially successful is the popularity of the stars in it.

Whichever way one looks at it, the "star" question is there, because examination of every successful play or film reveals that some strong drawing-power was responsible for the box office receipts, and that if it was not the leading player, then it was the author, or the producer, or the title, or even the effect of efficient exploitation of the production.

A production which is sufficiently startling and magnificent to justify the banging of the publicity drums, could easily be the "star" attraction, and so also could a title which is a household word.

A title, for example, like "On the Dole" would probably have box office appeal in itself. By all this, I am only trying to prove that to succeed in films, or even in the theater, you must have a "star," and that if the magnet is not human, then there must be a substitute.

I believe in the star system, because filmmaking is a business, and as a director I cannot afford to lose the money I am putting into my business.

The world may complain that film stars are paid money which makes cabinet ministers' salaries look like pocket money, but, believe me, every penny he or she is paid is worth it to the producer, otherwise the producer would not pay it.

Stars are paid according to what they bring into the box office, and if they bring in £20,000, then no one can blame them that they are paid accordingly.

Maurice Chevalier once had a three-year contract signed at £500 a week the first year, £750 the second, and £1,000 a week the third. So successful was he, however, that halfway through the contract his salary was raised from £750 a week to £2,500 a week, and he was worth every penny.

At one theater it was reckoned that "if full" the theater would hold £900 a performance. When Chevalier played there they played twelve performances a week, and every performance was packed. The theater thus gained £10,000 a week, out of which Chevalier was paid £5,000 as his share.

It is all really a question of supply and demand. The public demand their stars and the films supply them. When the public cease to demand, then the films will cease to supply, but I do not think this will happen yet, and after all why should it?

There is a very good psychological reason for "star worship": it fills some inherent need of which I see no reason why the public should be deprived. I know it is cynically labeled "sob stuff," but does anybody really care what it is labeled?

After all, is not sheer artistic emotion something to be proud of and not ashamed? There is little enough glamour in the drab business world of many of the audiences: why then should they be blamed for wanting it in their relaxation?

Moreover, aren't we forgetting one rather important fact: that a star only attains stardom because he or she has proved his or her worth and ability on the screen or stage.

The critics who argue that "the play's the thing" and "it's good acting and not names that count," seem to forget that a star's "name" still has some connection with his or her acting.

The public which says, "Let's go and see So-and-So's film tonight," say that because they know that "so-and-so's" film and acting is always worth seeing, and the same applies to the stage.

Those names that you see in electric light over the theaters and cinemas are all names who have proved their salt to both the producer and the public.

And if the public had seen, as I have done, the reverse of the picture, those bitter struggles to stardom—the disappointments, the sheer hard work, the poverty often coupled with starvation at the beginning, the courage and pluck and determination to win through—I do not think they would grudge them the electric lights.

Stardom is not won easily. I know people whisper about the power of the publicity drum, but no amount of publicity can create something which is not there, and a star who is only a child of publicity will not last.

And I do not think that anyone can say the "star system" means that the production as a whole is neglected. If they do, then let them spend a day, or two days, on the sets and see the infinite trouble, labor, and patience that is expended on one single shot. I have known a producer throw to £40,000 of work away and start production again from a fresh angle!

You cannot destroy the star system, because at rock bottom it is the public who create and acclaim the stars.

The Enjoyment of Fear

Alfred Hitchcock

I suppose the proper way to begin a piece on the enjoyment of fear would be to prove that such a thing exists. Can fear be enjoyable? Or even pleasant? I was discussing this point with an old friend not long ago.

"Fear," he said, "is the least pleasant of all emotions. I experienced it when I was a boy, and again during both wars. I never want my children to experience it. I think it entirely possible, if I have anything to say about it, that they'll live their entire lives and never know the meaning of the word."

"Oh," I said, "what a dreadful prospect!" My friend looked at me quizzically. "I mean it," I went on. "The boys will never be able to ride a roller coaster, or climb a mountain, or take a midnight stroll through a graveyard. And when they're older"—my friend is a champion motorboat racer—"there'll be no speedboating for them."

"What do you mean?" he asked, obviously offended.

"Well, now, let's take the speedboat racing, for instance. Can you honestly tell me that the sensation you get when you cut close to a pylon, or rough water, with a boat riding close on one side and another skidding across in front of you, is anything but fear? Can you deny that a day on the water without fear, without that prickly sensation as the short hairs on your neck rise, would be an utter dead failure? It seems to me that you pay lots of money a year for fear. Why do you want to deny it to your sons?"

"I'd never thought of it quite that way," he said. And he hadn't.

Few people have. That's why my statement, made in all sincerity, that millions of people every day pay huge sums of money and go to great hardship merely to *enjoy* fear seems paradoxical. Yet it is no exaggeration. Any carnival man will tell you the rides that attract the greatest clientele are those that inspire the greatest fear. It is self-evident that the poloist, the steeplechaser, the speedboat racer, and the fox hunter ride for the thrill that comes only from danger. The boy who walks a tightrope or tiptoes along the top of a picket fence is looking for fear, as are the auto racer, the mountain climber, and the big-game hunter.

And that is only the beginning. For every person who seeks fear in the real or personal sense, millions seek it vicariously, in the theater and in the cinema. In darkened auditoriums they identify themselves with fictitious characters who are experiencing fear, and experience, themselves, the same fear sensations (the quickened pulse, the alternately dry and damp palm, etc.), but without paying the price. That the price need not be paid—indeed, must not be paid—is the important factor. Take, for example, one of the classic fear situations: the legendary, though now sadly obsolete, circular band-saw approaching the bound and gagged heroine. If this distressing contretemps were to exist in real life, the emotional experience of the helpless young woman as the saw approached would be anything but pleasant. Even if one merely viewed a real person thus jeopardized, it would be most displeasing. The suburban matron whose eyes all but pop out of her head with ecstatic excitement as she watches the cinematic blade approach the cinematic neck would no doubt faint dead away if she encountered a similar problem in her home. Why, then, does she enjoy it in the movies?

Precisely because the price will not be paid and she knows it. The saw will never reach its intended target. The plot may, and indeed should, indicate that the heroine's rescue is totally impossible. But deep in the subconscious mind of the spectator is the certainty, engendered by attendance at similar dramatic works, that the totally impossible will occur. The hero, though we have just been made aware that he lies unconscious at the bottom of a pit, surrounded by rattlesnakes, boiling oil, and the smell of bitter almonds, will appear in time to reverse the action of the saw and trap the villain. Or the saw will break down. Or it will appear that the villain has carelessly neglected to sharpen it—or, if it is an electric saw, to pay his electric bill. Fear and fear not, that is the essence of melodrama. Fear: the saw may dismember the ingénue. Fear not: it won't.

Fear in the cinema is my special field, and I have, perhaps dogmatically, but I think with good cause, split cinematic fear into two broad categories—terror and suspense. The difference is comparable to the difference between a buzz bomb and a V-2.

To anyone who has experienced attacks by both bombs, the distinction will be clear. The buzz bomb made a noise like an outboard motor, and its chugging in the air above served as notice of its impending arrival. When the motor stopped, the bomb was beginning its descent and would shortly explode. The moments between the time the motor was first heard and the final explosion were moments of *suspense*. The V-2, on the other hand, was noiseless until the moment of its explosion. Anyone who heard a V-2 explode, and lived, had experienced *terror*.

Another example, one that has been experienced by most of us, may make the distinction more definite. Walking down a dimly lighted street in the late hours of the night, with no other people about, a person may find his mind playing strange tricks. The silence, the loneliness, and the gloom may set the scene for fear.

Suddenly a dark form thrusts itself before the lonely walker. *Terror.* It does not matter that the form was a waving branch, a newspaper picked up by a gust of wind, or simply an oddly shaped shadow unexpectedly coming into view. Whatever it was, it produced its moment of terror.

The same walker, on the same dark street, might have no inclination toward fear. The sound of footsteps coming from somewhere behind might cause the late stroller to become curious, then uneasy, then fearful. The walker stops, the footsteps are not heard; the pace is increased, so also the tempo of the thin sounds coming out of the night. *Suspense.* The echo of his own steps? Probably. But suspense.

On the screen, terror is induced by surprise; suspense, by forewarning. Let us suppose, to make all this clear, that our plot is concerned with a married woman residing in Manhattan and engaged in amorous dalliance with a young cad.

The young cad learns that his inamorata's husband is in Detroit on business and immediately proceeds to the lady's apartment. The two are there engaged in activity as compromising as the censors will permit. Suddenly the door is flung open. There stands the enraged spouse, gun in hand. Net result: terror. There is no suspense whatsoever in the sequence, for the possibility that the husband might be in the vicinity was never hinted by the lovers, and the audience, identifying itself with them, must share their shock at the husband's entrance.

Now, how could we play that incident if we wished to create, not terror, but suspense? Remember our rule: terror by surprise, suspense by forewarning. Very well, we begin with the two lovers in the hotel room. The husband, we learn from the less personal fragments of their conversation, is presumed by them to be in Detroit. Then we see the husband alighting from an airplane. But what is this? This is not Detroit, but New York! For the benefit of those who are not familiar with the two airports, we incorporate a significant glance at an identifying sign at the airport or, perhaps better, at the license plate of the cab as the husband gives the address of the hotel.

Now back to the two lovers. Note that, in this telling, the audience cannot identify itself with the lovers, because the audience knows what the lovers do not, that the husband is on his way and may trap them. But the audience cannot identify itself with the husband either, for the audience knows what he, poor fellow, only suspects: his wife is unfaithful. Now we go back and forth between the lovers and the husband. They continue their lovemaking. The husband alights from his cab. The cad straightens his tie and prepares to depart. The husband begins to mount the stairs. Will he arrive in time? Will the cad make good his escape? What will happen if he does not? These are the questions that the audience asks itself, and whether or not the husband arrives in time, a suspenseful situation has been created.

It is obvious from the above that suspense and terror cannot coexist. To the extent that the audience is aware of the menace or danger to the people it is watching—that is, to the extent that suspense is created—so is its surprise (or terror) at the eventual materialization of the indicated danger diminished. This poses a pretty problem for the director and for the writer of a motion picture. Shall the terror be diminished to enhance the suspense; or shall all suspense be eliminated by making the surprise complete and the terror as shocking to the audience as to the fictional participants?

The terror-suspense dilemma is normally resolved by compromise. There are several situations in a motion picture; the ordinary, and I think best, practice is to play most of the situations for suspense and a few for terror. Suspense is more enjoyable than terror, actually, because it is a continuing experience and attains a peak crescendo fashion; while terror, to be truly effective, must come all at once, like a bolt of lightning, and is more difficult, therefore, to savor.

However, one conflict in making pictures in which fear is a major element cannot be compromised. That is the conflict between the validity of the plot and situations and the implied guarantee given the audience that it shall not "pay the price" for its fear. To the roller-coaster operator that is a simple problem; it means that, although in appearance the ride must be as terrifying as possible, it must, in reality, be completely safe. The pleasant fear sensation experienced by a roller-coaster rider as the car approached a sharp curve would cease to exist if he seriously thought for one moment that the car might really fail to negotiate the curve. The audience at a motion picture is, of course, entirely safe from that point of view. Though knives and guns may be used on the screen, the audience is aware that no one out front is going to be shot or stabbed. But the audience must also be aware that the characters in the picture, with whom they strongly identify themselves, are not to pay the price of fear. This awareness must be entirely subconscious; the spectator must *know* that the spy ring will never succeed in pitching Madeleine Carroll off London Bridge, and the spectator must be induced to *forget* what he knows. If he didn't *know,* he would be genuinely worried; if he didn't *forget,* he would be bored.

What all this amounts to is this: as the audience sympathy for a character is built up, the audience assumes that a sort of invisible cloak to protect the wearer from harm is being fitted. Once the sympathies are fully established and the cloak is finished, it is not—in the audience opinion, and in the opinion of many critics—fair play to violate the cloak and bring its wearer to a disastrous end. I did it once, in a picture called *Sabotage.* One of the characters was a small boy, with whom the audience was encouraged to fall in love. I sent the boy wandering about London with what he supposed was a can of film under his arm, but what the audience knew full well contained a time bomb. Under this set of circumstance, the lad is protected by his cloak from premature explosion of the bomb. I blew him up anyway, along with several other passengers on a bus he happened to be riding.

Now, that episode in *Sabotage* was a direct negation of the invisible cloak of protection worn by sympathetic characters in motion pictures. In addition, because the audience knew the film can contained a bomb and the boy did not, to permit the bomb to explode was a violation of the rule forbidding a direct combination of suspense and terror, or forewarning and surprise. Had the audience not been informed of the real contents of the can, the explosion would have come as a complete surprise. As a result of a sort of emotional numbness induced by a shock of this kind, I believe their sensibilities might not have been so thoroughly outraged. As it was, the audiences—and the critics, too—were unanimously of the opinion that I should have been riding in the seat next to the lad, preferably the seat he set the bomb on.

The Television Broadcasting Age

LESSON EIGHT

Anti-Communism and Hollywood

HUAC, the Blacklist, and the Decline of Social Cinema

Brian Neve

The Origins of the Blacklist

The Hollywood Blacklist had its origins in the 1947 decision of the House Committee on Un-American Activities (HUAC) to hold hearings on communism in Hollywood. The committee had been formed in 1938, but only became a standing committee of the House of Representatives in 1945, at the prompting of notorious anti-Semitic Congressman John Rankin of Mississippi. Thereafter, in the years of an emerging Cold War politics, HUAC became a vehicle for politicians who opposed the New Deal tradition of social democracy and reform. The committee followed the example of the Joint Fact-Finding Committee of the California legislature (the Tenney Committee), which had held hearings on Communist influence in Hollywood since 1943. The November 1946 elections had returned Republican majorities to both houses of Congress, while the ground for ideological conflict within the film capital had already been prepared by the founding in 1944 of the Motion Picture Alliance for the Preservation of American Ideals (Motion Picture Alliance).[1]

The Motion Picture Alliance, which included such figures as Sam Wood, Walt Disney, and Lela Rogers (mother of Ginger Rogers), drew attention to what its members saw as left-wing propaganda in wartime film and the left-leaning influence of, in particular, Hollywood screenwriters. Many key members had strong associations with William Randolph Hearst, who had used his media outlets since the mid-1930s to publicize his anti-Communist position, while the Alliance also included veterans of the conservative fight against studio recognition of the Screen Writers Guild (achieved in 1940). The emergence of the Cold War and President Truman's executive order of March 1947, establishing a loyalty program for the executive branch, established an image of domestic subversion within government, while bitter industrial conflicts of 1945–1946 further polarized Hollywood politics. There was union-related violence at Warner Bros. and other studios as the Conference of Studio Unions (CSU) became involved in a prolonged dispute with both the studios and the International Alliance of Theatrical Stage Employees (IATSE). The CSU strike of 1946 was countered by a studio lockout, and by December 1946 IATSE had taken firm control of the Hollywood crafts unions. With the defeat of the CSU, Roy Brewer, the new West Coast head of IATSE, emerged as a powerful Motion Picture Alliance figure. He testified to HUAC in 1947 about what he saw as Communist responsibility for the labor disturbances.[2]

Not only Alliance members encouraged the House Committee to investigate Hollywood communism. During the first year of J. Parnell Thomas's chairmanship of HUAC, 1947, the Committee developed a close relationship with the FBI, which had collected extensive information on Hollywood communism with the aid of numerous informers. Amongst the studio moguls it was Jack Warner who stoked the fires of the anti-Communist crusade by providing the committee, meeting covertly in Los Angeles in May 1947, with horror stories of Communists working at his studio. Warner Bros. had been the most socially conscious of the Hollywood companies, but Jack Warner had been strongly influenced by the picket line violence at his studio in 1945.

It was in October 1947 that the formal hearings took place in Washington, D.C. In the first week there was testimony from "friendly" witnesses, mainly from the Motion Picture Alliance, as well as from defensive studio bosses, of whom the most cooperative was again Jack Warner. The second week was reserved for the testimony of nineteen more witnesses who were, for the most part, both screenwriters and Communists. (Edward Dmytryk and Adrian Scott seem to have been included at the last minute because of their responsibility, as director and producer, for the recently completed film attacking anti-Semitism, *Crossfire*, 1947).

With widespread liberal and industry fears of a blacklist, there was strong general support for the principle of the First Amendment on which these initial nineteen witnesses had agreed to stand. In particular, liberals Philip Dunne, William Wyler, and John Huston had organized the Committee for the First Amendment, and arranged for a planeload of stars to visit Washington prior to the second week of hearings. Yet the First Amendment strategy was implicit rather than explicit in the testimony of the ten "unfriendly" witnesses—Alvah Bessie, Herbert Biberman, Lester Cole, Edward Dmytryk, Ring Lardner Jr., John Howard Lawson, Albert Maltz, Samuel Ornitz, Adrian Scott, Dalton Trumbo—who were called on to testify before the hearings were unexpectedly suspended. Several of them became involved in a shouting match with Chairman Thomas, and all followed the example of the initial witness, screenwriter John Howard Lawson, in refusing to answer questions as to their membership in the party. The Hollywood Ten were each cited for contempt of Congress. HUAC publicized apparent evidence of their Communist affiliations (for example, Lawson's leadership role in the party was widely known), and therefore liberal support for the unfriendly witnesses' First Amendment rights collapsed in a few weeks. Some liberals were shocked at the performance of the Ten, while others—for example, Humphrey Bogart, who had traveled to Washington with the Committee for the First Amendment—came under fierce studio pressure to publicly denounce communism.

Eric Johnston, president of the Motion Picture Producers Association (MPAA), and spokesman for the producers and their boards of directors, had originally resisted any blacklist, but with the committee producing evidence of Communist membership, he quickly came to terms with the strength of the opposition. On 24 November the House of Representatives voted overwhelmingly for the citation of the Hollywood Ten for contempt of Congress. On the same day Johnston convened a meeting of studio producers and executives at the Waldorf-Astoria Hotel in New York. Their discussions led to the drafting, by a committee of five including Dore Schary, of the so-called Waldorf Statement, declaring that the studios would dismiss those of the Hollywood Ten under contract and would not re-employ any of them "until such time as he is acquitted or has purged himself of contempt and declared under oath that he is not a Communist." The statement continued: "We will not knowingly employ a Communist or a member of any party or group which advocates the overthrow of the Government of the United States by force or by any illegal or unconstitutional methods."[3] This statement essentially instituted a blacklist, although the full implementation would have to wait three years for the appeals of the Ten to be exhausted. (It is interesting to note, that although much discussion of the blacklist centers on the "Hollywood Ten," an eleventh man, Bertolt Brecht, also testified, denied being a Communist, and immediately left the country for Europe. Additional "unfriendly" witnesses who agreed not to cooperate with the committee but who were not called to testify in 1947 were Richard Collins, Gordon Kahn, Howard Koch, Lewis Milestone, Larry Parks, Irving Pichel, Robert Rossen, and Waldo Salt.)

There were soon indications that in the wake of this decision the studios were becoming more wary of social topics. Eric Johnston argued in 1947 that "We'll have no more films that show the seamy side of American life," while the same year William Wyler suggested that in the "current climate" he would no longer be allowed to make *The Best Years of Our Lives* (1946).[4] Yet the late 1940s saw various forms of social cinema, from the much celebrated social problem films *Crossfire* (1947) and *Gentleman's Agreement* (1948), to the cycles of films that would later be classified as semi-documentary and film noir. Location shooting allowed inexperienced but ambitious directors a degree of freedom from traditional studio supervision and also contributed to a greater sense of real life being recorded on film, while crime thrillers often allowed a political critique to be expressed in a disguised (and deniable) form. The unexpected re-election of Harry Truman in November 1948 was even taken as evidence that "liberal days were here again," encouraging studio heads to give the go-ahead to a group of films that raised and articulated (however belatedly) a set of liberal positions and ideas on race. What is more difficult to assess is the impact of the darkening national and international political situation, with the emergence of a Cold War agenda and an international specter of "Red Fascism" at the expense of the dominant concerns of the long Roosevelt era. With a series of economic and other shocks to the established studio system, including the decline in audiences from 1947 and the culmination of the administration's anti-trust action in 1948, it was increasingly clear that the established industry leaders and producers had to plan for change.[5]

Writers were notoriously low in the Hollywood pecking order, yet subsequent scholarship has done much to establish the impact of liberal and left-wing writers in important areas of film in the Depression years, during the war, and for a time after the war. The broad agreement of liberals and radicals on an anti-fascist and progressive agenda (especially during the late thirties and the war years, when the American Communist Party encouraged such an alliance) was seen as a "Popular Front." By the late forties this unity was in rapid decline (symbolized by the collapse of rank and file support for the Committee for the First Amendment), but the left-wing writer and director Abraham Polonsky referred to this time in the changing Hollywood system as providing "interesting" opportunities for a "thirties" generation of socially minded artists. This group of Depression era writers and especially directors were gaining a tentative foothold in the industry. Their distinctive social and aesthetic goals constituted a perceived threat to the producer-dominated studio system with its "pure entertainment" ethic. The search for postwar subjects, the wartime experiences of filmmakers, the trend toward independent production, and the opportunities for location shooting had all seemed to increase the range of issues and images in postwar cinema. Yet the deepening association in the public mind of the American Communist Party with a Soviet Union that was now a key international enemy of the United States meant that the days of the Popular Front alliance between radicals and liberals were numbered. Albert Maltz's appeal to John Huston in 1949, calling for an alliance against the forces of reaction on the basis of "common Jeffersonian principles," was in vain. Arthur Schlesinger, standard bearer for a new anti-Communist liberalism, a "vital center," was nearer the dominant current of intellectual thought, while those in Hollywood with radical associations were increasingly looking over their shoulders. When in 1950 the Supreme Court declined to review the cases of Dalton Trumbo and John Howard Lawson, appealing on behalf of the Hollywood Ten, the blacklist already implicit in Eric Johnston's statement was ready to be implemented.[6]

While some key social problem films, from *Crossfire* to *Gentleman's Agreement* and *Pinky* (1949) were successful at the box office, not all of them were seen as suitable for the increasingly important foreign market, either in economic or public relations terms. The decline in domestic audiences placed greater emphasis on the maintenance and expansion of foreign markets for American films. As Richard Maltby points out, the industry's need for State Department help in exploiting these markets hindered Hollywood's "social conscience" by obligating an increasingly "optimistic portrayal of the American way of life." Frank Capra, who had used radical and liberal writers in constructing his ultimately affirmative vision of America, commented in 1947 that: "Our job will be to make all criticisms expressed add up to praise—and I say it's going to be tough."[7] Only three weeks before the Waldorf Statement Dore Schary had called for renewed thought to be given to the "effect of our pictures abroad."[8] By the early 1950s, with the involvement of the CIA in America's international image, this would become an even more important consideration.

HUAC, McCarthyism, and the Blacklist

The effect of the new Cold War agenda on Hollywood can be seen in terms of the decision by the Supreme Court in 1950 not to review the appeal by Hollywood Ten members Dalton Trumbo and John Howard Lawson against the 1947 "contempt of Congress" conviction. In 1949 Justices Frank Murphy and Wiley B. Rutledge had died within two months of each other. With two other justices, they had been seen as a solid voting bloc on the Court in favor of civil liberties, giving First

Amendment issues preferred status in their deliberations. Yet by 1949 the pressures on President Truman were such that he filled the two vacancies on the Court by appointing conservative justices who were prepared to give more weight to issues of national security. In May 1950 the refusal of the reconstituted Court to review the case brought on behalf of the Ten led to them all serving prison sentences of six months to a year during 1950–1951. In a speech in New York in June 1950, before serving his sentence, Ring Lardner Jr. had commented that a Court with "Murphy, Rutledge, Douglas and Black could be counted on to slap down the demagogues." The next year, in the Dennis case, the same Court upheld the conviction of the leaders of the American Communist Party under the Smith Act for advocating the overthrow of the United States government. This case virtually outlawed the Communist Party, as well as legitimating the "anti-communist crusade" that was to follow."[9]

By 1950 the country was in the grip of something like a national panic over what was seen, at all levels of society, as a plausible domestic and international threat of communism. By February, when Senator Joseph McCarthy began his period in the limelight with his notorious speech in Wheeling, West Virginia, he was in part reacting to the conviction of Alger Hiss, the former State Department official and Roosevelt aide who had been accused by HUAC in 1948 of passing secrets to a Communist spy ring. To cultural historian Richard Pells, the conviction of Hiss lent credence to "the theory that all communists should be regarded as potential foreign agents." Later in 1950 the war in Korea began and Ethel and Julius Rosenberg were arrested on a charge of conspiracy to commit espionage, further fueling the obsession of the FBI and professional blacklisting organizations with Communists as actual or potential spies.[10] Indeed by this time domestic communism was seen largely in terms of an actual or potential Soviet threat to the interests of the state, rather than as a movement of radicals with varying degrees of relationship with the national Communist leadership.

In May 1950 the Motion Picture Alliance called for a "complete delousing" of the film industry. Its new president, John Wayne, felt that producers had not delivered on the commitments of the Waldorf Statement, and Alliance members welcomed what seemed to be an impending second wave of Congressional intervention. In June a booklet on the left-wing affiliations of television and radio personnel, *Red Channels,* was published, while in September Harry Warner addressed 2,000 Warner Bros. employees and executives on a sound stage about the Communist threat, making it clear that he wanted no Communists at the studio. In the summer there was also a protracted battle between liberal and conservative factions of the Screen Directors Guild over a plan, urged on the Guild membership by arch anti-Communist Cecil B. DeMille during the absence from the country of Guild President Joseph L. Mankiewiez, to introduce a mandatory oath for existing and new members affirming non-adherence to the Communist party. To DeMille, who was finally forced to back down in an epic membership meeting, the "question we are asking is, are you on the American side or on the other side."[11]

As anticipated, in March 1951 the House Committee resumed its Washington hearings on communism in the film industry. In effect, in the period from 1951 to 1953, the blacklist that was announced in 1947 was enforced. The core group of those who then found themselves unemployable by the main studios were those known by the authorities to have been Communists, and who, on being subpoenaed, declined to cooperate with the committee. Given the fate of those who pleaded the First Amendment in 1947, those unwilling to cooperate with the committee by naming names, were advised to invoke the Fifth Amendment against self-incrimination. While the committee and the FBI knew the names of present and past Communists, the naming of names by former members of the Communist party, together with a recantation of past beliefs, was a ritual required of those who wished to return to work. While witnesses may have left the party many years before, most still regarded their public identification of previous friends and colleagues as Communist party members as a process of informing that was morally repugnant. Many ultimately took part in what historian and journalist Victor Navasky later called "degradation ceremonies," or the naming of names, because this is what was required for them to be able to work again in the film industry, using their own names.

Those who declined to answer questions on the party membership of others invoked the Fifth Amendment. But in effect such a stance was taken as evidence that the individual had something to hide—in terms of present or past party membership—and they found themselves unemployable in the studios that were a party to the Waldorf Statement. Those who cooperated added names to the blacklist, unless the individuals concerned could clear themselves either before the committee, or through other clearance mechanisms soon to be established. In the hearings held in Washington from 1951 to 1953, over 200 Communists were named. In the first two years of the new bout of hearings Larry Parks, Richard Collins, Budd Schulberg, Edward Dmytryk (reversing his position as one of the original Hollywood Ten), Elia Kazan, Clifford Odets, and Sterling Hayden (who later declared himself ashamed of his testimony) were among those who became "friendly" witnesses, while Howard Da Silva, Abraham Polonsky, Paul Jarrico, Carl Foreman, and Lillian Hellman were among those who took the Fifth in the same period. Robert Rossen testified in 1951 about his own party membership but declined to name others, but in 1953 he returned to the committee as a friendly witness. The blacklisted actor Mickey Knox remembers Rossen telling him at the time that: "I did a terrible thing. I named my friends. But I have to work." Some blacklisted writers continued to work covertly, usually at a fraction of the salary, and often on unpromising assignments, while others moved abroad. Using fronts was not an option for directors (or actors), and an important group of directors interested in social or political themes, a number of whom had begun to develop reputations in the late forties, also looked for work abroad. The group included Joseph Losey, Jules Dassin, John Berry, Bernard Vorhaus, and Cy Endfield.[12]

While the studios' blacklist was generated essentially by the House Committee, with the complicity of those who gave it names, a number of private organizations exploited and expanded the process in the early 1950s for a mixture of commercial and ideological motives. American Business Consultants, formed in 1947 by ex-FBI men, marketed books and newsletters, in particular *Red Channels* (1950) and *Counterattack,* to employers and advertisers interested in the leftist associations of those in the entertainment industry. Other muckraking publications, including *Alert* ("A Weekly Confidential Report on Communism and How to Combat It"), available from 1951, and organizations including Aware ("An organization to combat the Communist conspiracy in the entertainment world"), set up in 1952, also touted sensational allegations. But by far the most influential organization in this period in expanding the blacklist and helping to create a wider "graylist" was the American Legion. The Legion with its 3,000 branches produced the most credible threat to picket theaters playing non-conforming movies, and its leadership and publications, including *Firing Line,* had a direct effect on the studios and their hiring policies.

In addition to the blacklist of over 200 Communists or ex-Communists, a graylist of a hundred or more artists with left or liberal associations operated in the early fifties. For example, Lewis Milestone, a "Popular Fronter" but not a party member, and a director who had bemoaned a state of "No pictures with messages" in 1949, spent the first half of the fifties in Europe in part because his presence on such a list made it difficult or impossible to get work. An issue of *Alert* in January 1951 referred to Milestone and Michael Blankfort, director and writer of *Halls of Montezuma* (1950) as "two notorious participants in Communist fronts and causes." The director Vincent Sherman was also on a graylist for eighteen months in the early fifties, in part because the magazine *Counterattack* was sending out confidential letters to his studio heads detailing his associations with alleged Communist fronts. The tenor of *Counterattack*'s campaign can be judged from other statements in their typewritten reports. One refers to "Isadore Scharf (pardon me, I mean Dore Schary)," an anti-Semitic reference to the studio head's full name, which was Isidore Schary. Another, in April 1951, suggests that the only way to "clear up the hundreds of Communists and pro-Communists" in the industry is to "get a boycott rolling against those producers and Moscow maggots in their casts."[13]

The American Legion never authorized a national boycott, although a number of right-wing groups further weakened industry resistance to the blacklist by picketing theaters that were showing suspect films. A group called Catholic War Veterans picketed *Born Yesterday* (1950) when it opened in New York. According to the film's star, Judy Holliday, whose political associations had been publicized by *Red Channels,* the placards read "While our boys are dying in Korea, Judy Holliday is instead defaming Congress." *Death of a Salesman* (1951) was picketed by a group called the Wage Earners Committee, calling attention not only to the supposedly subversive nature of Arthur Miller's original play, but to producer Stanley Kramer's "Record of coddling Reds and pinkos." Also

175

picketed was Joseph Losey's last-but-one American film, M (1951), presumably because of the left-wing associations of Losey and Waldo Salt, who contributed additional dialogue. (Salt was one of the Hollywood Nineteen. He had been subpoenaed by HUAC in 1947 but was not called to testify.) In addition, Ayn Rand's "Screen Guide for Americans," a pamphlet which in particular encouraged favorable screen treatment of business, was published by the Motion Picture Alliance. Blacklisting organizations were particularly hostile to what was seen as social realism. *Firing Line* ("Facts for Fighting Communism"), for example, warned its readers against the film version of *Death of a Salesman*: this "realistic picture of American Life," it argued, "will naturally be welcomed by Stalinists all over the world," and will give an "unflattering portrait of American life" to millions of foreigners. *Firing Line* also warned its readers about other distinctive if disparate films, including *Viva Zapata!* (1952), *Saturday's Hero* (1951), Chaplin's forthcoming *Limelight* (1952), and the liberal science fiction fable, *The Day the Earth Stood Still* (1951).[14]

The American Legion significantly increased the pressure by publishing an article by J. B. Matthews, "Did the Movies Really Clean House?," in December 1951. (Matthews, a fellow traveller turned anti-Communist, had been a star witness for HUAC in its first incarnation under the chairmanship of Martin Dies in 1938. A longtime Hearst associate, his voluminous study of the left-wing affiliations of Hollywood personnel had helped prompt Rankin's interest in a new investigation in 1945.) The studios and their financial backers were particularly frightened by the threat of American Legion picketing of theaters explicit in the Matthews article. There followed a reported "fruitful" meeting between the American Legion, Eric Johnston, and representatives of the key producing companies in March 1952. Out of this meeting, clearance procedures were established. These procedures involved the blacklisted artists writing explanatory letters to the American Legion, where "experts," including the veteran Hearst columnist George Sokolsky, actor Ward Bond, and union boss Roy Brewer, would separate the "liberal lambs from the Communist wolves." One studio that developed its own political screening program at this time was RKO Radio Pictures, with studio head Howard Hughes closing down production for three months in 1952 for this purpose.[15]

This pressure added to the woes of an industry already laying off workers in response to declining audiences and foreign markets. Yet in 1952 a group of anonymous screenwriters suggested that the continued investigations were seen by film executives as a mixed blessing, as not only were workers and unions "pacified, but the industry was enabled to 'slash employees pay-checks.' "[16] This argument seems to support the later interpretation that the blacklist was, at least in part, "good business" for the studios, enabling them to regain control over the entertainment marketplace after the economic and other "shocks" after the war. Jon Lewis has discussed the blacklist as a postwar business strategy adopted by an industry threatened by political regulation, declining audiences, and antitrust decisions, and he also sees anti-Semitism as a weapon used against both Hollywood Communists and the old-style studio moguls. The number of Hollywood liberals and radicals who were Jewish, and the fear of Jewish moguls that the investigations might encourage a wider anti-Semitism from WASP politicians in Washington, was a distinctive element of this era.[17]

Of those not called before the House Committee, many writers and directors were put under pressure to "clear" themselves by writing a formal letter to their studio employers. In July 1950 W. R. Wilkerson, in his "Trade Views" column in the *Hollywood Reporter,* wrote scathingly of "foreigners," including Billy Wilder and William Wyler, who had criticized the treatment of the Hollywood Ten. He argued that this "is no time for such claptrap and something should be done to muzzle them in the future." In his reply (published two days later) Wyler pointed out that open criticism of government was, "according to the principles on which our republic is founded," not only permitted but encouraged. Yet Wyler was finally pressed to write to the president of Paramount, Frank Freeman, in May 1954, making clear his "basic feelings and loyalties" and his "position in regard to the worldwide conflict between the Free World of the Democracies and the Slave States of the Soviet System." He drew attention to his sworn statement in the files of the Screen Directors Guild, showing that he had never been a member of the Communist party. He had supported an amici curae brief for Trumbo and Lawson in 1951, but by 1954, in a way that suggests the growing pressure on liberals to disassociate themselves from Communists, he was critical of the Hollywood Ten: "I was one of a group that urged them to deny or affirm membership in that party. I did that in the mistaken belief that members of the group were not members of that party."[18]

While Lillian Hellman (who herself took the Fifth Amendment) and Victor Navasky have written of the blacklist in terms of a simple moral distinction between those who named names and those who resisted, others have suggested a more complicated picture. Certainly many friendly witnesses mentioned disillusionment with the Communist party in their testimony—and party membership in the early fifties was in rapid decline. This may have weakened the resistance of some who went on to cooperate with HUAC. Most current and dedicated party members had little doubt as to what to do, but others, especially those who had been out of the party for some time, clearly balanced the unpleasantness of informing with a reluctance, to paraphrase Edward Dmytryk's words, to sacrifice career and family for a cause they had grown to dislike. Hellman's and Navasky's perspective has rather over-simplified the moral dynamics of the period, or at least under-examined the political dimension of the moral choices that artists faced at the time. The issues always appeared more morally clear-cut to those—the great majority of resisters—who were still committed to the party. Paul Jarrico, a screenwriter who was prominent in the Communist party and who was himself blacklisted, argued that, "for those who were generally pissed off at the party but reluctant to name names, the choice must have been difficult. For a person like me, a true blue red, the choice was easy."[19]

Social Content in Film

While inferences can be made from their previous credits about the effects of the times on some key blacklisted writers, directors, and actors, it is difficult to separate out the effects of the darkening Cold War atmosphere, the blacklist, and other changes in industry and society that were affecting the type of film being made. The concern with the image of America in foreign markets was certainly a factor that influenced the studios, as was the threat of picketing by the American Legion and other organizations. In a survey of the content of American films in the period 1947 to 1954, Dorothy Jones notes in particular a marked decline in social problem films from 1949 to 1952, with more emphasis on "pure entertainment," and in particular more anti-Communist films and war films of the "sure-fire patriotic variety." Jones also points to the Oscar winners of 1950–1952, *All About Eve*, *An American in Paris*, and *The Greatest Show on Earth*, as indicative of the type of product most favored by the Hollywood establishment.[20]

Other interpretations are generally consistent with this analysis, stressing a shift in the early fifties to Westerns, war films, and biblical epics, and to a perspective that was more often psychological than social. To blacklisted writer Walter Bernstein, psychology was in, social criticism was out, and Hollywood was becoming increasingly concerned to reflect the perspectives of a growing younger audience. At the time, the critic Manny Farber pointed to another development, a wave of "art or mood" films including *A Streetcar Named Desire*, *A Place in the Sun*, and *Sunset Boulevard* (all 1951); to Farber these "Freud-Marx epics" represented the social significance of the 1930s gone sour. Larry May, in his own study of what he sees as a cultural reconstruction of American national identity in the Cold War period, uses an analysis of thousands of film plots from the trade paper the *Motion Picture Herald* as a source of evidence on the key changes in theme from the 1930s to the 1950s. He charts a decline in unhappy (what he calls Noir) endings in the fifties, a rise in the focus on youth as an alternative to the adult world over the same period, and a fall in the incidence of depictions both of the rich as a moral threat and of big business as villainous.[21]

Certainly the early 1950s saw a tailing-off of the crime dramas now classified as part of the film noir cycle. Thom Andersen has written of a sub-group of noir films—he labeled them "films gris"—which was characteristic of the period 1947–1951. These films shared some of the stylistic features associated with film noir but dealt in particular with social issues and exhibited an awareness of class as a critical factor in American life. Such films looked back to the 1930s in their politics, and were increasingly viewed with suspicion by those concerned that Hollywood films affirm America to a global market. The writers and particularly the directors who were most responsible for this cycle of films were those most affected by the second wave of Congressional investigations. Jules Dassin, for example, directed *Thieves Highway* (1949) and *Night and the City* (1950) before becoming a victim of the blacklist and moving permanently to Europe. Nicholas Ray avoided the blacklist, but his work in the late forties, including *They Live by Night* (1949) and *Knock on Any Door* (1949), dealt with the problems of youth in a way that clearly relates, in retrospect, to Andersen's notion of work and the "psychological injuries of class." Ray also worked in part in Europe in the fifties, and was reportedly on a graylist for a time, while arguably making metaphoric reference to the blacklist in *In a Lonely Place* (1950) and *Johnny Guitar* (1954). The youthful rebels of the fifties became cultural icons, but were rarely linked to broader social forces. *The Wild One* (1954) appeared shorn of most of its criticism of business following PCA pressure, while the James Dean persona in Kazan's *East of Eden* (1954) and Ray's own *Rebel Without a Cause* (1955) is primarily defined in terms of conflicts within the family.[22]

Two other directors associated with some form of social drama who left America for Europe for political reasons were Joseph Losey and Cy Endfield. *The Prowler* (1951), from a script mainly written by Dalton Trumbo, certainly fits the main contours of Andersen's model. To Losey the film was about "false values": " '100,000 bucks, a Cadillac, and a blonde' were the sine qua non of American life at the time and it didn't matter how you got them—whether you stole the girl from somebody else, stole the money, and got the Cadillac from corruption." In an early scene a policeman, Webb Garwood (Van Heflin) is called to a baroque Los Angeles house to investigate a suspected prowler. He there begins a relationship with a lonely woman, Susan Gilvray (Evelyn Keyes), attracted to the lifestyle and social status that she represents. Class envy and sexual passion are blended, and writer and director, sharing a social perspective on the material, both contribute to what becomes, with a little help from the PCA, a social morality tale. Soon after the film's release Losey, anticipating the imminent delivery of a subpoena, left for London, while Trumbo began a period in exile in Mexico.[23]

Cy Endfield also moved to London, and one of his last American films is characteristic of the perspective and approach that was being marginalized by the politics of the time. *Try and Get Me! (The Sound of Fury)* (1951) was one of the last of the socially pointed noir films of the late forties and early fifties. Within a study of yellow journalism, crime, and mob violence, the film sets out a notion of false values, as family man Howard Tyler (Frank Lovejoy), desperate to find work, strays into petty crime and ultimate victimhood. The PCA suggested its usual "voice for morality," and warned against "any philosophizing that might seem to relieve your murderers of the blame for their crimes and put this blame on society generally." Yet the film still provides an unusual view of the pressures of unemployment on family and breadwinner, and it represents a dimension of film that Endfield and others might have explored further had circumstances been different.[24]

Perhaps the core figures of this small body of work, however, were the actor John Garfield and the radical writer-director Abraham Polonsky. Garfield received his training as an actor within the legendary Group Theatre in New York in the thirties, gaining prominence following his role in Clifford Odets's *Awake and Sing* in 1935. The actor had helped to set up Enterprise Pictures on leaving Warners in 1946, and had appeared in two key late-forties films with political significance, the upbeat *Body and Soul* (Robert Rossen, 1947) and the dark *Force of Evil* (Polonsky, 1948), both from Polonsky scripts. It was Garfield who had insisted on the reinstating of Hemingway's black character in *The Breaking Point* (Michael Curtiz, 1951), providing what Thomas Cripps calls a "bold stride towards a humane portrayal of interracial comradeship." Although the FBI knew Garfield was not a Communist, he was subpoenaed in March 1951 and then harassed further when he talked of his own political affiliations but refused to discuss others'; he was pushed into a magazine recantation of his political views before he died of a heart attack in May 1952. Polonsky, writing about Garfield, said that the "Group trained him, the movies made him, the Blacklist killed him." The director of *Force of Evil* had written a typically witty and politically informed script for *I Can Get It for You Wholesale* (Michael Gordon, 1951)—informed in particular by his concern with sexual double standards and the pervasive effects of capitalist values—before returning from a trip to France to face HUAC. Tracked and wiretapped by the FBI, Polonsky took the Fifth Amendment in April 1951 at a hearing at which the chair, the conservative Republican Harold Velde of Illinois, described him as "a very dangerous citizen." In the mid-fifties Polonsky worked anonymously on a number of scripts, as well as writing a series of "You Are There" teleplays for CBS television, and a novel, *A Season of Fear,* dealing with the blacklist. His banishment from film following the hearing raises questions about how his highly integrated art and politics might have developed ill 1960s absence of a blacklist. As it was, Polonsky remained on the blacklist until late in the sixties when he received screenplay credit (his first since 1951) for *Madigan* (Don Siegel, 1968) and returned to directing with *Tell Them Willie Boy Is Here* (1969).[25]

A cycle of films released in 1949 and 1950 brought a new and liberal perspective to the question of race prejudice in America. The so-called "message cycle," including *Pinky* (Elia Kazan, 1949) and *Intruder in the Dust* (Clarence Brown, 1949), came to an end more because it had run its course than because of any pressure on producers in this area. Joseph Mankiewicz's *No Way Out* (1950), with Sidney Poitier in his first feature film role, was the most forthright of the cycle. Thomas Cripps has suggested that the "central metaphor of integrationism" in these films influenced the later themes of the civil rights movement.[26]

After 1950, according to film historian David Eldridge, the changed political atmosphere made it "difficult for politically and socially sensitive films to get made in this period." CIA monitoring of the social content of the movies, certainly in 1953, shows the U.S. government's strong concern with America's movie image (and especially with foreign perceptions of America).[27] From different positions, reactionaries, conservatives and "corporate liberals" influenced the blacklist and the movie agenda in the early fifties. As Jonathan Munby argues, Eric Johnston's desire for an end to Depression memories and for affirmative images of a new America of economic abundance and class consensus all too easily aligned with the distinct resentments and agendas of the Motion Picture Alliance and HUAC.[28]

Throughout the 1950s, studios and producers were wary of scripts that might attract the attention of the professional blacklisters. Bernard Vorhaus, soon to be blacklisted, remembers trying to interest two studios in a social problem story and finding that such topics, unpolitical but "critical of certain conditions," were seen at the time as "suspect." Cy Endfield felt that the box-office success of darker "social" films, including his own *Try and Get Me!* and Billy Wilder's *Ace in the Hole* (also called *The Big Carnival,* 1951) was damaged by a change of public mood at the onset of the Korean War. The studios were particularly sensitive about American social content in films pitched at foreign markets, while in any case, by the middle of the decade the relative prosperity was throwing up problems that seemed quite distinct from those of the 1930s and the war years.[29]

Another blacklisted writer, Michael Wilson, who wrote the script for *Salt of the Earth* (1953), contributed several articles to *Hollywood Review* on the impact of the contemporary political mood on screen content. Into the vacuum created by the collapse of the humanist strand in filmmaking, Wilson argued, had come a series of films set in World War II that glorified the services. In 1954 he complained that not only had anything even remotely resembling the Mr. Deeds character (in Frank Capra's *Mr Deeds Goes to Town,* 1936) vanished from the screen, but also that the "fascist personality" was replacing the romantic hero. Capra's decline in the fifties may indicate the natural eclipse of a career, but it may also reflect the problem of marketing his populist fables in a Cold War era which was sensitive to anything that looked like social criticism. Only the Western retained some ability to criticize, with *High Noon* (1952) and *Silver Lode* (1954) making oblique reference to contemporary politics, and Anthony Mann's *The Far Country* (1954), presenting serious social reflection in a story from America's mythic past.[30]

Those who cooperated with HUAC and returned to filmmaking after a time away frequently found it difficult to re-engage with familiar genres. The agenda had moved on, as can be seen in the different tones created by Fred Zinnemann, in his film based on James Jones's best selling novel *From Here to Eternity* (1953) and by Edward Dmytryk in *The Caine Mutiny,* a major box-office success of 1954. Dmytryk had served his six-month jail term as one of the Hollywood Ten, but had then "cleared" himself by reappearing as a cooperative witness before HUAC in April 1951, denouncing the Communist party. *The Caine Mutiny* establishes a situation in which the audience supports the naval rebellion, but then the conclusion reverses the whole tone of the story and affirms the principle of obeying authority as a primary obligation. National security undercuts the notion of justified opposition to a tyrant. Another writer-director returning to Hollywood, Robert Rossen, had been a key figure in socially relevant filmmaking since the late thirties, with key credits including his script for Warners' *They Won't Forget* (1937) and his direction of *All the Kings Men* (1949). He returned to filmmaking after his 1953 cooperative testimony with the melodrama *Mambo* (1955) and the epic *Alexander the Great* (1956), but only really returned to the social milieu of his pre-HUAC film career with *The Hustler*, in 1961. As Thomas Schatz argues, the shift in Hollywood themes can be judged by the return of Howard Hawks and John Huston to Warner Bros. as producer-directors in the mid-fifties, nearly a decade after *The Big Sleep* (1946) and *Key Largo* (1948). Hawks returned to make *Land of the Pharaohs* (1955) while Huston, a key figure in the early resistance to HUAC, made *Moby Dick* (1956). Huston's films following *The Asphalt Jungle* (1950), in which crime is examined in class terms, lack the social and political implications (and associations) of virtually all his early work.[31]

The Case of Elia Kazan in the Early 1950s

Elia Kazan was one of a number of artists who arrived in Hollywood from outside, very often from New York theatrical and/or political circles. An extraordinary template for such a career development had been set by Orson Welles at the beginning of the 1940s, with his unprecedented contract at RKO and renowned opening production (*Citizen Kane*, 1941). Later in the decade Abraham Polonsky, Jules Dassin, Joseph Losey, Nicholas Ray, and Elia Kazan also embraced a film industry in which the old studio controls were beginning to weaken. Kazan established a reputation at Twentieth Century–Fox in the late forties by successfully directing both prestigious social problem films and semi-documentary productions. As the 1950s dawned there were signs that Kazan had begun to downplay any overt political associations, but there was every indication that he wanted to work on more independent and ambitious film projects.

Kazan's goals for this new phase in his career were artistic more than explicitly political, but he was conscious that his political associations—his two-year Communist party membership in the mid-1930s—made him vulnerable to any renewed Congressional investigation. Like Welles and others of his generation, Kazan was conscious of the ways in which working in Hollywood involved a conflict between notions of film as art and film as entertainment. For example, the conservative editor of the *Hollywood Reporter,* W. R. Wilkerson, had welcomed the Waldorf Statement as a means of purging the industry of a "thirties" generation of well-educated and serious-minded filmmakers who favored "realism" and felt that entertainment was not enough. In a 1951 letter to Jack Warner, Kazan noted that "from the thinly veiled hints to us in some of Billy Wilkerson's editorial remarks, I gather that his opinion is that *Streetcar* is not the kind of picture he thinks the industry should be making."[32] With *Viva Zapata!*, his "Mexican horse epic," Kazan was again subject to industry pressure via Darryl F. Zanuck's overall supervision, although the location shooting and his own relationship with John Steinbeck as writer were consistent with the director's striving for greater independence.

The intense sensitivity at this time of Zanuck and his studio to the political meanings that might be attached to films is well demonstrated by the debates on the script of *Viva Zapata!* in early 1951. At the time there were political threats to two of Kazan's projects. While Zanuck was asking whether this was "the moment to tell the story of a Mexican revolutionary hero?," another figure in Kazan's immediate social and political milieu, Arthur Miller, was withdrawing from a planned project based on events on the New York waterfront, following political interference and cold feet at Columbia Pictures. Kazan seemed to feel that with *Viva Zapata!* he could handle the studio and make an acceptable compromise, and that the finished film would be broadly consistent with Steinbeck's— and his own—notion of the Mexican revolution. The political pressures of the time clearly led to changes in the script, though the notion of a repudiation of power by the peasant leader can be found in early drafts, and "opposition to communism" remains only a secondary sub-theme in the final version of *Viva Zapata!*[33] In December 1950 Zanuck was worried that audiences (and professional anti-Communists) would associate Zapata with communism: "I hope people don't get the impression that we are advocating revolt or civil war as the only means to peace." The most noticeable of the later script changes was the enlargement of the role of the professional revolutionary, Fernando, in order to balance the sympathy for a revolutionary leader with an explicitly anti-Stalinist motif. The composer Alex North, whom Kazan had brought to Hollywood to score *A Streetcar Named Desire*, wrote critically to his friend that Darryl Zanuck seemed to be the "'strong' man in this version," and that the latest script suggested to him a "post Korean War version with all the not too subtle innuendoes."[34]

Politically, as Richard Slotkin suggests, Steinbeck and Kazan defended a populist idea of the people of Morleos against both the "strong man" dictatorships of Diaz and others and the "left-wing" opportunism of Fernando. However one resolves the debate which any historical reconstruction invites, the film does make the Mexican peasantry a key part of the drama, at times invoking Eisenstein, in ways that are unusual in American cinema.[35]

Viva Zapata! was completed but unreleased by the time that Kazan first appeared before the House Un-American Activities Committee, in January 1952. He answered questions on his own Communist party membership, but refused to give the names of others. The film was released in February, and in a letter in the *Saturday Review of Literature* in early April Kazan discussed how the "political tensions of the present time bore down on us—John Steinbeck, and Darryl Zanuck and me—as we thought about and shaped a historical picture." He pointed out the significance of the "Communist mentality" of the Fernando character, and referred to Zapata as "a man of individual conscience," who led his people "out of bondage and did not betray them." A week later Kazan returned to the House Committee, this time naming eight former members of the Group Theatre as Communists. In an unprecedented paid advertisement in the *New York Times* he argued that those in possession of facts concerning "a dangerous and alien conspiracy" had an obligation to let the facts be known "to the public or to the appropriate Government agency." He supplied the committee with a self-serving account of his career and productions, a list that ended with a reference to *Viva Zapata!* as an "anti-communist picture.[36]

There are those, including historians of the period, who see the film's portrayal of Zapata and his movement as "still subtle, powerful and true." Yet at the time, and in particular in the light of Kazan's testimony, some saw the film as conservative in its implications about the possibility of successful popular revolt. John Howard Lawson, for example, critiqued the film's conservative message as follows: "If power is an absolute source of corruption, if it must be renounced by every honest leader, the people are doomed to eternal submission."

Zanuck was disappointed with the box-office returns for *Viva Zapata!*, and the episode strengthened his resolve to move towards a policy of "strictly entertainment films." Concerned with foreign revenues, Zanuck stressed the importance of color productions and also the new medium of CinemaScope—both of which were arguably less suitable for social realist subjects. Kazan, in his first film after his testimony, and arguably as part of his "clearance," accepted a studio assignment from Zanuck, going to Germany to make *Man on a Tightrope* (1953), a drama about the efforts of a traveling circus to escape to the "West" from Communist Czechoslovakia. Unsatisfactory to mainstream audiences, to his peers, and to Zanuck, who cut the film, *Man on a Tightrope* represented Kazan's lowest point before the resurgence represented by *On the Waterfront* (1954).[37]

The raw material for Kazan's next film was provided by events on the New York waterfront in the early 1950s. The inequities of the hiring and employment methods on the docks, including the notorious "shape up" (in which longshoremen were daily forced to assemble before a union hiring boss, who would only choose a portion of them to work the shift), had been widely documented by journalists and commissions, as had the corrupt practices of unions and employers. After Kazan's project with Arthur Miller fell through, Kazan's wife had urged him to contact screenwriter and novelist Budd Schulberg.

Molly Day Thatcher, daughter of a Wall Street lawyer and granddaughter of the president of Yale, had married Kazan in 1932, and their relationship centrally affected his work and career decisions. It was Molly Kazan who had, by the 1950s, developed a principled anti-Communist critique, and who wrote her husband's notorious *New York Times* advertisement. As Navasky shows, family circumstances impinged on how people reacted to the challenge of HUAC. The lasting relationship between

Schulberg and Kazan was also an example of the way the politics of the time reshuffled artistic associations and alliances. Schulberg had himself been in the Communist party in the late thirties and chose to appear before HUAC as one of the first of the new round of friendly witnesses in 1951, having been named before the committee by screenwriter (and former member of the Nineteen) Richard Collins. Schulberg presented himself as a strong "premature anti-Stalinist" (to use a phrase he used later, in talking to Navasky), pointing to the silence of American Communist Party members in the face of the injustices in the Soviet Union and Communist Eastern Europe.

The script that Schulberg produced with Kazan, based on close relationships with the real rebels on the New York waterfront and the Catholic priests who supported them, was rejected by Twentieth Century–Fox and the other studios before Sam Spiegel agreed to an independent, New York-based production.[38]

Kazan had used the phrase "man of individual conscience" in relation to *Viva Zapata!*, but the term is also central to *On the Waterfront*. For all Schulberg's committed research (including his work with those who testified to the New York State Crime Commission) and the use of real New York locations (in the bitterly cold winter of 1953), the film drifts, under Kazan's direction and with Marlon Brando's central performance, from the sociological to the personal and even existential. In preparing for the film Kazan made it clear that he saw the film not as a documentary but as Terry Molloy's story, a subjective account of a personal journey toward redemption and dignity. The intensity of this perspective, Brando's ability to internalize and represent it, and the effectiveness of Schulberg's overall contextualization of this story, are what distinguish the final film.

While Schulberg has denied the intent to make the film a metaphor for the "naming names" ritual that both he and Kazan had taken part in, Kazan has at various times suggested that his own approach to the material was in part influenced by this traumatic experience. (Steinbeck had referred to "'the Congress thing' having torn him apart"). Kazan at the time refuted the idea that the film represented an apology or defense, suggesting that "if we'd been trying for that, we wouldn't have had Brando's brother killed. Brando gave his evidence because he was angry. How's that an apology for us?" On the other hand, he admitted that "any experience the artist goes through he uses in his work."[39]

Kazan's work with Brando—and for all the actor's "genius" one cannot but give credit to this focused direction, to what later in his career Kazan called his own "transference of emotion" to the character—helped give the film an impact that even those who bitterly opposed its politics were forced to recognize. Here was a film, and a hero, that drew on the thirties traditions of class and the common man while also constructing an interior sense that was suggestive of a new and more uncertain politics. The film was a commercial success and swept the Academy Awards, although there were those who were quick to denounce what they saw as the "informer as social hero" motif for the times. John Howard Lawson wrote of the film's "anti-democratic, anti-labor, anti-human propaganda," and saw it as emblematic of the "influence of McCarthyism on American film production." The British critic and director Lindsay Anderson devoted an article in a British film journal to what he called the unconsciously fascist implications of the film's ending, while Navasky's notion that the Waterfront Crime Commission was an "analog for HUAC" also pegs the film back to this issue.[40]

For all the self-serving behavior of this period—and Kazan has broadly admitted that he essentially named names because the cost of his continued silence, in terms of his career prospects in film, became too great for him—commentators sometimes underplay the gathering force of the liberal discontent with the Communist party and the autonomy of elements of anti-Communist feeling. Kazan's friend Joseph L. Mankiewicz spoke in 1950 of the liberal as an additional victim of McCarthyism, being "slandered, libeled, prosecuted and threatened with extinction." It is common to talk of the turning of film from social to psychological themes in the fifties, and to see Kazan's work as a key example of this trend, although the centrality of psychology in dominant notions of acting in the thirties progressive theaters is clearly as important an influence on Kazan's early career as radical politics. There is little doubt that his testimony and contribution to *On the Waterfront*, in some combination, dramatize his newfound Americanism, and his new distance from the immigrant outsider's perspective that had first led him to politics in the thirties.

In *East of Eden* (1955) Kazan retreated into history, although James Dean's role and performance had a contemporary social and cultural resonance, suggesting the way postwar economic and social change was producing new icons and identities. *Baby Doll* (1956), Kazan's second film collaboration with Tennessee Williams, is arguably more socially pointed than his first. Often seen as a trifling black comedy of sexual jealousy, the fierce reaction of the Catholic Legion of Decency and of Cardinal Spellman indicated that the washed clean, post-testimony Kazan was still provoking anger. Viewing the film now it is certainly possible to see background as foreground, and to make a case that the watching, amused black characters are indicative of the civil rights revolution that was still to come on the film's release. As for *A Face in the Crowd* (1957), with Kazan reunited with Schulberg, this satire starts with the 1930s common man but then shows his manipulation and destruction in an emerging marketing culture in which celebrity sells toothpaste and right-wing politics alike. There are echoes of 1930s and 1940s progressivism, but no credible vision of change; the people eventually see through the co-opted and corrupted Lonesome Rhodes (Andy Griffith), but there will be others to take his place.[42]

A Fight Back: *Salt of the Earth*

Salt of the Earth (1954) was a remarkable attempt by blacklisted artists to fight back through the medium of film. While in the short term the film reached only a small general audience, in the longer term it successfully reached specialized audiences—people who knew the film was ahead of its time. Paul Jarrico, Herbert Biberman, and Adrian Scott (the producer of *Crossfire*) were involved in the formation of the Independent Productions Corporation (IPC), in September 1951. (Jarrico, a leading figure in Hollywood Communist Party circles in the early 1950s, had pleaded the Fifth Amendment before HUAC earlier that year; Biberman and Scott were members of the Hollywood Ten.) Simon M. Lazarus, who had himself taken the Fifth Amendment before HUAC, became the corporation's president, seeing the possibility of good financial returns by tapping into the considerable talents of blacklisted artists.[43]

While the producers at IPC at first considered several projects, they soon focused their attention on one particular set of events as a suitable subject for their opening production. In the fall of 1950, Local 890 of the International Union of Mine, Mill, and Smelter Workers (Mine–Mill), based in Bayard, New Mexico, went on strike against the Empire Zinc Corporation, a subsidiary of New Jersey Zinc, the largest zinc producer in the United States. A distinctive feature of the strike was the fact that Mexican Americans constituted an overwhelming majority of the strikers; the union was viewed as supportive of their civil rights. Affiliated with the Communist party, Mine–Mill had (in 1950) been one of a series of left-wing unions recently expelled by the CIO. James J. Lorence has documented the process that led IPC to base its film on the protracted strike in New Mexico, and also the unique way in which the members of the Local became part of this creative process. Another feature of the strike which impressed producer Paul Jarrico was the key role played by the women. He may also have seen parallels between the strikers and blacklisted film workers. Jarrico saw the project as a "crime to fit the punishment" (of being blacklisted) and defined the crime as an effort to depict the "dignity of women, labor and a racial minority." The filmmaking process was from the beginning closely monitored by the FBI, "for whom the progress of *Salt of the Earth* became an obsession."[44]

Writer Michael Wilson had been successful in the early fifties with his shared (Academy Award winning) screenplay for *A Place in the Sun* (1951) and his script for *Five Fingers* (1952), but by 1952 he had been blacklisted. Director Biberman and Jarrico considered but finally disregarded a critical assessment of Wilson's script by John Howard Lawson.[45] The union, Mine–Mill, became the producer, with the members of the Local being widely consulted on the script and production process. Biberman rejected the notion of Anglos in key roles, in this sense making the film a challenge to dominant Hollywood conventions concerning the representation of ethnicity. Five professional actors were used, including Mexican actress Rosaura Revueltas in the key role of Esperanza Quintero, and Will Geer, one of the first actors to take the Fifth and face the blacklist, as the Sheriff. For all the other roles, including Esperanza's husband Ramon, local non-professionals were used.

Shooting began in early 1953, and the production immediately led to political controversy. On 24 February 1953, on the floor of the House of Representatives, Congressman Donald Jackson suggested that the picture was "deliberately designed to inflame racial hatreds and to depict the United States of America as the enemy of all coloured people." The film, he continued, would "do incalculable harm" if shown abroad, and so should be suppressed.[46] This declaration produced an enthusiastic response from Howard Hughes on how the industry could and should ensure that the film was never shown. Columnists were quick to point out that this Communist movie plot was taking shape not far from Los Alamos, where the atomic bomb had been tested, and the film's production and subsequent distribution were subject to sustained harassment. Near the end of shooting Revueltas was arrested by the Immigration and Naturalization Service, with the result that the only shots of the film's main character in the climax of the film were close-ups shot in Mexico and smuggled across the border.[47] Roy Brewer refused Lazarus's request for a studio crew, and IATSE pressure made it difficult for the company to obtain a good theater for the New York premiere. The film played in only thirteen movie theaters out of the nation's 13,000 before its last first-run theatrical showing in September 1954.

The script contains some rather undigested chunks of political rhetoric ("This installment plan, it's the curse of the working man") and Juan Chacon, as Ramon, cannot quite convey the increasing importance of the domestic struggle in the Quintero household to the resolution of the general conflict over class and ethnicity. The script offers an unfolding dialectic during the extended strike, as the women, and particularly Esperanza, overcome setbacks and gain in confidence and social power. Revueltas underplays a key line to her screen husband: "I'm going to bed now. Sleep where you please, but not with me." Striking images are the exception, but include the first view of the women as a collective force, gathered on a hilltop like "Indians" in a John Ford Western, and the recurring and defiant circles of the picketing miners and their wives. There is also a pointed intercutting between Ramon and Esperanza, with the husband being beaten by the police and the wife in labor. The film provides a moving and stirring celebration of the ideals of its creators, and the issues (from sanitation and hot running water to Mexican identity, sexual politics, and class solidarity) are remarkable for their time.

The emphasis on class in *Salt of the Earth* is perhaps most forced, while the involvement of the Anglo organizer is underplayed, but it was certainly unfair to argue, as Pauline Kael did in her contemporary review, that the film was "as clear a piece of Communist propaganda as we have had in many years." The American Legion echoed this view, attacking the film in its newsletter as one of the most "vicious propaganda films ever distributed in the United States," seeing it as designed for a "hate America" campaign in Latin America.[48] The film, with its rousing score by blacklisted composer Sol Kaplan, reads now as more of a timeless moral fable than a semi-documentary. The Esperanza role is perhaps over-reverent and stylized, but the film does record an otherwise unreported area of postwar life, untouched by the growth of a consumer society. Its energy, commitment, and sensitivity to ethnic, class, and feminist issues, which were either marginalized or below the level of consciousness in 1950s America, make it a crucial icon of the blacklist era.

Conclusion

By the mid 1950s the political climate was beginning to moderate, and the cycles of anti-Communist and Korean war films were in decline.[49] The blacklist as an institution also began to crumble in the late 1950s, with Dalton Trumbo's efforts in particular contributing to its demise. Trumbo's Academy Award for *The Brave One* in 1957, under the assumed name Robert Rich, helped demonstrate the absurdity of the blacklist, given the vibrant black market in scripts, many of them made into films by King Bros. and released through United Artists, which was never a signatory to the blacklist. Yet lives were ruined and changed forever, and for some, such as Abraham Polonsky, the effects of the blacklist carried on into the late 1960s. Script credits were even more tardily adjusted; it took thirty years or more for Michael Wilson and Carl Foreman to receive proper public credit for their script for *The Bridge on the River Kwai* (1957).

The blacklist was part of an intense period of history in which American national identity was adapted for a new era of American Cold War leadership, and in which, in Arthur Miller's phrase, the oxygen "went out of the air" for certain ideas. The languages of class, populism, and social criticism became suddenly suspect, and all sorts of artists decided, like the actress Judy Holliday before the McCarran (Internal Security) Sub-Committee in 1952, to no longer say "Yes" to anything "except cancer, polio, and cerebral palsy."[50] For a particular 1930s generation of ambitious and talented artists, liberals or radicals, the dream had been one of greater artistic autonomy in terms of both the process and content of filmmaking. This collective dream was badly weakened by the events of the early 1950s.

Other factors changed the film agenda, including the decline of the "B" picture, the growing importance of the foreign market, and the industry's shift to forms and spectacles designed to repulse the threat of television. The language of cultural individualism was also becoming as relevant as any class agenda to many in the audience, especially as economic growth and suburban spread proceeded and the reconstituted film industry stumbled towards niche marketing. Yet the blacklist process ruined lives, silenced voices, and tarnished many survivors, and it contributed to the decline of a democratic and cosmopolitan strain in American popular culture. Depression memories dimmed, class consensus replaced class conflict, and authority and domesticity became new watchwords. Even Orson Wells, perhaps the most shining of Popular Front stars, and whose independent leftism left him unscathed by HUAC, if not by the FBI, failed to find an accommodation with the industry.[51] His *Touch of Evil* (1958), with its dark, morally complex perspective on the ordinary corruptions of public life, now seems to echo some of the forms and concerns that the blacklist helped to marginalize from the new and affirmative consensus in American cinema and life.

Notes

1. Thomas Schatz, *Boom and Bust, The American Cinema in the 1940s* (New York: Charles Scribner's Sons, 1997), p. 307; Walter Goodman, *The Committee* (London: Secker & Warburg, 1968), pp. 173–174; on the Tenney Committee, chaired by Jack B. Tenney, see David Caute, *The Great Fear, The Anti-Communist Purge Under Truman and Eisenhower* (London: Secker & Warburg, 1978), pp. 77–78.

2. Schatz, *Boom and Bust,* pp. 307–313; Louis Pizzitola, *Hearst Over Hollywood: Power, Passion and Propaganda in the Movies* (New York: Columbia University Press, 2002), pp. 405, 409–411; on the significance of the labor disputes of 1945–1946 see Gerald Horne, *Class Struggle in Hollywood, 1930–1950, Moguls, Mobsters, Stars, Reds, and Trade Unionists* (Austin: University of Texas Press, 2001), p. 218.

3. Curt Gentry, *J. Edgar Hoover, The Man and the Secrets* (New York: W. W. Norton, 1991), pp. 353–354; John Cogley, *Report on Blacklisting 1–Movies* (New York: The Fund for the Republic, 1956), p. 11; Larry Ceplair and Steven Englund, *The Inquisition in Hollywood, Politics in the Film Community, 1930–1960* (Berkeley: University of California Press, 1983), pp. 209–225, 261ff.; Lee Server, *Robert Mitchum: "Baby, I Don't Care"* (London: Faber and Faber, 2001), pp. 137–138; *Variety,* 26 November 1947, p. 3. Howard Suber, "The Anti-Communist Blacklist in the Hollywood Motion Picture Industry," Ph.D. dissertation, UCLA, 1968, pp. 24, 26, 285.

4. Eric Johnston, in Murray Schumach, *The Face on the Cutting Room Floor: The Story of Movie and Television Censorship* (New York: Da Capo Press, 1975), p. 139; Wyler, 26 October 1947, William Wyler Special Collection, Academy of Motion Picture Arts and Sciences, Margaret Herrick Library.

5. Carol Traynor Williams, *The Dream Beside Me: The Movies and the Children of the Forties* (Rutherford: Farleigh Dickinson University Press, 1980), p. 203: Les K. Adler and Thomas G. Paterson, "Red Fascism: The Merger of Nazi Germany and Soviet Russia in the American Image of Totalitarianism, 1930's–1950's," *American Historical Review,* 75, April 1970, pp. 1,046–1,064.

6. See Thorn Andersen, "Red Hollywood," in Suzanne Ferguson and Barbara Groseclose, eds., *Literature and the Visual Arts in Contemporary Society* (Columbus: Ohio State University Press, 1985), pp. 158–165; Paul Buhle, "The Hollywood Left: Aesthetics and Politics," *New Left Review,* 212, 1995, pp. 101–119; on the culture of the Popular Front, see Michael Denning, *The Cultural Front: The Laboring of American Culture in the Twentieth Century* (London: Verso, 1996), pp. 4–21, 26–27; Abraham Polonsky, interviewed in Eric Sherman and Martin Rubin, *The Director's Event: Interviews with Five American Film-Makers* (New York: Atheneum, 1970), p. 10; Albert Maltz to John Huston, undated, Huston Collection (1949 HUAC folder), Academy of Motion Picture Arts and Sciences; Arthur Schlesinger Jr., *The Vital Center: The Politics of Freedom* (Boston: Houghton Mifflin, 1949).

7. Richard Maltby, "Film Noir: The Politics of the Maladjusted Text," *Journal of American Studies,* 18, 1, 1984, p. 64; Capra in Larry May, *The Big Tomorrow, Hollywood and the Politics of the American Way* (Chicago: University of Chicago Press, 2000), p. 202.

8. Dore Schary, *Variety,* 5 November 1947, P: 1.

9. Morton J. Horowitz, *The Warren Court and the Pursuit of Justice,* (New York: Hill and Wang, 1998), pp. 56–59; Ring Lardner Jr., 19 June 1950, Ring Lardner Jr. Collection, Folder 239, Academy of Motion Picture Arts and Sciences; Ellen Schrecker, *Many Are the Crimes: McCarthyism in America* (Boston: Little Brown, 1998), p. 190

10. Schrecker, *Many Are the Crimes,* p. 154; Richard Pells, *The Liberal Mind in a Conservative Age: American Intellectuals in the 1940s and 1950s* (New York: Harper and Row, 1985), p. 272.

11. Suber, p. 37; on Wayne and the Motion Picture Alliance in the early fifties see Randy Roberts and James S. Olson, *John Wayne, American* (Lincoln: University of Nebraska Press, 1995), pp. 339ff; Harry Warner, *New York Times,* 10 September 1950; Kenneth L. Geist, *Pictures Will Talk: The Life and Films of Joseph L. Mankiewicz* (New York: Charles Scribner's Sons, 1978), pp. 173–206; Cecil B. DeMille, 18 October 1950, in Folder on Screen Directors Guild, 1950, George Stevens Collection, Academy of Motion Picture Arts and Sciences.

12. Suber, p. 38; Rossen, see Patrick McGilligan and Paul Buhle, eds., *Tender Comrades: A Backstory of the Hollywood Blacklist* (New York: St. Martin's Press, 1997), p. 377; Victor Navasky, *Naming Names* (New York: Viking Press, 1980), pp. 319–321.

13. Lewis Milestone, *New Republic,* 31 January 1949, pp. 12–17 and Lewis Milestone Collection, Folder 171/172, Academy of Motion Picture Arts and Sciences; *Alert,* 4 January 1951, 154; on Milestone, Lewis Milestone Folder, Hedda Hopper Collection, Academy of Motion Picture Arts and Sciences; Vincent Sherman, *Studio Affairs: My Life as a Film Director* (Lexington: University Press of Kentucky, 1996), pp. 246–247; *Counterattack,* undated, on Vincent Sherman; *Counterattack,* Communication 447, 2 April 1951; *Counterattack,* Communication 556 (on Schary), 3 October 1951, Box 14, Harvey Matusow Papers, 1950–1955, University of Sussex.

14. Ayn Rand, *Screen Guide for Americans,* The Motion Picture Alliance for the Preservation of American Ideals, Beverly Hills, California, undated; *Firing Line,* 15 March 1952, on *Death of a Salesman,* Matusow Papers, University of Sussex.

15. J. B. Matthews, "Did the Movies Really Clean House," *The American Legion Magazine,* December 1951, pp. 13–14, 49–56; Suber, pp. 44–48; Robert B. Pitkin, "The Movies and the American Legion," *The American Legion Magazine,* May 1953, pp. 14–15, 39–44; Cogley, *Report on Blacklisting,* p. 131; on Hughes, *New York Times,* 7 April 1952.

16. "X," "Hollywood Meets Frankenstein," *Nation,* 28 June 1952, Folder 230, Ring Lardner Jr. collection, Academy of Motion Picture Arts and Sciences.

17. Jon Lewis, "'We Do Not Ask You to Condone This': How the Blacklist Saved Hollywood," *Cinema Journal,* 39, 2, (2000), pp. 4–12, 17–18. Clancy Sigal, "Hollywood During the Great Fear," *Present Tense* 9, 1982, pp. 45–48.

18. *Hollywood Reporter,* 7 April 1952; W. R. Wilkerson, "Trade Views," *Hollywood Reporter,* 25 July 1950, p. 1: Wylers reply, *Hollywood Reporter,* 27 July 1950; Wyler to Frank Freeman, 3 May 1954, William Wyler collection, Political File, Folder 5.

19. Navasky, *Naming Names*; Lillian Hellman, *Scoundrel Time* (Boston: Little Brown, 1976). Paul Jarrico quoted in Michael S. Ybarra, "Blacklist Whitewash," *The New Republic,* 5 and 12 January 1998, p. 23: on Navasky see Andersen, "Red Hollywood," in Suzanne Ferguson and Barbara Groseclose, eds., *Literature and the Visual Arts in Contemporary Society,* pp. 158–165; Edward Dmytryk, *It's a Hell of a Life But Not a Bad Living: A Hollywood Memoir* (New York: Times Books, 1978), p. 146.

20. Dorothy B. Jones, "Communism and the Movies: A Study of Film Content," in Cogley, *Report on Blacklisting,* pp. 220, 282.

21. Richard Slotkin, *Gunfighter Nation: The Myth of the Frontier in Twentieth-Century America* (New York: Atheneum, 1992), pp. 347–348; Walter Bernstein, *Inside Out: A Memoir of the Blacklist* (New York: Alfred A. Knopf, 1996), p. 177; Farber, "Movies Aren't Movies Any More," *Commentary,* June 1952, in Farber, *Negative Space,* 1971, pp. 71–83: May, *The Big Tomorrow,* pp. 204, 273–293.

22. On the notion of film gris, see Andersen, "Red Hollywood," in Ferguson and Groseclose, pp. 183ff.

23. Michel Ciment, ed., *Conversations with Losey* (London: Methuen, 1985), pp. 90–93.

24. Breen to Robert Stillman, 3 May 1950, "The Sound of Fury," Production Code Administration collection, Academy of Motion Picture Arts and Sciences.

25. Thomas Cripps, *Making Movies Black: The Hollywood Message Movie from World War II to the Civil Rights Era* (New York: Oxford University Press, 1993), pp. 252, 259; on Garfield see Robert Sklar, *City Boys: Cagney, Bogart, Garfield* (Princeton, N. J.: Princeton University Press, 1992), pp. 203ff., and Polonsky introduction in Howard Gelman, *The Films of John Garfield,* (Secaucus, N.J.: The Citadel Press, 1975), p. 8; Paul Buhle and Dave Wagner, *A Very Dangerous Citizen: Abraham Lincoln Polonsky and the Hollywood Left* (Berkeley: University of California Press) pp. 10–11.

26. Cripps, *Making Movies Black,* p. 220.

27. David N. Eldridge, " 'Dear Owen': The CIA, Luigi Luraschi, and Hollywood, 1953," *Historical Journal of Film, Radio and Television,* 20.2, 2000, p. 155.

28. Jonathan Munby, *Public Enemies, Public Heroes: Screening the Gangster from Little Caesar to Touch of Evil* (Chicago: University of Chicago Press, 1999), pp. 211, 217.

29. Bernard Vorhaus, interview with Brian Neve (BN), 15 October 1987; Endfield, interview with BN, 18 December 1989; on Endfield see Jonathan Rosenbaum, *Movies as Politics* (Berkeley: University of California Press, 1997), pp. 323–337.

30. Michael Wilson, "Hollywood and Korea," *Hollywood Review,* 1, 1 January 1953, pp. 1, 3–4; Wilson, "Hollywood's Hero," *Hollywood Review,* 1, 5, April–May 1954, pp. 1, 4; Adrian Scott, "Blacklist: The Liberal's Straightjacket and It's Effect on Content," *Hollywood Review,* 2, 2, September–October 1955, pp. 1, 3–6.

31. Thomas Schatz, *The Genius of the System: Hollywood Filmmaking in the Studio Era* (New York: Pantheon Books, 1988), p. 439; James Naremore, *More Than Light: Film Noir and Its Contexts* (Berkeley: University of California Press, 1998), p. 130.

32. W. R. Wilkerson, in *Hollywood Reporter,* 2 December 1947, cited in Joseph Foster, "Entertainment Only," *New Masses,* 66, 1948, pp. 21–22; Elia Kazan to Jack Warner, undated, Warner Bros. collection, University of Southern California.

33. Arthur Miller, *Timebends: A Life* (London: Methuen, 1987), p. 308; Elia Kazan, *A Life* (Andre Deutsch, 1988), pp. 413–415; Zanuck, Memorandum, 26 December 1950, *Viva Zapata!*, Archives of Performing Arts,. University of Southern California; Jonathan M. Schoenwald, "Rewriting Revolution: The Origins, Production and Reception of *Viva Zapata!*," Film History, 8, 1996, p. 120.

34. Zanuck, Memorandum, 26 December 1950, *Viva Zapata!* Archives of Performing Arts, University of Southern California; Alex North to Elia Kazan, undated, Alex North collection, Academy of Motion Picture Arts and Sciences.

35. Slotkin, *Gunfighter Nation*, pp. 418ff.
36. Elia Kazan's testimony, 10 April 1952, and on *Viva Zapata!* as an "anti-communist film," in Eric Bentley, ed., *Thirty Years of Treason: Excerpts from Hearings before the House Committee on Un-American Activities, 1938–1968* (New York: Viking, 1971), pp. 484–495; Kazan's letters to the *Saturday Review*, 5 April 1952, 24 May 1952.
37. John Womack Jr., *Zapata and the Mexican Revolution* (Harmondsworth: Penguin, 1972), p. 565; John Howard Lawson, *Film in the Battle of Ideas* (New York: Masses & Mainstream, 1953), pp. 38–50; Aubrey Solomon, *Twentieth Century Fox: A Corporate and Financial History* (Metuchen, N. J.: Scarecrow Press, 1988), p. 71, 86.
38. "An Interview with Budd Schulberg," *Tikkun*, 15, 3, May–June, 2000, p. 11; Navasky, *Naming Names*, pp. 239–246, 306–310.
39. John Steinbeck to Annie Laurie Williams, 17 June 1952, in Elaine Steinbeck and Robert Wallsten, eds., *Steinbeck: A Life in Letters* (London: Pan Books, 1979), pp. 450–451; Brian Neve, "The Personal and the Political: Elia Kazan and *On the Waterfront*," forthcoming in Joanna E. Rapf's edited collection on the film, Cambridge University Press, 2004; Elia Kazan, *New York Post*, 30 August 1954.
40. John Howard Lawson, "Hollywood on the Waterfront," *Hollywood Review*, I, 6, November–December 1954, pp. 13–14; Lindsay Anderson, "The Last Sequence of *On the Waterfront*," *Sight & Sound*, 24, 3, 1955.
41. "Mankiewicz Pleads the Cause of the Liberal in the US," *Daily Variety*, 15 September 1950, p. 6.
42. See Sam B. Girgus, *Hollywood Renaissance: The Cinema of Democracy in the Era of Ford, Capra, and Kazan* (Cambridge: Cambridge University Press, 1998), pp. 155–176; see the case made by Philip C. Kolin, "Civil Rights and the Black Presence in *Baby Doll*," *Literature/Film Quarterly*, 24, 1, 1996, pp. 2–11.
43. James J. Lorence, *The Suppression of Salt of the Earth: How Hollywood, Big Labor, and Politicians Blacklisted a Movie in Cold War America* (Albuquerque: University of New Mexico Press, 1999), p. 54; Tim Miller, "Class Reunion: *Salt of the Earth* Revisited," *Cineaste*, XIII, 3, June 1984, p. 33.
44. James J. Lorence, *The Suppression of Salt of the Earth*, pp. 54–55; Paul Jarrico in Griffin Fariello, *Red Scare: Memories of the American Inquisition, An Oral History* (New York: W. W. Norton, 1995), pp. 281–283.
45. Lorence, *The Suppression of Salt of the Earth*, pp. 91–96.
46. Congressman Donald Jackson, in Gordon Hitchens, "Notes on a Blacklisted Film: *Salt of the Earth*," *Film Culture*, 50/51, Summer/Fall 1970, "Report on Blacklisting," p. 79.
47. Howard Hughes, "Notes on a Blacklisted Film," *Film Culture*, pp. 80–81.
48. Pauline Kael, "Morality Plays Right and Left," in Kael, *I Lost It at the Movies* (Boston: Little Brown, 1965), pp. 331–346; Lorence, *The Suppression of Salt of the Earth*, p. 130.
49. Trumbo to Hugo Butler, June 1955, in Trumbo, *Additional Dialogue: The Letters of Dalton Trumbo* (New York: Bantam Books, 1972), p. 322.
50. Caute, *The Great Fear*, pp. 519–520; V. Rajakrishan, "An Interview with Arthur Miller," *Theatre Journal*, 32, 2, May 1980, pp. 196–204. Testimony of Judy Holliday, 26 March 1952, *Subcommittee to Investigate the Administration of the Internal Security Act and Other Internal Security Laws*, Committee on the Judiciary, U.S. Senate, 82nd Congress, U.S. Government Printing Office, 1952, p. 166, Matusow Papers, University of Sussex.
51. Welles was in Europe from 1947 to 1955. On the FBI interest see James Naremore, "The Trial: The FBI vs. Orson Welles," *Film Comment*, 27, I, January–February 1991, pp. 22–27

Making the Film: Contemporary Accounts on Salt of the Earth

Breaking Ground

by Paul Jarrico and Herbert J. Biberman

I. When our company was formed two years ago, we agreed that our films must be based in actuality. Therefore, we were entering an arena of art to which we as craftsmen brought little experience and in which we found little precedent to guide us. It was clear that the best guarantee of artful realism lay not in fictions invented by us but in stories drawn from the living experience of people long ignored by Hollywood—the working men and women of America.

And so we searched for stories that would reflect the true stature of union men and women. We dug into material dealing with minority peoples, because we believed that where greater struggle is necessary, greater genius is developed. We looked for material that might record something of the dynamic quality women are bringing to our social scene.

Salt of the Earth, originally the third project on our schedule, seemed the best embodiment of the elements for which we had been striving. A true account of the miners of the Southwest and their families, predominantly Mexican-Americans, begged to be told without the hackneyed melodramatics which so often destroy honesty in the name of excitement. It was not the many abuses and hardships suffered by these people that loomed so significantly out of the material—it was their humanity, their courage and accomplishment. We decided that these Americans, at once typical and exceptional, could best be realized on the screen by the simplest story form of motion picture: a love story of two mature and decent people.

Michael Wilson, author of the story, had come to know these New Mexico miners during a long and bitter strike they waged against a powerful zinc company in 1951 and 1952. The story idea was born out of his first visit there, and he then wrote an extended outline, or, in movie parlance, a treatment of the story. Mr. Wilson returned to the mining community with this treatment, where it was read, discussed and criticized by a score of miners and their wives. With this guidance in authenticity he proceeded to write the first draft screenplay. When it was completed, again we followed the procedure of group discussion and collective, constructive criticism. By rough estimate, no less than four hundred people had read, or heard a reading of, the screenplay by the time we commenced production.

Perhaps it was our determination that the people in this film be life-size that led to our second decision. We asked the miners and their families to play themselves rather than be enacted by others.

These decisions brought the writer, director, crew and cast face to face with intricate problems of realistic form and content. How could we by-pass the pitfall of naturalism—a mere surface record of actual events—and emerge with an imaginative work of art that was still true in detail? How could we best blend the social authenticity of documentary form with the personal authenticity of dramatic form? What range of characterization should be given individual roles whose enactment would be undertaken by non-professionals? How could we capture the quality of speech of these bilingual people and yet make the picture completely intelligible to an average English-speaking audience? How could we make the amazing heroism of these people not only stirring, but *believable* and *inevitable?*

This last problem was particularly important to us, because only if we solved it could our picture help engender in an audience a belief in its own capacities, a confidence that what these people had done could be done again. We hoped that our film might become a cultural stimulus to other trade unions and minority groups, and convince them that they could tell their own stories through the medium of film.

High hopes! And vast problems. Certainly we cannot boast of having solved all these aesthetic questions. But we do think we have broken new ground. If our film can illuminate the truth that the lives and struggles of ordinary people are the richest untapped source of contemporary American art, and if it can demonstrate that such films can be made by these people themselves, then it will have achieved a basic purpose.

II. It is against this background of intention and dedication that the attacks upon this picture during the course of production must be seen. We had been shooting *Salt of the Earth* since January 20th, Inauguration Day. The production was sponsored by the International Union of Mine, Mill and Smelter Workers, and our cast included hundreds of its members and their families. Even after a storm of hysterical publicity burst over us, thousands of our neighbors and associates in the Silver City area assumed we had a right to be there.

A false assumption, said Congressman Donald Jackson. On February 24th, this California Representative delivered a speech in the halls of Congress, in which he said:

> . . . *Mr. Speaker, I have received reports of the sequences filmed to date . . . This picture is deliberately designed to inflame racial hatreds . . . [It] is a new weapon for Russia. For instance, in one sequence, two deputy sheriffs arrest a meek American miner of Mexican descent and proceed to pistol whip the miner's very young son. [They] also imported two auto carloads of colored people for the purpose of shooting a scene depicting mob violence.*

As a direct result of Congressman Jackson's speech, our leading lady was arrested, members of our cast and crew were physically assaulted, and a vigilante committee warned us to leave "within twelve hours or be carried out in black boxes." We defied the deadline, demanding and receiving the protection of the New Mexico State police, and finished our work on March 6th. After we did depart, however, and the protective police as well, the attacks on our Mine-Mill brothers and sisters continued. Two union halls were set afire, one of them burning to the ground. Also razed by arson was the home of a union leader, Floyd Bostick, who had played a role in the film. His three young children narrowly escaped the flames.

Without reading the script, or asking to, without seeing the film, or waiting to, an incendiary Congressman had spoken.

His fury can be understood only if one recognizes how unprecedented it was for manual workers and cultural workers of our country to collaborate, and what promise for a more truly democratic future such a collaboration holds. In organizing for independent production, we had one basic aim: to place the talents of the blacklisted (both those who had worked in films and those who had never been given the opportunity) at the service of ordinary people. There were indeed Negroes in this production: an assistant to the director, an assistant cameraman and two technicians—all in categories of work never available to Negroes in Hollywood.

Simon Lazarus, a respected motion picture exhibitor, had formed Independent Productions Corporation to back us. Money was borrowed from liberal Americans, it being understood that none of us who wrote, directed or produced the film would receive any remuneration until the loans were repaid.

In the wake of the Silver City storm, Mr. Lazarus was himself hailed before the Un-American Activities Committee and asked to divulge who the backers were. He refused to answer personal questions and thus could not be forced to inform on others. He did, however, volunteer to tell the Committee what our film was about. But the investigators were not interested. They did not want to investigate, but to prejudge and censor.

The efforts to prevent *Salt of the Earth* from being made began long before the spectacular assaults in Silver City, and continued long after our location shooting was completed.

Consider, as a pre-production problem, a crew. In Hollywood, most motion picture technicians belong to the International Alliance of Theatrical and Stage Employees (AFL). West coast head of the IATSE is Roy M. Brewer, who inherited his protectorate over Hollywood labor from two gangsters, William Bioff and George E. Browne. A zealous adherent of Congressional witch-hunters, Brewer has understood that his civic responsibility to enforce the blacklist goes far beyond his trade union responsibility to see that his men get jobs. That, no doubt, is why he refused to let us hire an IATSE crew. As a trade paper reported it later:

> *Simon Lazarus, named as prexy of the company, approached Roy M. Brewer, the chairman of the AFL Film Council, about nine months ago, seeking assurance from him that he could make a motion picture using the "Unfriendly Ten." Brewer yesterday recalled he flatly told Lazarus he would prevent such a project in every legal way possible.*—Daily Variety, February 25, 1953

"Legal" was an afterthought. What Brewer said was that he would see us in hell first.

We gathered a union crew despite Roy Brewer. Some were members of his own IATSE. Some had been expelled from the IATSE for opposing Brewer's rule. There were Negroes, denied membership in the IATSE because of its Jim Crow policies. Every member of our crew carried a union card.

As for post-production problems, the would-be censors of the picture have tried to sabotage it in every way. They have demanded that all laboratories close their doors to us, warned technicians not to help us—lest they find themselves blacklisted. Failing here, we expect they will extend their intimidation to film exhibitors when the picture is ready for release. Meanwhile, Congressman Jackson has been needling the Departments of State and Commerce to find some obscure statute which might forbid the export of this picture. No such statute exists, but we would be naive to think that the legality of our endeavor will give the bigots pause.

III. Will the film be shown? We have no illusions about the fight that lies ahead. Of this we are certain—the harrassment will continue, and we will need many allies to defeat the censors and saboteurs. Naturally, the degree of support we eventually get will depend on the end product—the finished film. If trade unionists someday discover that this picture is the first feature film ever made in this country which is of labor, by labor and for labor; if minority peoples come to see in it a film that does not tolerate minorities but celebrates their greatness; if men and women together find in it some new recognition of the worth and dignity of a working class woman—then this audience, these judges, will find ways of overcoming the harrassment.

But to reach these judges, we must first get past the *pre-judgers*. To reach these eventual allies, we need immediate allies—for whether the people are to praise this film or damn it, they must first have the right to see it. That is why we appeal to everyone who is morally concerned with free communication to help provide the atmosphere and the place in which *Salt of the Earth* can be shown and judged on its own merits.

Reflections on a Journey

by Rosaura Revueltas

I don't remember much of that flight from Mexico City to Ciudad Juárez. As the plane droned north toward the border, I was oblivious of the passengers around me, completely absorbed in my thoughts of the experience that lay ahead—the making of *Salt of the Earth*. I had waited so long to do this picture; production had been postponed several times because of various difficulties—but now at last I was on my way to Silver City.

In a way it seemed I had waited all my life to do this picture. My own mother was a miner's daughter. As a child I learned of the miners' hardships, their joys and sorrows; and I grew up wondering why these people on whom the wealth of nations depended were among the worst paid workers in the world. From the day I became an actress I longed to play a role that would honor my people. And now such a role had been offered to me—for these miners of New Mexico were *my people,* even though they lived across the border.

The plane droned on. I closed my eyes and thought of Esperanza, the miner's wife I was to portray in the picture. I was still thinking of her when we landed, and took the airport limousine to El Paso.

There were several Mexican students with me in the limousine. At the border we handed over our documents to the U.S. inspector. He glanced at our vaccination certificates, seemingly the only thing that interested him, returned our documents and waved to the driver to proceed. That was all.

I spent the night in an El Paso hotel, and the next morning, when checking on my plane reservation to Silver City, showed my papers to the airport clerk to make certain that they were perfectly in order. It seemed a little strange to me that my passport had not been stamped at the time of entry. I was assured that this technicality was of no importance; I could always prove my date of entry with my validated airplane ticket, as well as the fact that I had crossed the border in an airport limousine with other passengers (whose passports also had not been stamped).

So I gave the matter no further thought. From the moment I stepped off the plane at Silver City, to be met by a delegation of miners' wives, I was engrossed in the creative work before us. Even when the first attacks against our picture appeared in the press I felt no danger to my own status. We were within a week of our goal when two agents of the Immigration Department visited the lodge in Silver City where the cast and crew were staying. They wanted to see my passport. I showed it to them. In their cold, polite manner they told me they needed to inspect it and would return it to me in a few days.

Work on the picture went forward as usual for the next three days. On the fourth day, returning to the lodge from our location set, I found the same two agents waiting for me. This time they had a woman with them—a matron. They had come to arrest me on the grounds that my passport lacked an admission seal. They told me it was nothing serious, that I could return to work the next day if a $500 bond were posted in El Paso. Nevertheless, they forced me to leave immediately in their car, without dinner, and all the way to El Paso they kept interrogating me. Was I a Communist? Weren't the people I was working with Communists? Wasn't this a Communist picture? For the first time I began to feel frightened. Not for myself, but for the picture. Some powerful man or men were out to kill our picture.

Paul Jarrico, our producer, had followed us to El Paso in his car in order to post my bond. But no sooner did the authorities see that I was about to go free again than they revoked the original warrant of arrest, issuing a new one that stated I was to be held without bail.

That first night I was installed in a hotel room, and two guards set their chairs right outside my door. For the next ten days and nights these two "shadows" or their replacements never left me. I drew small comfort from the thought that this arrangement was preferable to jail. In a way, these shadows made the situation more ominous; I had committed no crime, yet I was their prisoner nonetheless.

But by the time of the first hearing I had regained my hope of an early release. I had great confidence in my attorney, Mr. Ben Margolis, and felt that as long as I had him at my side nothing could go wrong. But the first bad sign was the exclusion of my friends from the hearing. Many of them had come from Silver City and other towns, and although the hearing was supposed to be public, they were not admitted. Then, in the hearing itself, I saw my attorney win argument after argument and yet lose on the basic plea—that I be released on bond pending a formal judgment on my status. And I began to realize that the forces trying to stop the completion of our picture were more powerful than I had imagined.

Those last days in El Paso I recall only as a confused and evil dream. There were other hearings, protests, appeals—much of them in a legal jargon I didn't understand. But this much I did understand, and remember:

I heard a government attorney describe me as a "dangerous woman" who ought to be expelled from the country. At other times he referred to me as "that girl." Since he had no evidence to present of my "subversive" character, I can only conclude that I was "dangerous" because I had been playing a role that gave stature and dignity to the character of a Mexican-American woman....

I remember the face of the government attorney, or "prosecutor" I guess you would call him, and the nervous smile that contorted his lips, and the way his hands trembled. And I thought it strange that he, who represented Law and Authority, should be so frightened—while my friends in Silver City, who were undergoing intimidation and violence, were not nearly so scared as he....

Perhaps that is why I did not feel a sense of defeat when the decision was made that I return voluntarily to Mexico. My attorney and friends still believed that I would be vindicated in the higher courts—but a further appeal would take time. Meanwhile, production in Silver City had been completed except for a very few scenes involving me, and the company could not afford to keep the crew waiting indefinitely for my release. And so I agreed to re-cross the border.

It wasn't a happy leave-taking. There were bitter memories I could not leave behind. But I also carried home with me the spirit that had made this picture possible, the determination that would see it completed, and the inner assurance that a handful of ignorant and frightened men could never prevent its being shown to the peoples of the world.

On Location

from a Crew Member's Diary, by Jules Schwerin

Silver City, Jan. 13, 1953. Flew in from El Paso Sunday... this is a beautiful country of rugged mountains, semi-arid tableland and the bluest sky I've ever seen... weather is ideal for shooting now but old timers here say it's capricious and we may have snow or wind-storms without warning....

Jan. 16th. The miners and their families have given us a warm welcome... for them it has been a difficult year, waiting for this picture to get under way... some of them doubted that they would ever get to tell their story, but now it can be told, by *them,* playing themselves....

Jan. 20th. Most of the crew has arrived... I am struck by the remarkably high level of capacity of these men, many of them distinguished technicians with long records of outstanding achievement... the relationship developing between the crew and the miners is a wonderful thing to watch... a real spirit of brotherhood, each group learning from the other... every day more miners pitch in to help the crew, some of them after a grueling eight-hour day in the mines. Our construction team can take pride in the fact that the miners find our mine-head set authentic. They are amused by the film technique of building "wild" walls and partially constructed rooms, but they are quick to catch on to all the technical phases of movie-making....

Jan. 21st. The first scene with dialogue was shot today, the scene of the beef between the mine foreman and the men. Everyone was tense. One miner kept muffing his lines. He apologized, explaining that the actor-foreman reminded him of a real foreman he had known, and added: "He gets me so damn mad I forget my lines." If we can sustain this kind of reality, a few muffed lines won't matter....

Jan. 30th. The local theatre was filled yesterday with union people, coming to see the first "rushes" of the picture. When the mining families saw themselves on the screen, they howled and cheered and laughed... it was a catharsis... many of them tell us now, "we're not going to be alone anymore." And we of the crew know how deeply they feel this and are glad we are with them....

Feb. 4th. We're having real difficulty in casting "Anglo" roles. Two remarkable men have been cast as the principal deputy sheriffs in the picture. They are friends of the union, and hate to play these parts, although recognizing the necessity of someone being a heavy. They resent wearing the garb of the typical deputy, lest some union man mistake them for the real McCoy. Casting strikebreakers is even more difficult. "Anglos" sympathetic to the miners simply don't want to play these roles, while those who are "neutral" are afraid to sign up for work as extras lest local employers accuse them of being sympathetic to the union.

Feb. 10th. Our schedules must undergo daily changes to accommodate for the mobilization of actors, particularly in mass scenes. Most of the families have no telephone service... distances are fantastic . . . they live in various mining communities, ten, fifteen, twenty miles apart . . . organizing a baby-sitting-and-jitney-service for a hundred people is really something . . . and it would be impossible without the Ladies' Auxiliary of the union . . . we are all impressed by the stamina and courage of the women and the relaxed nature of their children . . . as a result of the strike, the women have moved closer to equality in the home and a fuller participation in union affairs. The results of that victory are seen now in the way women assume responsibility for matters formerly reserved to men. . . .

Feb. 16th. Despite the provocations and slanders of Congressman Jackson and the local vigilantes the community is surprisingly calm . . . many people in Silver City in no way connected with the union continue to offer us gratuitous services . . . the Catholic priests have been friendly and helpful . . . the union men say they expected these attacks would come . . . what a marvelous experience to work with such confident, courageous people!

Feb. 20th. Attacks on the picture are becoming more vicious . . . the local union-haters are beginning to mutter about mob action . . . tradespeople in Silver City who have been friendly to us are starting to retreat a little . . . some of those who have extended service to us are receiving anonymous threats by telephone. . . .

Feb. 24th. It isn't enough that we're in the vortex of a political storm whipped up by creatures who don't know what the picture is about—even the weather's against us. A snow blizzard swoops in on us, and trying to be flexible, we adapt the scene to shoot it with snow. Suddenly the sun comes out and the snow melts before we can even get a master scene. So we return to the original plan. Suddenly a wind storm comes up that makes the set look like the Gobi Desert. And so it goes. . . .

Feb. 27th. Immigration agents arrested Rosaura last night As they led her off, we all stood around feeling angry and helpless, and tried to act brave and unconcerned, assuring one another that she would be back tomorrow . . . but today we all worked harder than ever, with a new zest and a new grimness . . . the bond between the crew members and the union cast is stronger than ever . . . nothing can stop us now from finishing this film . . . our responsibility is great. . . .

March 1st. The union has decided to send Joe Morales to Washington to state the union's case, to see what can be done to stem the hysterical flood of lies, free Rosaura, and restore law and order . . . Joe, a charter member of the local, was chosen unanimously in a most unusual meeting, which was held on location, while shooting of the film continued in a nearby ravine . . . the meeting lasted all afternoon, with men slipping away from the deliberations to take their places before the camera . . . and because a few important voices were missing, the plan was submitted to one of the brothers who was sick at home, and another at work in one of the mines . . . conducted in the most parliamentary manner, this meeting was a demonstration of direct democracy . . . militant miners acting with calm and assurance, aware of the historic importance of what they had undertaken. . . .

March 4th. Today is "super-patriot's" day in Silver City. The vigilantes' campaign of intimidation is at last having its effect on the business community. All morning the loud-speaker in front of the leading theatre blared martial music, and toward noon the doors were opened for the showing of an anti-communist movie. All commercial establishments in town were "advised" to close shop and attend the movie—*or else*. All the same, stores kept their side doors open—to us. . . . The flag-waving hoodlums are threatening to lynch us, our star is still under arrest, and the weather stinks. So what do we do? We keep right on shooting the picture.

March 6th. The production is finished. We have a complete picture, except for a few shots of Rosaura . . . maybe when *the* picture is cut the editor can find a way of getting by without those shots of her . . . It was difficult to say goodbye. The usual guitar, the usual song, the usual laughter were absent. There was almost a fear of looking at one another—a look might have to start a farewell . . . the last scene was completed and our crew turned to face the miners and their families, our brothers and sisters, and all our affection, all of our admiration and respect for each other was shown in our embraces and unashamed tears . . . we had shared so much together, learned so much together . . . I hope that when the film is seen it will bring something of this closeness and understanding to other people. . . .

Union Made

by Juan Chacón

When our Union set out to make a movie about the lives of our people, most of us had an idea it might be attacked. My father has a little farm in this County, and I was born there. A lot of our great-grandfathers worked the mines here in the Southwest and had little farms of their own. My people, the Mexican-Americans, have tended the big crops, built the railroads and dug the ore that makes all this big, bare looking country so rich today.

In our Union here, Local 890 of the Mine, Mill and Smelter Workers, a lot of old timers remember the twelve hour day in the dusty wind of the open copper pit, or the heat of the underground zinc mine—twelve hours for two or three dollars a day. They remember the way the companies built houses for the Anglos while we were given shacks with water outside and no comforts inside except what we made with our own hands. They remember the way the miners who spoke Spanish would be put to work as "helpers" to the "skilled" Anglos—doing the same work for which the Anglo was paid twice as much. They remember the separate pay windows, separate washrooms, the separation even in the movies.

My own company, Kennecott, now admits this was the way things were, but they say, "Our policy has changed. Now it's separate, but equal." But don't ever believe it. There's no such thing as "separate but equal."

I never dreamed of being before a movie camera, much less of being a leading actor. But I was willing to play the role of Ramón in *Salt of the Earth* because this picture would give the world at least a little of the background of our past conditions. But this picture isn't *against*—it's *for*! It shows what we can do when we organize and we and Anglo workers organize together. The companies around here have always been afraid of Anglo-Mexican unity. For a hundred years our employers have played up the big lie that we Mexicans are "naturally inferior" and "different," in order to justify paying us less and separating us from our brothers.

Salt of the Earth helps to expose that lie. It shows that workers can get along regardless of religion, color or politics. It shows the gains we have made through the work of our Union. We don't have separate pay-rates anymore, and now we can move up to skilled jobs except where the craft unions keep us out. A lot of segregation still exists, because here in Arizona Kennecott keeps our housing apart from the English speaking miners—and that keeps a wall between us. They even have our kids go to different grammar schools.

But thank God for our Union and for the men who organized it. Back in the thirties, they were blacklisted, thrown off company property, and told to take their houses with them in thirty days or else. The funny thing is that's how the town of Bayard was born. Bayard was a junction in the highway and the jobless Spanish speaking miners dragged their wrecks here and started all over again. Later our Mine Mill Union won recognition and reinstatement for these workers. But what I meant was funny is that today Bayard is the center of the attack against our Union—and it all comes from some Anglo-American business men who settled here to "service" the town we built.

Since those early organizing days we have had many struggles for equality, the longest and bitterest of which was a recent strike against a zinc mining company that lasted fifteen months. The company seemed determined to make this strike a test, a show-down, an attempt to drive us "back into our places." When the company saw it couldn't starve us out, after eight months on the picket line, it got its anti-picketing injunction from a judge here. That's when our wives took over—and it was their idea. We finally won that strike, thanks to the courage and devotion of our women folks.

No movie in the world could tell the full story of those terrible months—and *Salt of the Earth* was not intended to be a documentary record of that particular strike. But I will say this—it is a true account of our people's lives and struggles.

One thing our picture won't show is the fun we had making it. And the headaches. After all, none of us here knew beans about movie making. But we did manage to lick most of our problems. Here's how we did it:

We organized a Production Committee composed both of people from the local union, the Ladies' Auxiliary and the motion picture company. This committee took up everything: the feeding of hundreds of people on the set, publicity, transportation, baby-sitting, equipment. But that was not all. This committee was a policy-making body, with the responsibility of seeing that our picture ran true to life from start to finish. Occasionally there were meetings in which the union people pointed out to our Hollywood friends that a scene we had just shot was not true in certain details. When that happened we all pitched in to correct the mistake. Most of these mistakes were made because the movie craftsmen had not lived through all our struggles; but they had all the heart and the good will in the world and that is how we managed to stand together and overcome the difficulties of making a movie with little money and many amateurs.

One of the most surprising things to us was that we found we didn't have to "act." El Biberman, as we came to call him, was happiest when we were just ourselves. So after a while, we stopped pretending and then, from the "rushes" we saw, the movie began to look better. We even picked up some Hollywood slang and got so we weren't surprised at all when El Biberman said, "Magnificent! Do it again!"

In making this picture we've shown again that no attacks or falsehoods can break our Union spirit, our willingness to work for what's right. We hope our picture will lead the way for other unions to do the same thing. Movies are the main form of entertainment for most people. That's why we figured the big-shots in the movie industry and the mining industry must have something in common—the need to keep alive the big lie about people. If ordinary people told their stories on the screen, think how the walls between us would be broken down! *Salt of the Earth* is our attempt to break through. We hope you see it.

LESSON NINE

Television's Impact on Hollywood

Introduction: Hollywood in the Home

Christopher Anderson

The transformation of the American motion picture industry following World War II has been viewed as a rupture, a crisis so grave that it forced the major studios to abandon or adulterate many of the practices that had virtually defined the Hollywood studio system since the 1920s. For those who worked within the film industry, the decade of the 1950s has been depicted as the decline and fall of an empire, a time of bewilderment in New York boardrooms and panic on Hollywood backlots. Screenwriter Robert Ardrey has described a scene in the exclusive Green Room at the Warner Bros. commissary during this era. Fresh from examining the latest sagging box office figures, Jack Warner burst into the dining hall, jabbing at contract producers and writers as they ate their lunches. "I can do without you! And you! And you! I can do without you!" he exclaimed as he strode defiantly among the tables. Suddenly face to face with Jerry Wald, by far the studio's most successful producer, Warner paused for an instant and then shouted, "I can *almost* do without you!"[1]

While such tales of temporary madness are probably apocryphal, they have fascinated fans, scholars, and even those who participated in the events, coloring memories of the era and shaping historical accounts. When once-powerful industry leaders such as Darryl Zanuck, Louis B. Mayer, and David O. Selznick fell from grace in the industrial reorganization of the 1950s, they perceived their enforced exile in epic terms, as a barbaric attack on Hollywood's glorious tradition. Selznick, in a letter to his friend and former partner John Hay Whitney, depicted the 1950s as the movie industry's Dark Ages: "Our old stomping ground, what is laughingly known as the motion picture industry, is very mixed up and unhappy. Whatever the weakness of the old and rugged pioneers, who are all disappearing from the scene almost simultaneously—what a hardy race they were!—their successors are pygmies by comparison. There is no leadership; all is chaos."[2]

Since stories of imperial decay draw their strength from nostalgia, it is no wonder that television, the era's new technology of mass entertainment, often played the antagonist in the mythic version of Hollywood's postwar crisis. And while television was not the sole cause of the changes that took place in Hollywood during the late 1940s and early 1950s, one can appreciate the movie industry's reported hostility toward a medium that threatened to displace the motion picture as the preeminent cultural commodity in twentieth-century America. Most hostile were the studio bosses; indeed, tales of Jack Warner's early animosity toward television are legendary. Studio personnel say that during the early 1950s Warner delivered an edict to producers at his studio, forbidding them to include television sets in the decor of Warner Bros. films. From our vantage point in a world saturated by television, it is hard to believe that a TV set could trigger such desperate measures from one of Hollywood's most venerable moguls, yet Warner was scarcely alone in voicing his animosity toward the industry's emergent competitor.

Throughout the early 1950s, the industry trade press debated whether television ultimately would reveal itself to be friend or foe of the movie studios. As television began its unprecedented expansion following World War II, revenues throughout the motion picture industry plunged dramatically. Warner Bros. suffered some of the worst losses, with net profits falling from a record

$22 million in 1947 to $2.9 million in 1953—a decline of nearly 90 percent in just six years.[3] Under conditions that threatened the very existence of the studio system, television served many in the Hollywood community as a convenient stock villain.

Yet Hollywood did not view television from a single perspective, or from a consistently antagonistic posture. In spite of the movie industry's legendary antipathy, the aversion of the major studios to TV actually lasted only a few short years during the early 1950s, and it was provoked not by fear of competition or ignorance of a new technology but by government decisions that essentially surrendered control of the television industry to the radio networks and erased any hopes that the studios had of forming competitive networks.

Even during the period when executives at the major studios demonized television, many independent producers and smaller studios embraced the opportunity to produce films for the new medium.[4] Long excluded from the lucrative profits guaranteed the major studios by their restrictive system of distribution and exhibition, independent producers looked upon TV as an open market, a new exhibition outlet beyond the stifling grasp of the major studios. Although the future of the telefilm business was far from certain in 1950, the atmosphere of opportunity among Hollywood's independent producers was similar to that of the film industry's earliest days, before the major studios dominated the business.

In network TV's early days, independent telefilm production companies were formed by a varied cast of entrepreneurs: émigrés from the major studios (Jerry Fairbanks), former B-movie makers (Hal Roach, Jr.), radio syndicators (Frederick Ziv), talent agencies (Music Corporation of America, or MCA), real estate investors (Lou Snader), oilmen (Jack Wrather), and, most prominently, actors (Bing Crosby, Jack Webb, Lucille Ball, and Desi Arnaz). In 1951 these producers began to leave their mark on the medium. During the fall of that year, Ball and Arnaz premiered *I Love Lucy* (1951–1957), the first filmed situation comedy to have a national impact. Webb followed later that season with *Dragnet* (1952–1959), the first successful crime series shot on film. Within a year *I Love Lucy* and *Dragnet* stood atop the network ratings as the most popular series on TV.

By mid-decade, as the television audience expanded, even old guard Hollywood leaders discovered incentives to produce for television. The month of October 1954 stands out as a key transitional moment in the relations between Hollywood's major powers and the TV industry. Early in the month, Columbia Pictures became the first major studio to produce episodic TV series when its TV subsidiary, Screen Gems, premiered *The Adventures of Rin Tin Tin* on the American Broadcasting Company (ABC) (1954–1959) and *Father Knows Best* on the Columbia Broadcasting System (CBS) (1954–1963). Within three days in late October, two of the film industry's top independent producers, David O. Selznick and Walt Disney, joined the migration to prime time.

Selznick made Hollywood's most auspicious debut with a two-hour celebration of electricity and American enterprise titled *Light's Diamond Jubilee*. The movie industry's most famous independent producer, Selznick had achieved a reputation for glamour and craftsmanship with such epic movies as *Gone with the Wind* (1939) and *Duel in the Sun* (1946). His prime-time debut extended this reputation to television by introducing to the medium such renowned movie talents as directors King Vidor and William Wellman, writer Ben Hecht, and actors Joseph Cotten, Helen Hayes, Thomas Mitchell, Lauren Bacall, and David Niven—and by featuring an unlikely performer in a commercial broadcast, President Dwight D. Eisenhower. Sponsored by the electric industry, this program capped a yearlong celebration of Thomas Edison's invention of the incandescent light bulb seventy-five years earlier. Thanks to the financial support of the electric industry, Selznick's extravaganza monopolized the airwaves as few commercial broadcasts ever have, appearing on almost every existing TV station and capturing the largest viewing audience in the new medium's history. On that Sunday night in late October, loyal viewers of NBC's (National Broadcasting Company) *Colgate Comedy Hour,* CBS's *Toast of the Town,* ABC's *Flight #7,* and the beleaguered DuMont Television Network's *Rocky King, Detective,* found their prime-time routines disrupted by this inescapable broadcast. In a year during which television viewers were confronted with a number of so-called spectacular, one-of-a-kind events, *Light's Diamond Jubilee* was still unique, the most ambitious program that Hollywood had offered television to that point.

Selznick's program attracted considerable attention, but Disney's premiere of *Disneyland* three days later was just as eagerly anticipated by television viewers. Disney had forged a reputation as the cinema's maestro of family entertainment; now his TV series promised to deliver what *Time* described as "the true touch of enchantment" to American homes. In spite of the technological limitations of the black-and-white TV set, especially its inability to reproduce animation's color spectacle, Disney expected the home video receiver to replace the movie theater as the portal to the Disney universe. In fact, as the title of the series suggests, *Disneyland* offered television viewers a reward that moviegoers couldn't share—privileged witness to the embodiment of "Walt's dream," the Disneyland amusement park then under construction. During the weeks that followed the premiere of *Disneyland*, the nation awoke to Walt's dream of an innovative amusement park designed expressly for the country's baby-boom families.

In reviews of the week's TV fare, critics recognized that the Selznick and Disney productions were milestones in the budding relations between the two media. "The two best TV shows of last week—and perhaps of this year," *Time* magazine reported, "originated in Hollywood and were created by veteran moviemakers."[5] Thus, by October 1954 filmed television production was no longer solely the dominion of companies on the distant fringes of the studio system but had become a viable option for the most well-established Hollywood producers. The major studios—led by Warner Bros., Twentieth Century Fox, and MGM—joined the field during the 1955 season. Over the next four years, Hollywood studios became the predominant suppliers of the networks' prime-time programming.[6]

The remarkable commitment by the major studios to television production can be illustrated with many examples, but the conversion at Warner Bros. was particularly telling. In January 1959, after decades in the movie business and only four years in TV, Warner Bros. found itself without a single theatrical motion picture in front of the cameras. The studio had not abandoned movie production, of course, but it had embraced series television, emerging as the single largest source of network series. Its eight different series—led by the hits *Cheyenne* (1955–1962), *Maverick* (1957–1962), and *Sunset Strip* (1958–1964) filled over one-third of ABC-TV's prime-time schedule and generated $30 million in annual revenue from network license fees alone. In order to meet the network's demand for programming, the studio had geared up its operations to produce the equivalent of a full-length feature film *each working day*. Even during periods when feature production slumped, TV production kept the studio bursting with activity. As a result, Jack Warner's early animosity toward the medium soon gave way to a pragmatic enthusiasm. "Television," he asserted during a speech in June 1959, "has been a very healthy influence on the motion picture industry. It's the ninth wonder of the world."[7] Warner's decade-long passage from antipathy to enchantment suggests just how much the stakes of movie and TV production changed for the major studios during the 1950s.

Of course, Selznick and Disney were not the first independent film producers who turned to television, nor was Warner Bros. the first major studio to embrace the new medium. But their emergence as suppliers of TV programming during the 1950s represents one of the most significant moments in the transition from the "Old Hollywood" of the studio era to the "New Hollywood" in which movie studios have become subsidiaries of transnational media and leisure conglomerates. The shift to television production in Hollywood—particularly by those producers with the heaviest investment in the Old Hollywood—marked television's emergence as America's principal postwar culture industry, while it also signaled a growing trend toward the integration of media industries. Since the movie studios began producing television, the diversification of media corporations into related fields and the consolidation of capital through corporate mergers have produced an environment in which the media industries are increasingly interwoven. Although these tendencies existed before the 1950s, the impulse toward integration rose markedly during that tumultuous decade and has become more pronounced in subsequent years. To appreciate the implications of the decision by the major studios to produce television, therefore, it is useful to view their actions as characteristic of a larger trend. The motion picture industry during the 1950s was less an empire on the verge of ruin than one struggling, under unsettling conditions, to redefine its frontiers.

Although Hollywood experienced changes during the 1950s, these weren't necessarily the seismic shifts described in the epic accounts of the industry's demise. Certain impermanent conditions had enabled the major studios to dominate the movie industry for more than a quarter of a century, but these conditions dissolved in the fluid social, political, and economic environment of post–World War II America. A number of converging forces propelled the industry into its postwar economic slump: the Supreme Court's 1948 *Paramount* decision, which ordered the major studios to divest themselves of their lucrative theater chains; heightened competition for the public's leisure and entertainment spending; demographic shifts in postwar American society; restricted foreign markets; and increased production costs in the industry.[8]

By the mid-1950s, in response to these conditions, the studio system had largely given way to independent production. The studios gradually phased out the standardized production of the moderate- to low-budget, formulaic films that had sustained the industry by providing a dependable means for meeting the fixed expense of studio overhead and the screen-time demands of exhibitors. This change meant dropping term contracts with creative personnel and reducing production at the studios. Instead, the major studios encouraged independent producers (many of whom were former studio producers, directors, or actors) to create individual, highly differentiated films that the studios would finance, distribute, and market. Under this strategy, the major studios appeared to be headed toward a new role as packagers, financiers, and distributors of independently produced feature films.

With the growth of the television audience during the 1950s, however, the television networks soon began courting the studios, trying to convince them of their potential importance as product suppliers which could profit from the networks' efforts to consolidate and expand power over advertisers and local affiliates. Studio telefilm production represented an alternative to the dominant mode of television production in the early 1950s, a system that had been imported almost directly from network radio. As in radio, advertising agencies purchased broadcast time in the network schedule and then produced live, New York–based programs to fill the time slots. Sponsors owned the program and often controlled the programming slot as though it were a franchise held at the sponsor's discretion. By turning to Hollywood studios and their existing production operations, the networks could step up their efforts to wrest control of programming from the agencies without themselves having to risk the heavy financial burden of program production. In addition, by investing in studio-produced telefilm series, the networks could guarantee themselves a portion of the residual profits that filmed series promised to deliver as "reruns" once they had completed their network run and passed into syndication.

The studios discovered that supplying television programs to the networks offered a new rationale for standardized, studio-based production. By shifting their mass production efforts into series television, a number of the major Hollywood studios were able to capitalize on *aspects* of the studio system even as the system itself changed. Thanks to its telefilm operations, Warner Bros., for instance, maintained term contracts with actors, directors, producers, and technicians, continued regular studio operations, and guaranteed a steady supply of product that was financed, produced, and owned by Warner Bros. until the entire studio was sold in the late 1960s. Thus commercial television, far from sounding the death knell of the Hollywood studios, offered a perfunctory salvation, an opportunity to reorganize and sustain established production operations when other social, economic, and political forces threatened to end the studios' established hegemony in the movie industry.

The studios probably would have survived in some form solely through a strategy of financing and distributing independently produced feature films, but television actually supported their continued dominance of the movie industry. At the same time, the TV networks embraced Hollywood-produced programming in order to consolidate their own control over the television industry. By the end of the 1950s, with the fates of the networks and studios deeply entwined, filmed television series emerged as the dominant product of the Hollywood studios and the dominant form of prime-time programming—a pattern that has remained unchanged for more than thirty years.

My goal is to make sense of this transitional period in the history of the motion picture and television industries by focusing on the transition into television production among Hollywood's most powerful studios and independent producers, those whose stake in the studio system had been the greatest. For both independent producers and major studios, the shift to TV was integrally bound up with other corporate strategies developed during the 1950s, including the studios' sponsorship of independent production, their commitment to big-budget blockbusters, and their diversification into other related fields. Among these strategies, the shift to TV was shaped not only by contemporary conditions but also by Hollywood's history of relations with the broadcasting industry. As this book examines the role of TV production in Hollywood's evolving corporate strategies, therefore, it also must ask how Hollywood producers envisioned television's value to the movie industry, both as a market and as a medium for symbolic expression. With different stakes and different experiences during the studio era, independent producers and major studios developed distinctly different conceptions of television, and those conceptions shaped the programming they produced.

Hollywood's emergence in television was not simply a matter of powerful movie producers' invading the TV industry and imposing their values and traditions on an underdeveloped medium. Indeed, the television industry already possessed a well-defined economic structure built upon the networks' ability to deliver viewers to advertisers by broadcasting regularly scheduled programming to a national audience. Movie producers who had grown accustomed to the ways of the studio system discovered that it wasn't going to be easy to adapt to a culture industry defined and controlled by other companies. In almost every instance, the corporate commitment to change was soon followed by the realization that change in the culture industries is more easily anticipated than managed. Consequently, the transition involved an active process in which movie producers haggled with networks and sponsors over economic relations, creative control, and program forms, while also attempting to conceptualize the organization and execution of TV production within their own companies.

First, the Hollywood studios had to negotiate the shifting relations of power in the TV industry, particularly since the networks enlisted the studios partially as a tactic for toppling the sponsors' control over production. In contrast to their impact on the movie industry, therefore, the studios had little hope of dominating the TV industry. Caught in a struggle between networks and sponsors, they seldom were able to dictate the terms under which they produced and distributed their programs. Their participation in TV played out in ways they scarcely anticipated, because it occurred under conditions they couldn't control, or sometimes even understand.

Second, as networks and sponsors debated the question of how to maximize the TV audience and the impact of advertising during the medium's early years, they experimented with scheduling strategies, program formats, and genres, producing different types of programming that constituted the experience of TV in a variety of ways. The decision to enlist Hollywood producers was an example of this experimentation. During the 1950s, Hollywood produced various types of programs for television, but ultimately helped the networks to define episodic series as the medium's dominant form. Episodic series were not necessarily what many of the studios had imagined producing when they began, but their participation in the industry ultimately reoriented their efforts in that direction and in many ways solidified the networks' commitment to the episodic series as prime time's dominant programming form.

Finally, Hollywood producers had to reconceptualize the studio system's established mode of production within the context of the television industry. To make this adjustment, they had to develop a system of production that responded to new technology (the TV set), a new form of distribution (network broadcasting), a new site of exhibition (the home), a new means of measuring popularity (ratings), a new commercial purpose (delivering viewers to advertisers), and new sources of revenue (network broadcast and syndication). Production practices had to be redesigned to take into account the demands of networks and advertisers, the economic restrictions of the medium, and negotiations with labor unions that also were attempting to adapt to the new medium. Narrative strategies had to be adjusted to the rapid pace of TV production, the conventions of episodic series, and the conditions of home viewing. The type of text most appropriate for these conditions was the subject of intensive, ongoing debate.

Although this article will discuss all of the major studios and a number of independent production companies, it will focus primarily on case studies of three different organizations—

David O. Selznick Productions and Walt Disney Productions, both major independent producers that functioned on the periphery of the studio system, and Warner Bros. Pictures, a fully integrated major studio during the studio era.

Each of these companies conducted its transition to television quite differently, and the variations capture the range of Hollywood's responses to the medium. Whereas independent producers like Selznick and Disney hoped to evade the restricted economic environment of the studio system via television, a major studio like Warner Bros. hoped somehow to sustain the status quo of the studio era. Dealing with networks and advertisers who endorsed distinctly different definitions of the medium, these Hollywood producers defined television in relation to the studio system, evaluating its potential in terms of whether it sustained or disrupted familiar notions of how to produce popular entertainment. They struggled to decide how to entertain, how to tell stories, and how to prosper in a medium they didn't control. At the same time, Hollywood producers also sought to define television in relation to the imagined outcome of the changes facing the movie industry. While each of these producers had participated for decades in the studio system, their widely varying forecasts for television's future led them along divergent paths. Why did each company choose its particular strategy for television production? How did it determine what kind of programs to produce? How did each define the relationship between television production and its ongoing film production? How did each company imagine television's role in the New Hollywood?

Because Selznick and Disney were independent producers, they had a degree of freedom in dealing with television that was unavailable to a major studio. Still, the transition to TV was more difficult for Selznick and Disney than for Warner Bros. because, as independent producers, they lacked the personnel and the financial resources demanded by television production. Selznick and Disney saw television as an opportunity for innovation, but even they had radically different experiences in TV. Selznick was hired by an advertising agency to deliver a particular program and, therefore, faced constant battles with his corporate patrons over conflicting ideas about how television should be produced. Disney signed his first contract with ABC, a network eager to be associated with Hollywood producers and one that initially shielded the producer from conflict.

For Selznick, years of negotiations with the major TV networks and elaborate plans to monopolize the field of television production ultimately generated a total of only two hours of prime-time entertainment, *Light's Diamond Jubilee*. While Disney was not interested in cornering the TV market, his first series, *Disneyland,* became the linchpin in a new strategy of diversification that ultimately vaulted his company into the ranks of major studios and launched the struggling ABC into competition with the other networks. Selznick produced the most heavily viewed entertainment program in the medium's early history but inspired few imitators in Hollywood. *Disneyland,* on the other hand, provided the catalyst for the major studios' involvement in TV, even as Disney distanced himself from the Old Hollywood by shifting into projects like his amusement park. Obvious questions arise: Why didn't Selznick's plans payoff? How did Disney prosper through TV even though his interests in television production were fairly limited?

The most firmly entrenched in the studio system of the three, Warner Bros. entered television inspired by the public relations success of the Disney program, which was invaluable in publicizing the studio's feature films and amusement park. Signing its first contract with ABC, Warner Bros. initially modeled its TV strategies after those of Disney, as did MGM and Twentieth Century–Fox that same year. But when it failed to duplicate Disney's ratings success, Warner Bros. responded to demands by the network and sponsors by shifting entirely to the production of episodic series. Within a few years, the majority of the studio's activities were oriented toward series production, leading many other Hollywood producers in the same direction. MGM and Twentieth Century–Fox were less successful in making the adjustment to series production; thus Warner Bros. became the leader in the major studios' shift into television. By the end of the 1950s, under conditions that it hadn't dictated, Warner Bros. provided an influential model for both the organization of TV production and the form of TV narrative. And yet during the early 1960s Warner Bros. was surpassed by a number of companies, as the studio failed to develop new series to replace its fading first generation. How and why did Warner Bros. become TV's largest producer only four years after creating its first series? What caused the studio's rapid decline at the very moment when television production elsewhere in Hollywood was booming?

The activities of these producers represent different strategies for Hollywood's interaction with television and for the TV industry's use of Hollywood during a period in which no single type of programming dominated prime time. Above all, this book attempts to explain why certain types of programs emerged under these conditions. Too few historians have acknowledged that broadcast programs are cultural texts produced within historically specific economic and social conditions to communicate some meanings to audiences. In most histories of television, the programs are fairly insignificant, envisioned less as symbolic forms than as the residue of economic relations or the reflection of social issues. But the rise of Hollywood-produced TV programming was motivated by more than economic decisions, and its consequences extended beyond the bottom line of network and studio profits.

The introduction into prime time of programming created by movie producers was one example of the experimentation in program forms taking place in television during the 1950s, as networks, sponsors, producers, policymakers, and audiences shaped television's role in American culture. Often identified as TV's "Golden Age" because of nostalgia for the prestigious anthology dramas and live comedies produced in New York during its early years, the decade of the 1950s was actually a period in which the TV industry entertained a wide range of program types as the medium extended from its original base in major cities and its relatively upscale initial viewership to an increasingly national audience.

The dramas and comedies of the Golden Age represented not so much the thwarted potential of network television as the dying gasps of a culture preserved from network radio, vaudeville, and the theater at a time when television was still only a metropolitan phenomenon. Selznick's extravaganza, on the other hand, represented one potential strategy in the networks' early efforts to construct the experience of television viewing for a *national* audience. His long-standing ambition to mount prestigious productions coincided with an early goal of networks and advertisers to define television viewing as "spectacular," an extraordinary national event delivered at once to homes across the country. By producing series television, Disney and Warner Bros. participated in an alternative programming strategy adapted from network radio, but one still oriented toward a national audience. In contrast with programming forms that traded on uniqueness, weekly episodic series encouraged an experience of television viewing as something ordinary, one component of the family's household routine.

The process by which Hollywood-produced programming came to dominate prime time can be seen as the consolidation of American television; the episode series that emerged became the template for TV narrative. Not until the major studios entered television did the medium reach the stage at which a single type of text characterized prime time in the same way that the feature film had come to typify the cinema. No more did Warner Bros. invent series narrative than did Desilu Productions with *I Love Lucy,* Freeman Gosden and Charles Correll with radio's *Amos and Andy,* MGM with its series of Andy Hardy movies, or Charles Dickens with his serialized novels. But the appearance of a major movie studio like Warner Bros. as the leading producer in television signaled the emergence of the episodic TV series as the medium's central expressive form. The rise of telefilm series produced in Hollywood represented the consolidation of a particular type of text that has dominated prime-time television ever since. Because this happened in Hollywood during the 1950s, one cannot understand how American television developed without asking how the process was affected by changes in the movie industry during the postwar years. In many ways, the history of American TV is the history of Hollywood TV.

Considering that all of the major studios had shifted into television production by the late 1950s, it is surprising how little attention has been paid until recently to the relations between the film and broadcasting industries. The tendency to treat American cinema and television as discrete cultural institutions is one of the fundamental issues that need to be addressed in an attempt to understand the rise of television production in Hollywood. Traditionally, histories of American cinema and broadcasting have been organized around a series of familiar narratives that form the framework for understanding the development of movies, radio, and television. One of the most well-rehearsed narratives depicts the broadcasting and motion picture industries as antagonists locked in a struggle over the hearts and minds of a fickle public. Accounts of the interactions between the motion picture industry and the broadcasting industry generally adopt a structure that traces the movie industry's initial disdain for radio and television, followed by its antagonism after the unexpected success of those two media, and finally its reluctant acquiescence to the new order of commercial entertainment forged by broadcasting's popular appeal. One early article succinctly represented this narrative structure, with its movement from conflict to resolution, as a tale of "complacency, competition, cooperation."[9]

The persistence of this historical narrative is evidenced in the writings of media scholars who see the rise of commercial television as the most apparent explanation for what they perceive to be the artistic decline of the American cinema since the studio era. Critic Todd Gitlin, for instance, has argued that the decay of the American cinema can be measured by the stages in the movie industry's capitulation to television. He bemoans the fact that "television, the bastard child of the movies and radio, has triumphed over its parents, leaving Hollywood to revel in revenues, publicity, passable product, and past glories." Suggesting that contemporary movies have become bleak, Gitlin describes the history of the American cinema since World War II as a gradual contamination in which "the thread—or sewage—of mainstream television runs through the whole process."[10]

During the past decade, however, a number of historians have demonstrated that this influential master narrative has obscured the symbiotic relationship that has existed between the motion picture and broadcasting industries since the founding of national radio networks during the 1920s. The publication of Michele Hilmes's *Hollywood and Broadcasting,* William Boddy's *Fifties Television,* and the anthology *Hollywood in the Age of Television,* edited by Tino Balio, signaled the full emergence of this revisionist movement in media history. This movement not only questions common assumptions about relations between the media by demonstrating their nearly continuous engagement over the years, but it also raises serious doubts about the usefulness of any media history that isolates cinema and broadcasting from one another or from the other cultural institutions in a particular era.[11]

While the boundaries that separate the media at first may appear natural and self-evident, their existence is not based on any inherent differences in the nature of media technology, the structure of media industries, or the attributes of media texts. Examined on any of these levels, distinctions between the media quickly blur. Instead, the boundaries that separate the media in our culture are the products of discourse, including both the discourse generated by the media industries and that produced by scholars and critics. As historian Carolyn Marvin notes, "Media are not fixed natural objects; they have no natural edges. They are constructed complexes of habits, beliefs, and procedures embedded in elaborate cultural codes of communication."[12] In other words, media are cultural constructs created, distinguished, and sustained by the social meanings ascribed to them. Traditional histories have drawn discrete boundaries around individual media by concentrating on a limited range of issues. Film history has tended to focus on the production and distribution of feature films; broadcasting history usually has emphasized technical innovation in electronics manufacturing, government regulation, and the economics of network broadcasting.[13] Above all, traditional histories have implied that the two media are distinctly separate, shaped by different historical forces while in pursuit of conflicting goals.

In practice, however, the motion picture and broadcasting industries seldom disguised their many alliances, and the general public seemed to have recognized the interpenetration of the media as soon as movies and radio began to share the stage as the country's most prominent forms of popular entertainment. During the late 1920s and early 1930s, every major studio attempted to form its own radio network, and both of the existing major radio networks sought entrance into the movie business. Will Rogers, the top-ranked box office star of the early 1930s, also was one of radio's most popular performers. Director Cecil B. De Mille's period of greatest box office success coincided with his appearance as the host of *Lux Radio Theatre* beginning in 1936. In his memoirs, De Mille recalled the radio show as "the experience which brought me closer to the American people than anything else I have ever done." By offering Hollywood's most popular stars in abridged audio adaptations of contemporary feature films, *Lux Radio Theatre* attracted thirty million movie-going listeners each week and brought Hollywood's glamorous aura across the threshold of the American home. During De Mille's decade-long tenure with the series, every film he directed appeared among the ten top-grossing films of its year.[14] Recognizing radio's promotional value, the studios also adapted successful radio programs for the silver screen—for example, the 1937 Warner Bros. feature *Hollywood Hotel,* a musical based loosely on the radio series hosted by newspaper columnist Louella Parsons.

By the time both the movie industry and network radio reached the height of their popular and commercial success in the 1940s, Hollywood celebrities appeared regularly on their own programs or on those, like *Lux Radio Theatre,* designed to promote feature films. Performers like Bob Hope and Bing Crosby consistently dominated the era's rankings of top movie and radio stars, and it is no coincidence that Hope, Crosby, and De Mille were all under contract to Paramount, the studio most committed to economic investment in the broadcasting industry during the studio era. Together, the films of these three radio celebrities accounted for two-thirds of Paramount's top-grossing motion pictures during the 1940s, the studio's most profitable decade during the studio era.[15] It thus seems possible that the popular success of movies and radio during the 1930s and 1940s depended at least partially on the fact that the media were not isolated from one another but were perceived as complementary experiences in which stars and stories passed easily from one medium to another.

As these brief examples suggest, the tendency to depict the cinema and broadcasting as isolated cultural institutions obscures their long-standing interdependence. Nowhere is this tendency more evident than in relation to the issue of advertising and commercial sponsorship, a point at which the studios' interests seem most distinct from those of broadcasters and yet one at which their interests frequently coincide. Because the movie industry must justify a policy of paid admissions while the commercial sponsorship of radio and TV programs makes them appear to be available free of charge, the movie industry has a stake in differentiating the two media, in making it seem unquestionable that movies have greater intrinsic value than TV programs and thus warrant audience "investment" at the box office. This pervasive distinction—circulated throughout the culture by film industry marketing, the popular press, scholars, and critics—has been articulated along a number of familiar lines: the cinema's technological superiority (the movie industry's marketing of technical innovations such as CinemaScope, 3-D, and Dolby sound), its greater capacity for spectacle or verisimilitude (press reports about lavish budgets and special effects or about an actor or director's fanatical obsession with "accuracy"), its relative freedom in depicting sexuality and violence, or the creative license provided to some of its directors. These criteria and others have been used at one time or another to mark the cinema's difference from television.

The most conveniently mapped boundary between the cinema and television, however, has been drawn over the issue of commercial sponsorship. During the convergence of the movie and television industries in the 1950s, for instance, a number of Hollywood movies expressed a distinction between the media by lobbing satirical bombshells at television's commercial motives. This critique of television appeared in satires like *Callaway Went Thataway* (1951), *It's Always Fair Weather* (1955), *A Face in the Crowd* (1957), and *Will Success Spoil Rock Hunter?* (1957). In its surprisingly elitist echoes of the contemporary "mass culture" debate, the relatively consistent representation of television in these movies seems more a product of the Frankfurt School than of Tinsel Town. Television, as depicted in these films about the TV and advertising industries, is a merchant of false consciousness, a medium irredeemably compromised by its devotion to advertising. The TV producers, celebrities, and advertising agency personnel who populate these stories are twisted by greed or flawed by cynicism, but their flaws are hidden from the TV viewers within the narrative. The TV audiences imagined by these movies are oblivious to the false appeals taking place on the TV screen and to the machinations taking place just offscreen.

As cinema spectators, however, moviegoers are able to recognize such dissimulations because the movie narratives provide privileged access to the characters' motives, revealing the hidden schemes that are masked by commercial television's obsession with surface detail. Indeed, these films construct a preeminent position for the cinema by representing the medium's epistemological superiority over television. Noticing this narrative motif in subsequent films depicting the institutions of television, Colin MacCabe has described it as "cinema's ability to make visible what is invisible to television." Through a variety of narrative strategies, films that represent television often stress "the opposition between the knowledgeable position we occupy as viewers in the cinema compared with the ignorance of the television audience."[16] This motif implicitly argues that the cinema is superior to television, not because of inherent technological advantages but because of television's commercialism, which inhibits its ability—or willingness—to depict social reality accurately.[17]

Movie industry discourse has often implied that the cinema exists in an autonomous sphere outside the corrupting influence of the marketplace, an idea best expressed by MGM's famous slogan, *ars gratia artis*. Along with the studio's unmistakable roaring lion, MGM's assertion of artistic autonomy served as the trademark for the particular cultural commodity that MGM marketed—feature films carrying the connotation of aesthetic quality. The irony of an entertainment corporation's advancing the doctrine of art for art's sake is obvious. As Theodor Adorno has noted, however, the disavowal of commercial impulses recurs throughout modern mass culture: "Vestiges of the aesthetic claiming to be something autonomous, a world unto itself, remain even within the most trivial product of mass culture. In fact the present rigid division of art into autonomous and commercial aspects is itself largely a function of commercialization. It was hardly accidental that the slogan *l'art pour l'art* was coined in the Paris of the first half of the nineteenth century, when literature really became large scale business for the first time."[18] Likewise, the studios' efforts to position their films within an autonomous aesthetic sphere developed from marketing strategies designed to differentiate their product from that of competitors. This practice continued even after the major studios themselves began to produce television films, and the seperation of the media had become harder to define, because the studios still had to justify the distinction between the films they produced for television broadcast and those that could be viewed only in theaters.

In spite of the movie industry's attempts to separate itself from broadcasting's crass motives and obvious ploys, however, the American cinema has never strayed far from the call of advertising. "When the first movie cameraman shot the first street scene that included a shop sign," Charles Eckert has written, "all of the elements of a new advertising medium were implicit."[19] Even during the first decades of the industry, producers signed deals with corporate sponsors, agreeing to tout brand-name products in their films. Studios assigned personnel to facilitate interaction with advertisers and even created divisions to produce explicitly sponsored films. Although the studios were eager to generate revenue through advertising, exhibitors appreciated the need to distinguish the movie-going experience from commercial broadcasting (to justify paid admissions) and, therefore, resisted the presence of advertising in movie theaters. Fearing repercussions from angry exhibitors and alienated moviegoers, the major studios ultimately introduced a more sublimated type of advertising and forged a more discreet relationship with advertisers. Brand-name products entered movies through "product placements," agreements to showcase products subtly within the milieu of the narrative. More obvious commercial tie-ins were shifted outside of the narrative, to marketing campaigns and celebrity product endorsements that accompanied a movie's release. The cinema never became an advertiser-supported medium, but its aims have been relatively consistent with those of commercial broadcasters. Although some critics see product placements as a recent phenomenon that demonstrates the contamination of the cinema by television's influence, Eckert suggests that the silver screen has always been a type of "living display window" for consumer culture.[20]

The motion picture industry's long-standing alliance with commercial sponsors, often obscured by common conceptions of the cinema's aesthetic autonomy, provides a pertinent example of the convergence of movies and related social institutions. This convergence blurs the boundaries between narrative and advertising in movies—an accusation traditionally leveled at commercial broadcasting. And like commercial broadcasting, the cinema promoted the values of consumer culture, including an ideology in which the consumption of commodities is centered primarily in the home and the institution of the family.

The impulse of manufacturers and advertisers to cultivate the home as the primary arena of consumption led advertisers to Hollywood, but it also led Hollywood into the American home—at first tentatively via the domestic medium of radio, then wholeheartedly upon the arrival of television. Indeed, Laura Mulvey argues that the cultural shift from the public exhibition of movies to the domestic reception of television during the 1950s coincides with "the triumph of the home as point of consumption in the capitalist circulation of commodities." Measuring the significance of this development for American culture, Nick Browne writes, "The commercial development of television in the post–World War II years as a mechanism for reaching into the household represents a singularly significant moment in the development of the American economy and culture. Through television, American business has represented, penetrated, and constructed the family with an eye to its aptitude for consumption."[21]

Hollywood recognized television's ability to reach into the household, the privileged site of consumer culture, and was as eager as any manufacturer to place its products in the American home. After deciding to enter television production, the motion picture industry even participated in the cultural discourse that helped to define television as a domestic medium, identified with the values of home and family.[22] In announcing the decision of Warner Bros. to produce television programming, for instance, Harry Warner took great pains to distinguish the studio's TV product from its theatrical features. In this instance, he didn't focus on the relative budgets, production values, narrative strategies, or stars; instead, he emphasized the divergent social functions of the two media. Warner Bros. TV, he proclaimed, would emphasize the educational aspects of television, which "can accomplish social good that sound films have failed to accomplish. . . . In my opinion, proper programs can unite families—father, mother, children—at home, rather than separate them as the search for amusement and 'a good time' has done in the past."[23] How ironic it seems that Harry Warner, a man who made his fortune with the motion picture, could implicate the movies and other public amusements as forces for corruption, while imagining television as the entertaining savior of the American family.

From Cecil B. De Mille's radio show to television production at Warner Bros., the movie industry has sought through the electronic media to convey traces of Hollywood to the American home—an impulse that continues today in cable TV and home video. Whether it meant displaying consumer goods in cinematic narratives, marketing ancillary products identified with movie stars and stories, promoting feature films through broadcasting, or exhibiting its own films and series on TV, the motion picture industry consistently demonstrated an interest in colonizing the domestic spaces of social life, a trend that Edward Buscombe describes as "the privatization of consumption in general and of entertainment in particular."[24] The studios collaborated with broadcasters and advertisers throughout the studio era and were eager to join them in cultivating the potentially lucrative market of the postwar American home. The rise of TV production among Hollywood's major studios may have seemed like a radical departure for companies traditionally devoted to theatrical exhibition, but, in fact, it realized ambitions that the industry had harbored for decades.

Notes

1. Robert Ardrey, "Hollywood: The Toll of the Frenzied Forties," *The Reporter*, 21 March 1957, p. 30.
2. David O. Selznick to John Hay Whitney, 7 August 1958, Selznick Collection. All Selznick-related sources are found in this collection.
3. William T. Orr, personal interview, 28 October 1986, Los Angeles; Roy Huggins, personal interview, 25 May 1991, Los Angeles. Other studios established similar rules. A 1949 memo at MGM reportedly prohibited mention of the word "television" in that studio's feature films. See "Hollywood in a Television Boom," *Broadcasting*, 26 October 1959, p. 88. For a discussion of this debate, see Milton MacKaye, "The Big Brawl: Hollywood versus Television," *Saturday Evening Post*, 19 January 1952, p. 30; 26 January 1952, p. 30; 26 February 1952, p. 30; Warner Bros. Pictures, Inc., *Annual Report*, 1947–1953.
4. See William Lafferty, "'No Attempt at Artiness, Profundity, or Significance': *Fireside Theater* and the Rise of Filmed Television Programming," *Cinema Journal* 27, no. 1 (Fall 1987): 23–46.

5. "The Week in Review," *Time,* 8 November 1954, p. 95.

6. Leon Morse, "TV Film: The Battle for Power," *Television,* May 1959, pp. 47–49; "Six Major Studios Turning Out 37% of Webs Telepix," *Variety,* 1 July 1959, p. 36.

7. "WB's $30,000,000 TV Income," *Variety,* 24 June 1959, p. 77; Warner Bros. Pictures, Inc., *Annual Report,* 1957; "Warner Likes TV, Not Actors," *Variety,* 17 June 1959, p. 5.

8. For a discussion of this period in the film industry, see Tino Balio, ed., *The American Film Industry,* pp. 401–438; Janet Staiger, "Individualism versus Collectivism," *Screen* 24, nos. 4–5 (July–August 1983): 68–79.

9. Lawrence L. Murray, "Complacency, Competition, Cooperation: The Film Industry Responds to the Challenge of Television," *Journal of Popular Film* 6, no. 1 (1977): 47–68.

10. Todd Gitlin, "Down the Tubes," in Mark Crispin Miller, ed., *Seeing through Movies,* pp. 19, 48. Other articles in this anthology continue the argument that commercial television is either directly or indirectly responsible for a catalog of artistic and ideological offenses committed by the contemporary American cinema.

11. Michele Hilmes, *Hollywood and Broadcasting: From Radio to Cable*; William Boddy, *Fifties Television: The Industry and Its Critics*; Tino Balio, ed., *Hollywood in the Age of Television.* See also such early influential articles as Edward Buscombe, "Thinking It Differently: Television and the Film Industry," *Quarterly Review of Film studies* 9, no. 3 (Summer 1984): 196–203; Douglas Gomery, "Failed Opportunities: The Integration of the Motion Picture and TV Industries," *Quarterly Review of Film Studies* 9, no. 3 (Summer 1984): 219–228; Richard B. Jewell, "Hollywood and Radio: Competition and Partnership in the '30s," *Historical Journal of Film, Radio, and Television* 4, no. 2 (1984): 125–141; and Robert Vianello, "The Rise of the Telefilm and the Networks' Hegemony over the Motion Picture Industry," *Quarterly Review of Film Studies* 9, no. 3 (Summer 1984): 204–218.

12. Carolyn Marvin, *When Old Technologies Were New: Thinking about Electric Communication in the Late Nineteenth Century,* p. 8.

13. Robert C. Allen addresses this aspect of traditional broadcasting history in *Speaking of Soap Operas,* p. 96.

14. De Mille, always one of the industry's great showmen, relished the seeming ubiquity of a nationally broadcast program: "I liked the big [ratings] numbers but what the Lux program meant to me cannot be measured by any numbers. It meant families in Maine and Kansas and Idaho finishing the dishes or the schoolwork or the evening chores in time to gather around their radios. It meant the shut-ins, the invalid, the blind, the very young, and the very old who had no other taste of the theater. It meant people, not in the masses, but individuals, who did me the honor of inviting me into their homes." De Mille's exposure, including his signature statement, "This is Cecil B. De Mille saying good night to you from Hollywood," transformed his name into a trademark tantamount to the notion of the movie producer and helped to popularize the concept of authorship in the movie industry (Cecil B. De Mille, *The Autobiography of Cecil B. De Mille,* p. 347). For a more extensive description of the Lux program, see Bernard Lucich, *"The Lux Radio Theatre,"* in Lawrence W. Lichty and Malachi C. Topping, eds., *American Broadcasting: A Sourcebook on the History of Radio and Television,* pp. 391–394; and Hilmes, *Hollywood and Broadcasting,* pp. 78–115. For De Mille's earnings, see Douglas Gomery, *The Hollywood Studio System,* p. 42. For a thorough discussion of the entire era of Hollywood's involvement in radio, see Hilmes, *Hollywood and Broadcasting,* pp. 26–77.

15. Gomery, *The Hollywood Studio System,* pp. 42–44. For a discussion of Paramount's early ties to the broadcasting industry, see Jonathon Buchsbaum, "Zukor Buys Protection: The Paramount Stock Purchase of 1929," *Cine-Tracts* 2 (Summer/Fall 1979): 49–62. For a discussion of Paramount's subsequent investments in television, see Timothy R. White, "Hollywood's Attempt at Appropriating Television: The Case of Paramount Pictures," in Balio, *Hollywood in the Age of Television,* pp. 145–164, and Timothy R. White, "Hollywood's Attempt to Appropriate Television: The Case of Paramount Pictures" (Ph.D. dissertation, University of Wisconsin-Madison, 1990).

16. Colin MacCabe, "The Discursive and the Ideological in Film: Notes on the Conditions of Political Intervention," *Screen* 19, no. 4 (Winter 1978–1979): 37-38.
17. Representations of TV sets in 1950s movies often continued this critique by depicting TV viewing as a sign of social pathology. *All That Heaven Allows* (1955) contains a scene in which the emotional abandonment of the Jane Wyman character by her grown children is captured in the striking image of her face reflected back by the indifferent TV screen that her children have given her as a gift. Television viewing signifies the disintegration of traditional family and community relations in such movies as *Rebel without a Cause* (1955) and *Bigger Than Life* (1956). In these films, TV viewing isolates family members from one another and obscures the larger social conflicts that threaten the viability of the family.
18. Theodor W. Adorno, "Television and the Patterns of Mass Culture," in Bernard Rosenberg and David Manning White, eds., *Mass Culture: The Popular Arts in America,* pp. 474–475.
19. Charles Eckert, "The Carole Lombard in Macy's Window," Quarterly Review of Film Studies 3, no. 1 (Winter 1978): 4. See also Stuart Ewen, *Captains of Consciousness: Advertising and the Social Roots of Consumer Culture,* p. 73.
20. As Mary Ann Doane has argued, "The film frame functions, in this context, not as a 'window on the world' as in the Bazinian formulation, but as a quite specific kind of window—a shop window" (Mary Ann Doane, *The Desire to Desire: The Woman's Film of the 1940s,* p. 24). Jane Gaines inverts the metaphor to analyze the relationships among shop windows, motion pictures, and consumer culture. See "The Queen Christina Tie-Ups: Convergence of Show Window and Screen," *Quarterly Review of Film & Video* 11, no. 1 (1989): 35–60. Mark Crispin Miller mistakenly sees product placements as a recent phenomenon and uses this insight to argue that the encroachment of TV's values on the cinema is both symptom and cause of the decline of the American cinema in the 1980s. See Mark Crispin Miller, "End of Story," in Mark Crispin Miller, ed., *Seeing through Movies,* pp. 186–246.
21. Laura Mulvey, "Melodrama In and Out of the Home," in Colin MacCabe, ed., *High Theory/Low Culture: Analyzing Popular Television and Film,* p. 98; Nick Browne, "The Political Economy of the Television (Super) Text," in Horace Newcomb, ed., *Television: The Critical View,* p. 597.
22. For a more extensive discussion of television's contested meanings in relation to notions of home and family in the 1950s, see Lynn Spigel, *Make Room for TV: Television and the Family Ideal in Postwar America.*
23. Thomas F. Brady, "New Hollywood Enterprise," *New York Times,* 9 January 1949, sec. 2, p. 5.
24. Buscombe, "Thinking It Differently," p. 201.

A Face in the Crowd:
An Interview with Kazan

Jeff Young

Marcia Jeffries (Patricia Neal) takes her radio show, "A Face in the Crowd," to the local jail in Piggot, Arkansas, where she comes upon a natural-born storyteller, jokester, and singer whom she dubs "Lonesome" Rhodes (Andy Griffith). She recruits him as a permanent part of her show. Instantly his success and power grow. So do their feelings for each other.

Rhodes is signed up for a Nashville TV show, and he takes Marcia with him. Again, he is an immediate sensation. His popularity increases as he is seen to be a truthteller in a world of sham and lies. The public loves him for making fun of his sponsor. The sponsor does not and fires him. But by then Joey de Palma (Anthony Franciosa) has moved in and gotten him an audition with a national sponsor and a network in New York. He goes to say his goodbyes to Marcia. Instead they become lovers, and the threesome head for the big city, accompanied by Mel Miller (Walter Matthau), one of Lonesome's writers, whom he scorns for being overeducated.

By now, Rhodes knows his own strengths. He wins over the sponsors and gets his own show. He sticks to his guns when it comes to telling the truth where others lie or sugarcoat, and soon the entire country falls under his spell. But throughout his rise he becomes increasingly aware of his power, comes to enjoy wielding it and gets corrupted by it. He throws his money and his weight around, womanizes, drinks too much, and becomes an almost grotesque version of his former self.

Marcia, despite knowing his faults and suffering from his betrayals, is hopelessly in love with him. He, in turn, remains dependent on her despite—or perhaps because of—his incredible success. He promises to marry her; instead, he runs off with Betty Lou, a seventeen-year-old baton twirler (Lee Remick).

Lonesome's influence on public opinion and his salesmanship have become such a force that he is asked to guide a staunch, right-wing senator's campaign for the Presidency. His power to move an audience has evolved into the power to manipulate them. His love for his audience turns into contempt. He becomes a brutal, dangerous demagogue.

Marcia can no longer stand by and do nothing. Despite still loving him, she reveals his true nature by turning on a microphone in the TV studio's control booth. Lonesome's nastiest, most abusive remarks about his supposedly beloved audience are broadcast coast to coast. The outraged public immediately drops him, his power evaporates, and he is left alone to bellow into the night.

All of the characters in A Face in the Crowd *aroused ambivalent feelings. In spite of their failings, it was impossible to overlook the humanity in any of them. Tell me, first of all, what you wanted to make the picture about?*

I was trying to make a political picture, a warning about television and television personalities. "Listen to what he says. Think about it. Don't be taken in by what he is, or appears to be." Budd Schulberg and I were very close in our views of everything. We were both aware that television could be what it has, in fact, turned out to be, an almost hypnotic terrible force. We knew television was selling "personality" because we had Eisenhower up there on TV all the time. You looked at him, and there was

Grandpappy. And everyone wants to be nice to Grandpappy. But if you listened to him he was saying nothing. In the character of Lonesome Rhodes I wanted to show the ambivalence in someone who was almost evil, but who said and believed many things that were right at the same time. I wanted him to be seductive and say out loud things that other people didn't. For example, I think in his time George Wallace in some ways reflected the truth of what a lot of people were feeling. When he walked about tax loopholes for the rich, I didn't assume he was cynical. I took it that like a lot of poor white kids he was aware that there was an Eastern establishment of industrial-military forces that got vast privileges, though he didn't put it in those words. There was something about that little guy that everybody despised that I liked. I felt the same way about Huey Long. His roots were in Populism, the concerns of the common man. Budd and I wanted our hero to seduce his audience so that they would think, "Yes, I can see why he's got that power." Then gradually show that power corrupts and he becomes corrupted, but that he's in part aware of what he's becoming. There is a dualism about television. On the one hand, it can be very beguiling and can turn a man into a hell of a salesman. On the other hand, if you get very close and expose a man enough, sooner or later he's going to reveal who he really is. McCarthy, in my opinion, was hurt more by one incident than anything else. He was seen on television whispering smugly behind his hand to Roy Cohn during the Army hearings. That image was repeated time after time on the nightly news. We made up the plot of *A Face in the Crowd* out of those dual or dialectic realizations. On the one hand our hero seduced the American public. On the other hand he exposed himself so much to the American public that his real nature came through.

Was there any source material for all that?

Budd and I had such a good time doing *On the Waterfront* I said, "Let's do another picture together." He knew the kind of thing I was thinking about so he suggested a short story he had written called *Your Arkansas Traveller*. I read it and liked it and that was it. Then we spent literally months doing research. We went to Young and Rubicam product meetings and talked to advertising people. We went to Nashville a lot and got into the Nashville sound and the Grand Ole Opry. I hung around with a camera. We met a lot of stand-up comics, some of whom are in the picture. Every aspect of the film was carefully researched. It was about a phenomenon that was happening in America at that time. We were always talking about and looking out for native, grassroots fascism. One thing that a lot of people overlooked is that Fascism always had attractive elements of populism in it. Hitler's followers initially, the members of the National Socialist Party, were guys who were on the outs, who had no power or even jobs. Mussolini's party was made up of "the regular guys."

What was the aesthetic problem you set for yourself?

To be seductive and yet funny. I wanted to have an amusing picture and still have a lot of "warning" in it. I don't think I blended the styles quite right, I mean the satiric and the tragic. That's a very hard blend to achieve. I think I came close, but I don't think I achieved it.

Where do you think you failed?

I don't really know. I thought there would be more sympathy for Rhodes than there turned out to be. I saw the film again a year and a half ago. The house was full of kids, and they were stamping their feet. Maybe it was ahead of its time. You see there again, like in *East of Eden* and *Baby Doll*, I was trying to create a figure who was both attractive and a menace.

This was Andy Griffith's first film. Where did you find him?

He was a stand-up comic. He had no training or experience as a professional actor. But Budd and I heard his record, something about football, and when we talked to him, we both liked him a lot.

Given his inexperience, how did you work with him?

I showed him what I wanted a lot. Take for example the early scene in jail when the sheriff wakes Lonesome. I knew from my own experience that a lot of animals fight on their backs. It's their favorite position because they fight with their claws. I also knew that good street fighters always use their feet and legs. So in the scene I made Andy throw out a foot, and that gives him time to pull himself together. I illustrated that to him and he imitated me. It affected his voice and everything else and made him fierce. He understood it too. He's not a brawler, but every country boy has seen fights.

You actually acted it out for him?
I did it more and more though certain scenes I didn't have to illustrate. Nobody could beat him in front of a microphone. I did all kinds of things. In the big scene at the end of the film when he's up on the balcony, I got him drunk for two days. Somebody wrote an interview attacking me, saying that I got him drunk against his will. An absolute falsehood. Andy will tell you he wanted to be good and couldn't do it. When he got drunk, it was easier so he got drunk. I called it the Jack Daniels school of acting.

Did acting it out for Griffith embarrass him in front of the others?
No, they all liked Andy. And I'd made a big favorite of him. He didn't take it as an insult. He didn't know anything about directing, so he took it as if it were the normal way to work. I did have a talk with Walter Matthau, because I wanted him just as simple as he could be, to just walk through playing Mel Miller. Pat Neal I had to keep ambivalent. I had her keep her mind on the fact that Marcia loved Lonesome but was fighting it off.

Once again you use a relationship with a woman to reveal the central male character.
A man, in every phase of his life, is moved by the same things. You watch a man playing tennis and you see the way he's going to be in his work, how he treats his children, how he is in bed. You watch the way a man walks and you see where his tension is. It's all one piece. What he does on the social and political level, he's also going to do on the personal level. What's touching about Marcia is that she sees the good in Lonesome and thinks she can change him. She fights for the good in him and waits for the good in him to dominate. She's in a sense like a mother who keeps thinking, he's all right—in his heart I know he's okay. And in Lonesome's heart he was "okay," but too little and too late. Early on the viewer sniffs out that he is a rascal—a lovable one, but still a seducer. But Marcia contests your suspicions. The fact that she believes in him does two things. It keeps the ambivalence going. The audience thinks maybe she is right. Maybe the good will win out over the bad. They also watch the woman being fooled and fooling herself and are very touched by it, because she gives her whole life to him.

Did you set for yourself any kind of pictorial style?
I wanted it photographed very plainly. There were great technical difficulties. I had to open up the f-stop on the camera enough so that I could photograph what was happening on the TV monitor screens and still photograph people and get some sort of exposure on their faces. If you opened up too much, there would be too much light and all of their features would wash out. That was a very hard thing to balance. I also wanted a lot of cuts, which meant shooting more set-ups. I had worked with Harry Stradling on *Streetcar* and adored him. He was temperamentally a model to me of what a cameraman should be. He was always cheerful, nothing was too difficult for him. You could say to him at ten minutes to quitting time, "I need two more close-ups, Harry." And you'd get two more close-ups. He could do anything at any speed. Harry loved what he was doing abundantly.

Why the need for so many cuts?
The material always dictates the style. Here we had all kinds of physically big scenes with lots of extras. You just can't light everyone in a mob as if each were posing for a portrait. They're not going to be on screen that long. I wanted a slam-bang style, and I didn't want to be held up by a lot of fussing.

Let's go back to the narrative. Marcia gets Lonesome to do her radio program. He does a country-boy routine, and while he's doing it, you keep his voice going and cut to people listening to the show and responding to what he's saying. Later, Lonesome does a broadcast where he tells all the townspeople that the sheriff would make a good dog catcher; you cut to the sheriff's house with five hundred dogs on the lawn. In Memphis he does his first TV broadcast and again, it's a country boy up against the city slickers. In New York there's a broadly played audition scene in which Lonesome confronts the advertising executives and their client. You do it again when he sells the senator and gets involved in politics. In each of the scenes, the structure is almost identical. It is the outsider against the establishment. He has to win them over, and he does so by attacking or making fun of them. How do you play essentially the same scene so many times and avoid it feeling repetitive?

First of all I tried to make sure they were all funny and amusing. But the main thing was to make sure that it wasn't just plain repetition, that his behavior changed, that he got bolder and bolder and more and more destructive of the advertising and business customs from one confrontation to the next. The progression was based on Lonesome's increased awareness of his growing power and the pleasure he got from wielding it. His personality becomes increasingly synthetic. It comes to resemble more and more a kind of hayseed fascism: "know-nothingism," in effect.

Did you work with Schulberg on the script?

I worked with him all the time on the conception and on the ordering of the scenes, but I never wrote a word. My contribution was not in the verbal language, the dialogue, but in the language of film, especially in the language of sequence and climax. They are as much the director's prerogative as the writer's, so they have to be determined in collaboration. We worked out the basic movement of the story—what they used to call the continuity. Then I disappeared, and Budd wrote a complete first draft. Then I reappeared, and we worked over it.

Once you get into working over and over a script with the writer, how do you then separate yourself enough to be objective?

You begin to lose your objectivity immediately, but you no longer want to be objective. You want to be personal and egocentric. You become as one, and it can be a wonderful relationship. I would always speak absolutely candidly to Budd, just as I would later try to be candid with myself. It's harder to be objective when I work alone because I have no one to challenge me.

How do you keep your sense of invention from being exhausted?

Partly by involving myself in another project so desperately that I couldn't think of anything else. Also, you assert a will not to think of it, forget it, walk away from it. I did a play while Budd wrote the script. Objectivity can be a problem. You deal with it one way or another, the best you can. When you get a script finished, if you trust a couple of people, you can let them read it. You get very egocentric by that time. You have to be. Directing is an exertion of your will. That's why you've got to be steel inside as to your goal. Fortunately, I have had good relationships with authors. I protected them. I never picked up a pen. That's important. Don't scribble. Don't write lines. The director mustn't take away the screenwriter's identity as the "author." You try to get the best out of screenwriters by liberating them. Have them deal with the real problems rather than have them deal with pleasing you. I'm very strong and insistent so I have to be particularly careful that I don't say, "Do it my way." Indirectly, subtly, I eventually make my will known. But really and truly—I mean this— you do it as a suggestion. It's a subtle relationship. You don't want a writer just running around aping you and admiring you. You want someone who's strong and helpful. With really good authors it's especially important to deal collaboratively. They're on guard against a "writing director" and for good reason. In the old days in Hollywood the studios or the producers would have an author write a complete scene-by-scene scenario, and then they'd say, "Now that the structure is good, we need someone to do the dialogue." They'd fire the writer and get someone else to "dialogue it."

For all the big scenes in the film, there are many extremely intimate ones as well, for example when Lonesome tells Marcia about his childhood. It's the real beginning of his winning her over. How did you work through those intimate moments?

I always started very quietly in a scene like that and had the actors just talk and listen to each other. It's very important. She was always trying to see the good in him. I would give him the very simple action of just winning her or boasting. The main thing is to make the audience believe that these two people are interested in each other and that he wants her as much as she cares for him. Whether he does or not, I don't know. I never was convinced that Lonesome really wanted her, but he wanted everybody, whoever happened to be at hand.

What was the essence of his character?
He'd spent his life as an outsider, and that was the way he thought of himself. But when he gets down to it, he wants the same things the "in" people want. He's a very seducible guy with a very tough front. He's typical of many show business types. They look like rebels, but they're really not. That whole world is very seductive. Money and fame often come very quickly, but they're unstable. So you grab what you can as fast as you can. Lonesome is typical of a lot of actors, directors and writers who go into this very difficult profession. Show business people find themselves showing off a lot, selling themselves constantly. When you're uncertain of yourself, you're dependent upon other people to like you. Comics do that, clowns do that, politicians do that. They're all related to each other because they live by the approval of others. What Lonesome really seeks from Marcia is her approval even though he goes after it in a huffy, arrogant way.

She says that she likes the way he laughs. He replies that he puts his whole self into it just as he puts his whole self into everything he does.
He's really saying, "Go to bed with me, I'll put my whole self into that, too." And he's just gotten a first taste of power. He's gotten people to bring their dogs to the sheriff's front lawn, and Marcia asks him, "How does it feel to have the power to do this?" And "she" equals the audience. They're wondering about the same thing. You feel him liking it, enjoying it. And as soon as you enjoy it, power begins to corrupt you. It becomes power for its own sake. His ego is justified, and he says, "Ah, I've got them." He has a certain vengefulness because he's been on the bottom of society his whole life and all of a sudden he's on top. He enjoys that. We all suffer in this public relations civilization. The taste of our civilization is determined by columnists. And most of the critics are columnists. They're on a head trip, showing off their egos. So the whole thing is a big public relations ego competition.

Shortly thereafter an agent arrives who wants to take him to Nashville, who likens him to Will Rogers. You see him begin to wield another kind of power. He makes a pass at Marcia.
He does something that's absolutely typical of comics and singers. They combine their career push with a sexual push, directed at anybody who happens to be there for conquest. Getting a better deal for himself allows him to wink at Marcia, showing off to her.

In the scene at the train station, as he and Marcia are leaving Piggott, Arkansas, we see the worm in the apple. He's all smiles to the public, but privately he slams the locals.
By this time, the audience has gotten the idea; they know what he's likely to become, but that scene is Marcia's first big and maybe last good chance to pull away from Rhodes. He says, "Boy, am I glad to shake that dump." She is shocked, she should walk, be saying to herself, he's a phony, I made a mistake. But she does not. Instead she feels, "I can fix him." She's sick, you know—a little masochistic. She takes more abuse than any woman should all through the picture.

Did you give Neal that to ploy?
No, the script does that. You have to play against it. I made her really feel that she was in love with him, which is what women do. They rationalize. The word "love" is an umbrella. It covers a multitude of sins. It disguises what's really happening. You say you "love" someone, but you may want to dominate him, encourage him, or you may want his favor. When a man says he loves a woman, it may mean he loves to brutalize her, or it may mean she's got his conscience, as was the case here. Both women and men kid themselves sometimes. They use that word "love," and it excuses everything they do.

In getting her to play the scene, did you use an "umbrella" term or were you more specific?
   I told her, "You do love him, you feel he has so much good in him that you've got to see him through." It's got to be absolutely sincere. You do not direct the actress with the result you hope to get from the script. You give her something that will produce, combined with the script and the situation, the results you want. You don't tell Pat Neal he's going to destroy your life, but call him back. That's called "playing the result."

The film keeps you guessing because you're never quite sure about Lonesome.
   There's always some element of honesty in him. He's a truthteller in a hypocritical civilization.

In the first scene at the Nashville TV studio, Lonesome is terribly uncomfortable and you sympathize with his bewilderment. Then he makes a touching speech about being lost in the big city. It's done with an openness and innocence that's moving and intriguing because it plays off a moment of arch nastiness in which he calls Mel Miller, "Vanderbilt '44." When you have a complicated scene in which a character, played by an untrained actor, moves through different levels or pitches of behavior, what do you do?
   I told Griffith the whole thing is a fraud, and then I cast a real phony to play the director of the TV show. I always tried to make Andy feel that he was telling the truth, and that Lonesome's strength came from that. The whole problem with Andy was to make him more sincere, more believable and direct. The phoniness is created by the story as it develops and by the scenes as they're directed and laid out. Within that context of falseness, you make Andy believe that he alone sees and tells the truth. Even when Lonesome explains to Marcia why he married Betty Lou later in the picture, there is some element of truth in it.

But in that scene you're describing, he goes to Marcia. She doesn't come to him. He calls and barges into her room. Obviously, he needs something from her, he's not just being a decent guy.
   He needs her to believe in him. For a lot of men, the woman they are with when they first get successful becomes the talisman of their success. They have that woman connected with the idea "I made it with her." In this case Lonesome believes that his success is related to his worth, and Marcia has become not only his talisman, she's the container that holds success through a demonstration of conscience. He believes that if she thinks he is a good person, then he must be a good person. So it's very important to him that she continue to believe in him. But he's a complex being. He has very anarchistic and disruptive feelings too.

One of the ways he succeeds is by knocking the establishment. He knocks his sponsor, and they threaten to pull his contract. He goes back on the air and knocks them even more. Anthony Franciosa plays Joey, a flunky who works for the sponsor. He totally agrees with his boss to his face, but in the next breath goes behind his back and sets up a deal to sell Lonesome to national television in New York. When the sponsor does fire him, Lonesome goes back to say goodbye to Marcia. I guess he really goes back to spend the night with her.
   No he doesn't. He really is a very complex character and is never totally insincere. In the first place, he does a very honest thing when the sponsor says, "I'm going to fire you if you tell the truth about our product." He tells the truth even more. You've got to admire him for that, He really means, "I don't want any part of this, and I'm going back to my old life." And that's the moment when Marcia realizes that she can only hold him by going to bed with him. She feels that there's something terrifically truthful and alienated about his wanting to go home. But she calls him back, and what she says in a sense is, "I believe in you and anything I have is yours. You're worth more than I am, and I'll put my life on the line with yours." That's what a pure girl does. That's a beautiful scene. I also like the scene in the ad agency in New York that comes soon after. I thought it was hilarious. In the end what it came down to is that what you sell in America is not what's in the product but what's in the ad.

I disagree with you about that scene. I didn't think you did it very well.
   It was too broad?

Yes. It seemed to me that you were glib in the handling of those small parts. The people were reduced to clichés.
   Possibly so. The whole advertising world does appeal to my sense of the ludicrous. Sometimes when I think something is amusing, I let it go on too long or I go too far with it.

In a series of transitions you show Lonesome's rise and the sales of the product he's selling go up. It ends with an extreme close-up of his mouth in a big grin. You then cut to an enormous wide shot of a country estate in Connecticut—the General's house. The General owns the sponsor, Vitajex, and he knows he's got a valuable tool in Rhodes.
   Lonesome's gone on to a new plateau. He sold himself so well that now he's useful in a different way. New horizons of power are opened up.

It's a second-act curtain in a way. There's another set of transitions. Lonesome makes the cover of Life, Look *and the* Journal American. *It ends with him being given a penthouse suite. He's made it to the top.*
   And you feel that his latest success is the work of a bigger PR man, namely General Haynesworth. The General's plan is to give Lonesome political power and influence, to make him into a person who creates public opinion. It is sort of an anatomy of American power.

Again, as you said, Lonesome intertwines his career with his relationship with Marcia. He asks her to come over—he's desperate to see her, despite the fact that while he is talking to her, his assistant is hurrying another woman out of his apartment.
   That's exactly the point. Marcia is very hip. She knows about the other woman right away, and still she's tempted to be with him. Putting that other girl there was a brilliant idea on Budd's part. Lonesome's behavior is truthfully the way someone like him feels after he's had a night with a girl that he's found to be terribly boring. He may want another girl, the same type, three nights later, but there are moments of self-disgust and loneliness in that kind of screwing, and he thinks, Marcia's my real identity. I've got to have her.

He asks her to marry him. He says, "I need you . . . I'm in mighty tall grass . . . You're my lifeline to the truth." She responds, "Don't hurt me."
   That's her way of accepting. She knows she's going to get hurt. That's why she says it, of course. Many women who go into that kind of marriage know that. They're not fools. After she accepts his proposal, he shows her the lights of the city from his penthouse windows. We had much more in that scene which we cut. Budd had a great idea—that Lonesome would have a garden on his penthouse balcony. He says, "You can't keep anything alive up here. Dust in this city kills everything." It was his attempt to get back to the best, most honest part of him.

Why did you cut it?
   It didn't seem to work. Maybe we thought we'd said enough about how he was feeling. Throughout the picture Budd and I contrasted Lonesome's obvious enjoyment of manipulating people with his genuine reactions to the corrupt elements around him. Self-disgust is the most characteristic and typical reaction.

It's very believable that he wants to marry her, and that's why the next scene works. Marcia is sitting in his penthouse when in comes a woman who introduces herself as Mrs. Rhodes—Lonesome's wife whom he had never divorced. If she doesn't receive $3,000 a month, she's going to make it plenty hot for both of them.
   That's a classic scene in women's lives. Marcia conceals her pain. She has too much pride to let it show.

How do you approach a scene where actors have to conceal their feelings?

I did two things in that scene. First, I told Pat, "Don't give her the satisfaction she wants." And I told the other dame, "That prim little bitch sitting there is a phony." I made her believe that Pat Neal herself is a phony. So you deal in reality. It made the scene fun for the other woman.

Do you have to get them to feel the pain first, and then conceal it?

An actor is going to jump at feeling that. The problem is to get her to conceal it.

When Marcia comes to confront Lonesome, we see the nastiness in him. Lonesome and Joey are demonstrating a laugh machine to the General. What an idea that was.

That's Budd. I didn't tell Andy, "You're nasty now." Instead I said, "You're showing this machine off, it could put you at the top. And this bitch is being sour and making nasty cracks. You want to kill her." So he behaves as if she were actually disloyal. All the time you give the actor justifications for what he does. He's right to be sore at her, but she's also right. Drama is the opposition of two sides that are "right," or else the conflict doesn't amount to anything.

Lonesome Rhodes is now becoming a power freak and losing touch with the little people whose laughter made him. He replaces them with a machine, his artificiality has a correlative.

When you use an obvious symbol like that, you're walking a tightrope, and you've got to protect it in every way you can. One thing that helped a lot was that I played the antagonism between Lonesome and Marcia so the audience's total concentration wasn't on the business with the machine. She's resentful and thinks he's become a phony. She even looks at him differently. The scene could have been just a rather far-fetched gag. So it was essential to find a way to relate it to the central story. That's always important to remember. You should never say, "Now we're taking a hiatus and just having some fun." If there's a scene about an applause box it should mean something to the protagonist. As soon as you do that, you cover a multitude of sins because you're always on the main line and everything else is ornament, comment, device. The heart of this scene was the machine and the boss's reaction to it, but even more importantly it was about Rhodes showing off and trying to win him.

The text of that scene doesn't directly tell the main story.

So I interwove a subtext even if it was only expressed by the way Neal and Griffith looked at each other or the way she tagged along behind him. You don't have to have dialogue all the time to keep the story flowing. You tell the actors what's really going on underneath while they're doing whatever the hell they're doing. That happens all the time in life. When you're angry with somebody you avoid the anger. You don't run out and scream. You do something else. I avoid a confrontation unless it has to be settled or you just can't hold it in anymore so you blurt it out. I always give the actors something else to do if possible, otherwise you just get people talking to each other. The more you make it indirect, the more interesting the final explosion or confrontation is.

You keep changing about how much and/or how directly you tell things to the actors.

It depends on what you're getting from them. Their intuitions might be exactly right. There was an interesting article by Liv Ullmann in the *Times* the other day. She said Ingmar Bergman doesn't tell his actors much. He says you can talk a goddamn scene to death. A lot of young directors, who are aiming high, tend to do just that. I used to do it. The point is that to get what you want you may have to just say a single word. You may have given the direction the night before. You may have given it as you said good morning or as you shared your Danish pastry with them. You may do it in some indirect way that leaves them thinking. Or you may do it by explaining that the business they're doing is somehow redolent of the conflict. But you even try to give that direction indirectly because otherwise they're trying to satisfy you, whereas the point is to deal with their partner in the scene.

In the next scene Marcia goes into the writer's room where everyone is trashing Lonesome.

That scene is really about the intention of the girl. What is she going to do? She is confronted with the fact that these guys are saying terrible things about Rhodes that she completely agrees with. She doesn't know what to do, and it dramatizes her inner conflict. You don't see it directly. She doesn't protest. She even joins in knocking him to a certain extent but you know that she's also committed to the guy.... Why are you laughing?

I'm laughing at the precision of your recall. That scene was shot a very long time ago.

It's not just recall. It's a principle of directing. The way I see things, as I said, is that every scene in some way or other should deal with what's happening at the core of the story, or else don't have the scene.

The film shifts gear when we return to Piggott, Arkansas for the cheerleading contest.

One big decision we had to make when we went down to Piggott was how to shoot this huge scene. I decided to build a tower from which we photographed the high school band spelling out "We love Lonesome Rhodes." That cost a lot of money, but I decided the picture needed that kind of opening up. The spectacle also let you see things from Rhodes' point of view—how seductive it all is. Everyone is at his feet, and they really like him. That's America. Everything is PR. Also, it is tempting. Lee Remick, who played Betty Lou, was twenty-one and in perfect physical condition, really a bloom, just a perfect little bud of a girl. She's open and available to him. How could any man resist? Why should he? Of course it's easy to say he's being untrue to Marcia, but that's what makes life complicated and interesting. His appetite for adulation is without bounds. He's starved, like a lot of guys who have spent most of their lives at the bottom. They've been down so long that when they get up, they can't stop climbing.

Throughout the baton contest, Lonesome and Betty Lou keep giving each other the eye. Joey, now his manager, watches it happening. You can see him trying to figure an angle.

I was trying to show that Joey is jealous of anyone moving in on his hold on Rhodes, above all Marcia. What you have is a triangle with Rhodes in the middle. The temper of the times as expressed by Joey is on one side, and Marcia, the girl that thinks he's the only fellow that's saying certain truths out loud in public, is on the other side. He's pulled between the two so Joey is delighted to see him get locked in with Betty Lou. He sees it as a way of cutting Lonesome away from Marcia's influence. He's like some agents in Los Angeles who get between their clients and their wives and yet at the same time send their wives presents and do everything they can to flatter them. You see them slowly break up a marriage. You see, even in the baton scene, you're trying to say something that relates to the central story. Lonesome's a victim of the system. That's putting it in rather corny terms but that's what he is.

But isn't Marcia the real victim? In the following scene, she and Mel sit in a bar, drinking. An advertising man gives her a wire saying that Rhodes is off to Mexico, ostensibly to get his divorce in order to marry her. Despite all the things she knows bad about him, she's still hooked on him—we see it in her face.

I think what Budd did with Marcia there is immense. She's absolutely in agreement with every criticism made of Rhodes, and still she's loyal. It must be like a cold blade on her heart. If that's the result of psychoanalysis, it's unhealthy. It would be better if she killed him. She's killing herself this way. You see the same thing on the faces of Hollywood wives who have husbands like that. You see the cost.

When she goes to meet him at the airport, expecting him to marry her, he has his new wife with him. You shot Patricia Neal pushing through the mob to get to him in a way that she literally becomes a face in the crowd.

I didn't do that consciously, but if the basic idea of a film is valid, it will create those sorts of images again and again. The point of the shot was to show he wanted to hit Marcia as hard as he could. He needed to hit her pretty hard in order to make a final break with her.

Then he goes to Marcia and says, "I was afraid to marry you."

He visits her. That's important because it shows he has the guts to face her. He doesn't try to avoid it. I think that's Andy's best scene in the picture. That scene is essential because it saves Lonesome Rhodes from being just a sneaky, double-crosser. This way the audience can understand his feelings and why he married Betty Lou. I mean, who needs that idealistic busybody, which is what Marcia is, always telling him what he should be. Saving his life is really none of her damn business. He just wants to enjoy himself. Suppose he doesn't want to be the great savior of the American people? At the same time, Marcia's right, too, because he double-dealt her. That's the essence of the whole Stanislavsky system. You justify everyone's point of view. Drama is best when you're dealing with opposing feelings within the audience and they don't know who's right. Conflict doesn't mean a thing if it's mechanical and physical. It means something when the conflict is general, when it's not only between two forces but between values. That's what we face all the time in life. When you decide in favor of "A" you are not deciding in favor of "B." You're losing something when you decide. That's what makes a decision difficult; that's what drama is about. There's a loss and there's no way of getting out of it. There's no perfect solution. A wonderful thing happens in that scene. Again, I've got to give Schulberg a lot of credit. It's the most unusual, unexpected thing in the film. After Lonesome gets all through explaining himself, he says he'll take care of her. "I'm gonna give you a healthy slice of our whole operation . . . say ten percent of my end. . . ." And she explodes, "Giving me. Giving me! You're not giving me anything. A Face in the Crowd was my idea. The whole idea of Lonesome Rhodes belongs to me. I always should have been an equal partner. Well, now I'm going to be an equal partner. . . . And I want it on paper." Instead of being the nice, clean girl that crawls back to Piggott, Arkansas, she holds on even then. It comes out of the pain and desperation of his betrayal. It's a way of attacking him while still holding on to him.

Despite this personal setback, Rhodes continues gaining public power. He takes over the presidential campaign of right-wing Senator Fuller. To him it's just like selling any other product.

He's fully enjoying his power, now. When the General, who is again his sponsor, warns him to play it cool, he brushes him off, saying, "I'm a force."

He demands to have a new TV program, The Cracker Barrel Show—*as a platform for his ideas and he gets it.*

What's good is you think, "God, this is ridiculous, the satire is too much." But at the same time you have a feeling, maybe it's close to something that could really happen. It makes you think about it more than it would if it were less extreme. On the other hand, I could have made the Senator nicer and smarter and it wouldn't have hurt.

Marcia and Mel watch a broadcast of the new show on a TV set in a bar.

I was trying to dramatize the scorn that Rhodes by this point had for the people, which is what fascism really is. Democracy depends on some basic, indissoluble intelligence and goodness in people. It assumes that if you tell people the facts, they'll come to the right decision, which is part superstition and part hope. Here he's just manipulating them.

When Lonesome discovers that his manager has been screwing his wife, the confrontation is played out in front of a built-in soda fountain right in his living room.

I don't know who the hell it was Budd and I read about who had an ice cream fountain in her house where she made her own sodas and sundaes. We did the same thing with Betty Lou, and the image is obliterating—it reduces her to nothing. He kicks her out. He was getting isolated. He turned against the General, he turns against Joey. He's all alone.

So he runs right back to Marcia. He's literally taking off his clothes as he comes through the door, claiming that it was her he wanted all the time.

I hoped the audience wouldn't know how she would treat his overture. I wanted to keep it a surprise, so at the end of his long appeal to her, she goes into the closet—you think she's gone to put on a nightgown. Instead, she suddenly comes out with a coat on. She runs out of the building and it's raining. She hails a cab. The first one won't take her—a mundane detail about New York City, which keeps things rooted in reality. The next night at the TV studio, Lonesome behaves like a raving maniac, blowing his stack at everybody while Marcia watches silently from the control booth. We began to shift the focus away from Lonesome and onto Marcia. The audience begins to wonder what she'll do. It was very, very important to reveal the technology of the broadcast because we had to make Marcia's final act real and believable. As the credits begin to come up at the end of the show, she opens the sound pot so that the audience hears the scornful things Rhodes is saying about the American public. The others in the control room try to drag her away, but she holds on. It was a way to have her bring him down single-handedly.

With a sweet smile on his face he says, "Aren't they all stupid, just like sheep." While he's doing that, you cut to people all around the country watching him and reacting.
It's just like at the beginning of the film when he was in the station talking about homemade pie, and we showed the woman cleaning the inside of her oven and cooking a pie, only in reverse. That's worked in with another symbolic mechanical thing which is him going down on the elevator. We intercut between the shots of the numbers on the elevator going down and the shots of everyone, behind his back, taking him apart. The elevator boy says, "Lonesome Rhodes express, going down."

Then he goes to his own party. Nobody has shown up. He's all alone. Then you cut back to the control room. Marcia's still there. Mel persuades her to tell Rhodes that it was she who did him in.
I wanted the audience to feel her pain. She feels guilty. She's done a terrible thing. She's killed her man, her child.

Mel is very supportive, and he's obviously in love with her, but I began to dislike him.
A little bit. I tell the audience that he's absolutely right, he's strong and she should go with him, but at the same time there's a smugness about him. It's a little bit of my feeling about intellectuals leaking through, but his smugness was also essential to the story. If Mel hadn't been so absolutely sure of himself and his values and, thus, a bit pompous, we might only have felt disgust for Lonesome. We might not have seen that something good went down with Lonesome Rhodes. Without that ambivalence, the whole film wouldn't be worthwhile.

In the final scene, Rhodes is reduced to insanity.
I got Andy drunk to play it. We couldn't get it any other way. I wanted him out of control. He had to be a screaming and yelling maniac, ready to be taken away in a wagon. I didn't know how else to do it. It required a really great actor, and Andy had never acted before.

Granted he needs to be out of control, but you also gave him a lot of precise dialogue. He's raving and ranting up on the balcony until he quiets down. Then he races to Marcia, and starts raving again, until she says, "It was me." And he snaps. Instantly calm, Rhodes wishes her luck with Mel. It was very touching. Isn't it risky having an actor drunk when he has all that to do?
Those things were not all shot in the same half hour. He was only drunk when he was up on the balcony. After he played that scene a few times, he was conditioned by it. It was hard, but we did it. The picture ends as they drive off, and you hear his voice calling, "Come back." That was really walking a tightrope. Lonesome's all wrong. Everything the opposition says is true, and still in some way you maintain a modicum of sympathy for him.

I suspect that works partly because you, personally, have enormous affection for him.
I suppose having a thorough acquaintance with elements of corruption and things in myself that I don't totally approve of and admitting them helps. It's very important that a director doesn't within his own soul take a superior stance. I hate smugness, and anytime I can take a shot at it I do.

LESSON TEN

*The Birth
of the Blockbuster*

From Roadshowing to Saturation Release: Majors, Independents, and Marketing/ Distribution Innovations

Justin Wyatt

While a considerable literature addresses the aesthetics of the last golden age of Hollywood—1968–1975—accounts of changes in the industrial parameters (production, distribution, and exhibition) of those years are rare. Yet a strong relationship exists between the period's aesthetic and industrial changes. Aesthetic "products" are presented to suit the conditions of the overall market, and as the marketplace shifts across time, so does the product.

During the 1970s, film distribution practices for both the majors and minors in Hollywood altered substantially, revealing a steady shift toward the mass saturation release pattern still in place in 1997.[1] Through a review of these distribution strategies, I will illustrate the interdependence of aesthetic and industrial changes in the New Hollywood. Such an analysis also uncovers the relationship between the major studios and the independents. The innovations in film distribution can be traced directly to the margins of Hollywood, to those companies operating outside the studio system.

Searching for an Audience: Distribution, Production, and the Hollywood Recession

After the success of an increasing number of big-budget films released during the 1950s and early 1960s (such as *The Ten Commandments,* 1956; *Around the World in 80 Days,* 1956; and *Ben-Hur,* 1959), the studios began to focus on the large-scale, roadshow picture as the anchor of their distribution schedules. In many respects the roadshow picture was just another attempt to present film as different from television—or, to be more precise, as bigger, grander, and more spectacular than television. Roadshowing, with reserved seating, limited showings (usually ten or twelve per week), and lavish film subjects, transformed the act of moviegoing into a special occasion—an event. Of the components of the roadshow, a name cast and high production values (often linked to a large budget) were commonly accepted as the most significant for a successful engagement.[2] Studios furthered the practice through developing full-scale sales and publicity departments specializing in roadshow presentations.

Since these films could take months to open nationwide, roadshowing allowed studios to refine sales and advertising approaches. This method of distribution met several challenges, so the added time came in handy. Most obviously, studios incurred the greater expense of a hard-ticket engagement, which also necessitated limited (usually one matinee and one evening) shows per day. Roadshow engagements required additional box-office personnel, ushers, and support staff, creating larger "house nuts" (the cost of running the theater, which is routinely subtracted from the box-office gross before a percentage of the box-office revenues are returned to the studios). The increase in house nuts decreased studio profits on these films. Such a shortfall was exacerbated by the limited number of screenings.

Despite seemingly successful roadshow experiences with *The Bridge on the River Kwai* (1957) and *Lawrence of Arabia* (1962), Columbia Pictures executives, for example, felt so constrained financially by the traditional roadshow schedule of ten shows per week that, with the release of *A Man for All Seasons* in 1965, the studio increased the roadshow schedule to sixteen performances each week. Attendance at *A Man for All Seasons* also was bolstered by group sales that were attracted to the "event-quality" of the roadshow. Fund-raising groups were able to buy blocks of tickets at a 10–20 percent discount;[3] groups then would add an amount to raise funds for their cause or activity.

While these fund-raising activities helped roadshows to recoup a greater amount in a shorter period, the increased number of roadshowed films created a more competitive market for these "events." As Twentieth Century-Fox sales vice president Abe Dickstein commented, "If there's one thing that will kill the roadshow business, it's presenting films on a reserved-seat basis that just don't warrant this special attention."[4] To remedy this problem, studios resorted to elaborate advertising and publicity opportunities to establish a particular film in the marketplace. Columbia, for instance, was concerned about the lag between the completion of principal photography on the roadshow musical *Funny Girl* and its 1968 release date; the lengthy gap of almost a year between production and release could diminish press interest. Columbia and producer Ray Stark provided an array of impressive publicity materials during the interim: a five-minute collage of stills set to Barbra Streisand singing "I'm the Greatest Star," a fashion short made for women's clubs and merchandisers, a ten-minute documentary for theatrical release, a CBS-TV show titled "Barbra in Movieland," and a lengthier documentary, *This Is Streisand,* for the film's European release.[5]

Roadshows eventually began to target specific audiences.[6] United Artists helped to pioneer the "ethnic roadshow" through *Exodus* (1960) and *Cast a Giant Shadow* (1966), both films concerning Israel's battle for independence. Targeting the substantial Jewish population in New York City, UA set *Cast a Giant Shadow* as a roadshow attraction only in theaters there. The attempt to connect with a Jewish audience was furthered by scheduling extra holiday matinees during Passover,[7] Paramount, on the other hand, was credited with developing the youth roadshow with Franco Zeffirelli's *Romeo and Juliet* (1968); focusing on the film's young stars, Paramount scheduled a series of youth screenings and tie-ins with publications such as *Seventeen*. [8]

By 1968 the roadshow had become significant to every studio's yearly distribution slate. As *Variety* analyst Lee Beaupre reported, "Roadshow is the name of the game now being played by the majors. At current count 12 pix are expected to go out on hardticket in the last four months of this year, as compared to only 10 reserved-seaters during the previous 20 months."[9] While the emphasis on spectacle produced some large-scale hits, the bottleneck of expensive roadshows by the end of the decade proved problematic for the studios. As Darryl F. Zanuck, then head of Twentieth Century-Fox, commented in 1968: "We've got $50 million tied up in these three musicals, *Doctor Doolittle, Star!, Hello, Dolly!,* and quite frankly if we hadn't had such an enormous success with *The Sound of Music,* I'd be petrified."[10] Fox did, in fact, realize a substantial loss on these films, posting overall losses of $36.8 million in 1969 and $77.4 million in 1970. Other studios—MGM, Warner Bros., United Artists, Paramount—also suffered significant losses around the start of the 1970s. Conditions became so dire that from 1968 through 1971, total industry losses exceeded $500 million. [11]

This crisis indicated the poor fit between the youth audience, an increasingly important part of the filmgoing public, and Hollywood's focus on the large-scale roadshow film. This situation proved to be beneficial to independent companies, as some of the most financially successful youth films were produced outside the majors. Avco Embassy released *The Graduate* (the top-grossing film of 1968), and a small production company, BBS, produced *Easy Rider* for Columbia. Independent companies thrived by exploiting market segments ignored by the majors. These smaller studios were able to prosper in this environment through two methods: (1) by working with subject matter untouched by the majors and (2) by operating outside the traditional realm of the majors in terms of distribution. The independents were able to forge a market identity through these methods, but in the long run such innovations—both aesthetic and institutional—were subsumed by the major studios.

Independent Opportunities: Markets and Marketing Beyond the Majors

The margins of the major studios extended considerably in the era following the Paramount decision, a period during which the studios essentially became distributors.[12] With projects being set up on a case-by-case basis, and the old studio system unraveled, the majors began to lease their lots and cut back considerably. Distinctions between the "Big 5" (Loews / MGM, Fox, Warners, Paramount, RKO) and the "Little 3" (Columbia, United Artists, Universal) became blurred with these industrial changes. Smaller companies (for example, American International, Roger Corman's New World) maintained a presence through offering a clearly differentiated product such as the exploitation or teen film. Those companies presenting "typical" Hollywood fare, such as National General, Allied Artists, and Associated Film Distribution (AFD), primarily marketed their projects around stars and found the competition too fierce for long-term survival.

Art-house films thrived in urban centers, signaling a renewed interest in foreign nations and an apparent audience desire to view film as akin, under certain circumstances, to the high arts of literature, music, and drama. The art film benefited from the decreased production among the majors; as the industry trade paper *Variety* commented in 1953, "There is a feeling among the film importers that, with a general product shortage in the offing, imports from abroad—in both subtitled and dubbed versions—are heading into a somewhat brighter future."[13] While these art films were primarily foreign, a small number of independent American films also served this market throughout the period. By the early 1960s the art cinema had matured through the efforts of companies such as Cinema V, run by Don Rugoff. Cinema V, often cited as a model for such later 1990s' independents as Miramax and New Line, operated in part by establishing an identity based on its otherness from the major studios. This otherness—through products and business practices—greatly aided the continued presence of the art cinema.

Cinema V grew from Rugoff and Becker theaters, a chain started in 1921 by Don Rugoff's father, Edward, and Herman Becker. When the elder Rugoff died in 1952, the chain had just opened its first theater on the Upper East Side of New York, the Beekman.[14] After Becker's demise in 1957, Rugoff gained sole control of the company, and he began a quick expansion in the burgeoning world of art-house exhibition, building one of the first twin theaters, Cinemas I and II, in 1962, and controlling such prestigious theaters as the Paris, Baronet, Plaza, and Sutton, all on the up-scale Upper East Side. Added to other Cinema V houses in New York—the Murray Hill, Gramercy, Art, and Paramount theaters—Rugoff established himself as the premier exhibitor of art-house product. At the time, Rugoff claimed that the expansion responded to a greater visibility and awareness of art-house product in the United States: "Now I meet people who don't know I'm in the business and they start talking about movies as an art form. Much more so than plays or books or anything else. I think the movies have created more excitement in recent years than any other form of art. . . . I don't know if there's going to be enough product to go around. But I think that new theaters are going to stimulate the growth of moviemaking."[15]

Simultaneously, with the backing of a consortium headed by composer Richard Rodgers, Cinema V branched into distribution, starting with the British comedy *Heavens Above!* in 1963.[16] Sticking with a slate of art films, Cinema V was responsible for distributing such influential independent projects as Shirley Clarke's *The Cool World* (1963), Michael Roemer's *Nothing But a Man* (1964), Larry Peerce's *One Potato, Two Potato* (1964), and François Truffaut's *The Soft Skin* (1964). Structurally, the ties between distribution and exhibition were crucial to the success and longevity of Cinema V. With control of the art houses in New York divided between Rugoff, Walter Reade, Jr., and Dan Talbot (New Yorker Films), Rugoff was assured a market for his Cinema V product.

Despite several successes during the decade, though, the market for art film was product-driven. Given the discerning filmgoers at the core of the art-house audience, attendance for each film was key to the market. As a result, Rugoff eventually encountered some downtime in distribution, which by the early 1960s was remedied by a shift in demographic focus to the youth audience. Rugoff claimed by the mid-1960s that the teen and college set was "the future for Cinema V."[17] This strategy proved successful through two 1966 films: Karel Reisz's antiestablishment comedy *Morgan!* and Bruce Brown's surfing documentary *The Endless Summer*. With the surfing film, Rugoff scheduled an intermission even though the entire picture ran only ninety-one minutes; the entrepreneur believed that audience members would want the break to discuss the action and surfing styles depicted up to that point. This unusual practice illustrates the care with which Rugoff approached each project—seeking to maximize the uniqueness and marketability of each film.

In this manner Rugoff and Cinema V responded to the difference of each film from mainstream fare and then sought to exploit this difference as much as possible. This approach responded directly to the perceived lack of promotion given to imported and independent films during the period. As *Variety* described this problem, while imported films compare favorably in storytelling, human interest, and artistic merit, "they simply don't promote . . . . Their product is unsold in the land of sell. They remain hopelessly inferior competitors in the department of make-known and make-attend."[18] *Variety's* call for "special treatment" and "slow-build releases" was met by Rugoff, who clearly appreciated niche marketing.

Print advertising for the films became the primary focus for this treatment. Following a graphically simple, visually distinctive approach to visual marketing often associated with Saul Bass's film credits and advertising designs, Rugoff believed in simple, recognizable logos to distinguish each project. Even for those films playing at Cinema V theaters from other distributors, Rugoff reserved the right to reject the ad campaigns, and he reportedly discarded 90 percent of them in favor of his own designs.[19] Rugoff worked closely with the Diener, Hauser, Greenthal advertising agency in designing the Cinema V logos. Among the most memorable were a trio of silhouetted surfers on the beach for *The Endless Summer* (1964), an embracing couple for *Elvira Madigan* (1967), and, most provocatively, a hand with a scantily clad girl replacing the raised middle finger for Robert Downey's satire of the advertising industry, *Putney Swope (1969)*.[20] Once an image was shaped for the campaign, Rugoff "wild-posted" the ad across major cities playing the film, so that a visual reminder of the picture would appear in both ordinary and extraordinary settings.

Whenever possible, Rugoff was aware of the publicity benefits connected to these images. For the Dušan Makavejev film, *WR: Mysteries of the Organism* (1971), Rugoff fashioned an ad featuring a photograph of a young woman eating a banana. With the New York play date in December 1971, the photo and critical quotes were subordinated to a larger story attending the refusal of three Boston papers to advertise the film.[21] One paper, the *Record-American*, offered to run the ad if the word "organism" was omitted (because it seemed too close to "orgasm"). The *Globe* flatly refused to advertise the title at all, as did the *Herald Traveler*, which had a policy not to advertise any X-rated films. After Rugoff used the Boston ban to advertise the picture, a series of pieces appeared in the New York papers on the principles of cinema advertising, all of which mentioned the film. That Rugoff used the controversy to promote the film was hardly a secret or a surprise to his fellow exhibitors. As one observed at the time: "Latest ad ploy [for *WR*] comes after a number of varied campaigns, none of which seemed to have captured the essence of [the film's] sexual political satire." The attempt to create media controversy, a "media moment," around a current release was replicated many times by Cinema V.

The successful exploitation of the youth audience, albeit still within the context of the art cinema, proved instrumental to another lucrative market, one more amorphous and marginal—the adult film. Despite the reluctance of the independents, the MPAA Rating System instituted in 1968 acted as an economic benefit, effectively segmenting the marketplace for film. The "X" rating became synonymous with stronger adult (later pornographic) content. The consequences of the X rating for the majors were dire. Approximately 50 percent of theaters across the country refused to play X films, and as many as thirty large city newspapers, along with many television and radio stations, refused to advertise them.[22]

The MPAA Rating System, the growth of the art and underground cinema, "X" as a marketing tool, and the confusions around censorship, all served to nurture the adult film as a marketplace phenomenon. Growing from the tradition of art films that seemed to stretch the boundaries of free expression (*La Dolce Vita,* 1961; *And God Created Woman,* 1956; *Room at the Top,* 1958), the first adult features were supplied by European producers. Films from Sweden and Denmark were screened with subtitles in art houses, thus giving them an aura of class and sophistication. The economic power of the adult film became stronger toward the close of the 1960s, ranging from the foreign imports, such as *I Am Curious (Yellow)*, breaking capacity records in New York in 1969 and placing number one on *Variety's* Top Grossing Films Chart (November 26,1969), to the sexploitation films, such as *The Stewardesses, I, A Woman,* and *Therese and Isabelle.* (The possibility of any soft-core independent film reaching the top of the *Variety* chart currently is ludicrous, with the contemporary market for this product primarily dominated by videocassettes and cable.)

The increased visibility of the adult feature toward the end of the decade accompanied greater freedom in content. In 1968, for example, a case before the Maryland state censorship board demonstrated that exploitation features had progressed from upper torso nudity to full frontal nudity in features such as *Walls of Flesh* and *Savage Blonde.* As a trade paper reported on this transformation, "Time was when a nudie made exclusively for the exploitation house had the male retain some dress, usually a pair of shorts, and the female her panties."[23] The issue was extended even further with the U.S. distribution of the Swedish film *I Am Curious (Yellow)*. Featuring simulated sexual intercourse in medium and long shot, the film offered a mix of political, sexual, and social satire with a story centering on the "radical" life-style choices of Lena, a young Swede unbound by sexual and social conventions. Banned outright in Norway, Vilgot Sjoman's film was censored heavily in Britain, France, and Germany.[24] Grove Press picked up the American distribution rights, only to have the film impounded by the U.S. Customs Service. Until the U.S. Circuit Court of Appeals, Eastern District, ruled that the film could be shown uncut, Grove Press continued to maximize publicity around the movie through releasing a paperback copy of the script, with over 250 stills for those who preferred looking at the pictures. When the film finally was cleared for release, Grove was able to extract strong terms from exhibitors as a result of the media controversy; the distributor asked for $50,000 in advance and a 90/10 split favoring the distributor after recoupment of the advance.[25] The New York opening in March 1969 was phenomenally successful, with an opening week of $91,785 at two small theaters, the Cinema 57 Rendezvous and the Evergreen.[26] Within six months of release, the film grossed $4 million in fewer than twenty-five theaters. *I Am Curious (Yellow)*'s performance illustrates the power of publicity and the ability of one film to exploit the national dialogue over sexual freedom and expression.

Given that *I Am Curious (Yellow)* is a dry, didactic film, distinguished only by its sexually frank material, its box-office performance was extraordinary. As the reviewer for *Time* wrote: "If it were not for the sex scenes, *Yellow* would probably never have been imported. It is simply too interminably boring, too determinedly insular and, like the sex scenes themselves, finally and fatally passionless."[27]

By the end of the 1960s the market for adult film had branched into three distinct areas: adult dramas that incorporated increasingly explicit sex scenes and subject matter; softcore pornography often using X as a ratings attraction; and hardcore pornography that was limited to large cities and linked to hardcore bookstores and strip clubs. Softcore was distinguished from hardcore by the degree of "realism": soft involved simulated sex, while hard included insertion and orgasm shots. Reflecting the increased competition from mainstream cinema, the Presidential Commission on Obscenity and Pornography estimated that adult film receipts dropped 10 percent to 20 percent from 1969 to 1970 because of "increased competition from sexually oriented motion pictures playing outside the exploitation market."[28]

The majors responded to the more liberal climate by distributing a larger number of explicit films often made "palatable" by their association with adjoining art forms. Adaptations of *Goodbye, Columbus* (1969); *Portnoy's Complaint* (1972), and *Rabbit, Run* (1970)—all based on "serious" works of fiction—arrived on screen with the trades cynically describing their appearance as an attempt by the major studios "to broaden sexploitation."[29]

Cinema V and Continental continued to buttress their release schedules with adult-oriented dramas: *WR: Mysteries of the Organism, Ulysses* (1967), *Putney Swope,* and *Trash* (1970). These films all contained explicit material, yet were perceived as part of an "art cinema." The combined distribution and exhibition arms of both Cinema V and Continental aided these films that were alternately too strong, too esoteric, and too "foreign" for the majors, and too arty and too serious for the porn market.

The art and adult markets demonstrate the viability of independent cinema during the turbulent era in which the major studios were experiencing a considerable recession. These markets were able to thrive by stressing their difference from mainstream filmmaking and by targeting youth as a market segment. In addition, both markets prospered by focusing on advertising and separate exhibition opportunities rather than competing with the majors for circuit theaters. These lessons would be underlined even further with the burgeoning family market that was being served by independent distributors. Through acknowledging the innovations of these markets outside of their primary focus, the major studios eventually were able to regain their prominence. This comeback illustrates how innovations in the independent film world eventually filter through to mainstream studio moviemaking.

Distribution Shifts: Toward Four-Walling and Saturation Releases

While the markets for art and adult cinema were crucial for the independent companies of the period, perhaps the most significant innovation in distribution during the era can be traced to another segment marginalized by Hollywood, the family film. The practice of four-walling, in which the distributor rents the theater outright, was fostered greatly in the mid-1960s by American National Enterprises (ANE).[30] Located in Utah, ANE concentrated on family wilderness adventures starting with *Alaskan Safari* (1965). While four-walling had been done on occasion as far back as the silent era, traditionally the distributor and exhibitor split box-office receipts according to a predetermined formula (often a sliding percentage of the gross, favoring the distributor). The four-wall arrangement placed a greater onus on the distributor, since the exhibitor received the theater rental up front. The upside of the deal for the distributor was that, for a high-grossing film, it retained the vast majority of the box-office revenue.[31]

The form of marketing attached to four-wall projects, as practiced by ANE and similar companies such as Pacific International Enterprises and Sunn Classics, was fundamentally different from films distributed more traditionally. As the four-wall engagements were limited to one or two weeks, the films needed immediate audience awareness and interest.[32] The four-wallers relied heavily on saturation television ad campaigns targeted precisely at specific audience segments through market research conducted beforehand. Distributors of four-wallers needed to gauge their audience specifically. As Frederick Wasser recounts, "Surveys taught the producers that their prime customers were lower-income families with earnings in the ten to twelve thousand dollar range, two or three children, and limited schooling."[33] These companies fostered a market identity around the concept of family, attempting to establish an image in which the company name would become synonymous with family entertainment. The Walt Disney Company was often cited as a role model for this goal.[34]

While the studios might have downplayed the success of these companies as the consequence of aggressive marketing and their ability to serve a starved but small family audience, the case of Tom Laughlin's film *Billy Jack* (1971) could not be so easily dismissed. Tapping into concerns voiced by the young, *Billy Jack*'s eponymous hero (played by Laughlin) was a half-breed and a self-appointed guardian of Indian rights. Most of the film's action revolved around the hero's attempts to help a school on the reservation against the violent and racist residents of a neighboring town. *Variety* assessed the film's box-office potential on its release in 1971: "Film is strictly for selected situations where its chances are uncertain, but reception may benefit by feature also reflecting some of the troubles of present-day youth."[35]

As released initially by Warner Bros., *Billy Jack* garnered little interest. Laughlin, who believed that Warners did not adequately support the film in the market, filed suit, charging that Warner Bros. "didn't give the picture the proper 'push'."[36] Settling out of court, Warners agreed to a reissue and a renegotiated distribution deal with Laughlin. The revised deal stipulated an even split of both profits and costs for the reissue.[37]

While the new arrangement covered Warners in terms of advertising expenses, Laughlin was able to realize a much greater share of the revenue than under his previous deal. His approach with the reissue was to four-wall the film. Armed with much data about the specifics of each engagement, including demographics of the region, educational characteristics, population density, and ethnic composition, the goal was to saturate the airways with commercials aimed at different demographic groups.[38] Separate ads foregrounded romance, countercultural/anti-Vietnam War aspects, action, and martial arts—a varied campaign designed to reach a broad spectrum of moviegoers. A large number of theaters were rented within the region of the television signal, maximizing the convenience of attending the film. As Laughlin commented, "A filmgoer should be able, after being dunned relentlessly by the campaign, to fall out of bed and find a theater where *Billy Jack* is playing."[39] Rereleased on May 9, 1973, with a generous ad expenditure of $250,000 in Southern California under the four-wall approach to mostly second and third-run neighborhood theaters, *Billy Jack* grossed $1.02 million in the first week in sixty-two theaters from Santa Barbara to Bakersfield.[40] The gross represented a record box-office return for the region. Weekly figures were similarly impressive in such major markets as New York ($1.45 million), Philadelphia ($710,000), and Chicago ($600,000). Eventually the film reached more than $30 million in domestic film rentals.

Throughout the country the film was sold on a week-to-week four-wall basis. Exhibitors were reimbursed for their theater rental before the engagements started, and a uniform admission price ($2.50 for adults, $1 for children) was enforced at all engagements. While previously there had been a large number of four-wall family films, Laughlin's movie marked the first time that a PG film had been four-walled. The success of *Billy Jack* indicated that the four-wall method of distribution could be used successfully beyond the family market.[41] In addition, *Billy Jack* demonstrated that a failure in initial release could be reversed by the four-wall approach and, more specifically, by saturation television advertising targeting specific demographics. The extensive use of market research to gauge potential audience interest and demand enabled Laughlin and marketeer Max Youngstein to aggressively pursue many audience segments. The approach was built like a "military campaign," aiming for an audience from several independent segments rather than narrowly exploiting a single segment.[42]

Following Laughlin's lead, studios began to experiment with four-walling as a distribution method. At first, their attempts were limited to films that had proven financially disappointing in initial release: in 1974 Warners rereleased the Robert Redford film *Jeremiah Johnson,* Universal chose the May/December romance *Breezy* starring William Holden, and Avco Embassy attempted to resurrect *The Day of the Dolphin*. On the *Dolphin* rerelease, *Variety* described the effort: "Armed with newfound marketing ploys such as saturation video campaigns, four-walling, and tested and retested advertising campaigns, distributors [are] try[ing] anything short of shanghai-ing people off the street to improve grosses."[43]

Distributors eventually broadened the range of films released under four-wall situations. For instance, six months after its initial release, Warner Bros. four-walled its blockbuster *The Exorcist* as a means to rejuvenate the film late in its release.[44] Within the independent film world, distributors also began to four-wall films outside the family genre: art-house films (the 1953 Italian opera film *Giuseppe Verdi,* rereleased in 1974), religious/inspirational films (*The Hiding Place*), and even gay porn (Wakefield Poole's *Boys*).[45]

While four-walling grew as a market practice, a backlash developed within several industry sectors. Distributors began to complain that exhibitors' terms were inflated far beyond the house nut covering the theater's operating expenses. Laughlin stated that the theaters added "so much air" to the rental price that four-walling would start to become a losing proposition." Exhibitors, along with the National Organization of Theater Owners (NATO), feared that four-walling would become the primary arrangement between exhibitors and distributors. The concern was that exhibitors would be cut off from profits usually gained from hits (where the percentage split between exhibitor and distributor would benefit both if the film grosses well). As Paul Roth, NATO president, described four-walling, "That's not a marketing technique . . . it's an illegal sales technique, that would put the larger exhibitors who could afford to charge less rent, at an unfair advantage."[47]

Union projectionists demanded higher salaries for four-wall films, arguing that they should receive their slice of the four-wall windfall.[48] In the New York City case of *The Exorcist*'s four-wall engagements, the projectionists were able to secure a wage differential for the run, leading to the prediction that in the future four-walling would routinely lead to such "hidden" costs and thus no longer be as attractive to distributors.

Richard Moses, senior vice president for MGM marketing, argues that unrealistic theater rentals were not the only reason for the eventual decline of four-walling. He puts the blame on the distributors, which selected the wrong pictures for the venture.[49] Just as roadshows relied on event status, four-walled films needed to be *perceived* as special events. Admittedly, the hard-sell television approach may have created an illusion of difference that the films themselves did not warrant. Films with an exploitable premise, especially those with sensationalistic subject matter (witness the 1974 four-wall Sunn Family lineup: *Chariots of the Gods, Mysterious Monsters,* and *The Outer Space Connection*) that could be conveyed quickly and efficiently through the visuals in a television commercial, yielded most readily to the four-wall selling method.

Four-walling's overexposure can be gauged by the release pattern for Laughlin's next effort, *The Trial of Billy Jack* (1974). Surprising the industry greatly, Laughlin chose not to exclusively four-wall the picture, but instead relied on saturation bookings for the sequel. Given the extraordinary success of the original, Laughlin was able to extract strict terms from exhibitors for the sequel: a 90/10 split toward Laughlin and a minimum cash guarantee adjusted for a low house nut for each theater.[50] In cases for which Laughlin could not set deals on these terms, he chose to four-wall the film in a limited number of cities, as he did in New York, Philadelphia, and Phoenix.[51] Laughlin maintained that he did not want to four-wall the film in every location since exhibitors had been substantially padding their rental terms given the tremendous success of many four-wall films. For the vast majority of engagements, Laughlin negotiated standard, albeit stringent, contracts. *The Trial of Billy Jack* opened very wide, at 1,100 theaters, plus 180 four-wall engagements, on November 13, 1974. Box-office after the first week was $10.5 million; amazingly, given the terms of his deal, Laughlin was able to recoup the total negative and advertising costs within seven days.[52]

The major studios retained the most significant marketing components of the four-wall approach in their move to saturation releases: the heavy reliance on television advertising supported by market research and the pattern of wide distribution linked to the advertising. The shift to audiovisual marketing was crucial. Its significance can be noted by changes in the motion picture advertising budgets. From 1972 through 1974 the proportion of the average film's ad budget paid to newspapers dropped from 58 percent to 44 percent, while the amount paid to television in the same period jumped dramatically from 15 percent to 42 percent. [53] Addressing a convention of newspaper advertising executives in 1975, Jonas Rosenfield, Fox's advertising, publicity, and promotion vice president, blamed the poor reproduction of ads, discriminatory rate practices, and lengthy deadlines for the shift. Rosenfield used the example of the Fox action film *Dirty Mary and Crazy Larry* (1974) as a paradigm for effective film marketing. Produced at a negative cost of under $1 million, Fox allocated $2 million for national television advertising. The film grossed $32.5 million. Rosenfield commented that, if the marketing had focused on print instead of television, $6 million would have been the expected gross.[54]

This alteration in marketing was fostered by advertising agencies, particularly Grey Advertising, which had expertise in targeting specific demographic groups through network and local television ad buys. Columbia worked extensively with Grey Advertising in developing the campaign for the 1975 wide release of *Breakout,* a Charles Bronson action thriller about a split-second rescue from a high-security jail. Aiming to make every potential customer (particularly males 18 to 49) aware of the film prior to release, Columbia ran ads to hit 92 percent of the television households in the country and 84 percent of the entire 18–49 male target group. [55] To achieve this result, Grey used a technique known as "roadblocking" in which a *Breakout* ad ran the same hour on a designated night on every television station in the key New York market. [56] The goal was to exhaust the box office within two weeks rather than allow the film to play out across several months.

The Marketing Legacy of *Jaws*

While saturation release and television-oriented marketing were designed to diminish the effect of a critical response to a film (a hit-and-run sales tactic), the stakes were raised considerably that same year with Steven Spielberg's *Jaws*. The difference between *Breakout* and *Jaws* can be seen if we examine the marketing assets of the two films. While *Breakout* offered its star (Charles Bronson) as insurance of success, *Jaws* sported a presold property (Peter Benchley's best-selling novel released in paperback less than six months before the film's release). The marketing campaign for *Jaws* created a strong visual identity for the film: the image of the naked swimmer tiny in the ocean against the huge shark, jaws open and ready to attack its prey. Producers Richard Zanuck and David Brown, realizing the benefits of the book tie-in, actively promoted the print version of *Jaws,* even though they had no direct financial interest in those sales. Zanuck and Brown wanted to clearly establish the paperback cover image in the marketplace by the time of the film's release months later. As Zanuck commented, "We adapted the artwork from the book to the artwork in the film promotion. By the time we sneaked the film in Dallas, we didn't even need to name it in the ad. We put in the logo of the shark's teeth and the swimming girl and 3,000 came out in a hailstorm."[57]

Following from the earlier saturation and four-wall experiments, *Jaws* relied on television advertising to support opening wide (at 409 theaters) on June 19, 1975. Universal boasted "the biggest national TV spot campaign in industry history," substituting national for local television buys. Given the wide release, Universal realized cost advantages by buying national prime-time spots rather than buying a similar schedule on a market-by-market basis. Since the national television spot replaced the usual local television commercials, Universal demanded that exhibitors contribute to the national advertising based on potential local earnings; exhibitors therefore were charged between $175 and $400 depending on the number of theaters in a given market, a one-time charge as part of their deal with Universal.[58] The match of television advertising, presold property, and strong playability (*Time* aptly referred to the film as "an efficient entertainment machine") created the record opening-week gross of $14.31 million. By September 5 *Jaws* became the largest-grossing film in motion picture history up to that time, surpassing *The Godfather.* Not willing to toy with success, the foreign release of the film replicated the domestic pattern with heavy television advertising and wide simultaneous release. For example, *Jaws* was booked into more than a hundred theaters in Britain alone for the United Kingdom opening on December 26.[59]

The commercial performance of *Jaws* demonstrated many lessons to the film industry, not only reinforcing the power of large-scale national television advertising and wide release, but also illustrating the potential of a presold property and an early summer release date (it opened in June and played through Labor Day). By setting a new box-office record in such a short span of time, *Jaws* also redefined the concept of a blockbuster or breakthrough hit. In later years $100 million became a benchmark for the blockbuster. Spielberg's film also heralded the era of the high-concept film, that is, cinematic products with a narrative that could be boiled down to a single sentence and then marketed visually through print advertising and especially commercials.[60] These projects were oriented around marketing assets: stars, genre, an exploitable premise, all targeted toward specific demographics with the potential to cross over into other audience segments. The commercial equation was refined through several other films in the second half of the 1970s. These projects effectively extended the marketing and distribution opportunities of these high-concept projects.

A year after *Jaws,* Twentieth Century-Fox copied the strategy for its promotion of the horror film, *The Omen*. Launching the picture with a tie-in novelization and two weekends of nationwide sneak previews, the distributor also sank the equivalent of the film's negative cost ($2.8 million) into advertising. While the film was not based on a best-selling book, the producers generated their own $1.50 Signet paperback novelization by *Omen* screenwriter David Seltzer. Based on the sneak previews and extremely positive word-of-mouth, the paperback sold out in three hours in New York and Los Angeles.[61] The film's distinctive logo—three 6's inside the O of the title—was emblazoned across the paperback and all print advertising to establish the movie's identity. While its R rating, almost by definition, limited grosses to a modest degree, *The Omen* opened at 526 theaters and garnered rentals of $28 million, making it the third-highest grosser for the year.

Producer Dino de Laurentiis, obviously admiring the box office of *Jaws,* offered another man-against-beast tale, a remake of *King Kong,* for a Christmas 1976 release. Depending on the success of the original film and the forty-three years between the two versions, the remake of the original 1933 classic was a presold, property; bringing an immediate point of identification for potential audience members. De Laurentiis also heavily merchandised the film, choosing not to focus exclusively on the children's market. The promotional campaign for the film included licenses with obvious tie-ins (GAF Viewmaster pictures and 7-Eleven Slurpee cups) as well as more imaginative and esoteric ones (Jim Beam "King Kong" cocktails from a "commemorative King Kong" bottle). With a massive television advertising campaign running from December 12 until Christmas Day on national television (the film opened on December 17), de Laurentiis released the film to 961 theaters—more than twice the size of the *Jaws* opening. Given the similar themes, marketing angles, and distribution approach, the industry anticipated similar grosses between the Spielberg film and *King Kong*. As a *Variety* columnist asked after *Kong*'s opening weekend, "Can *Kong* best the Great White Shark of *Jaws* and become the biggest and fastest grossing film in the history of the biz?"[62] Although *King Kong* failed to reach that goal, the opening was robust (a $6.97 million weekend).[63]

The case of George Lucas's *Star Wars*, released initially on May 25, 1977, shifted the equation of the breakthrough hit further through an emphasis on merchandising and a box-office gross that eclipsed even *Jaws*. Lacking the presold properties of *King Kong*, *Star Wars* had to combat several marketing problems to establish a market identity. First, market research tests showed that the title alone connoted a science fiction film about a conflict in outer space, a concept that appealed to a limited audience (males under twenty-five years of age).[64] To counter that notion, Twentieth Century-Fox through its advertising positioned the film as space fantasy, with a strong element of human relationships and adventure; the studio's campaign centered on human characters in the foreground and space hardware in the background. The ad line ("A long time ago in a galaxy far, far away") was designed to evoke "a future world with the romanticism of fairy tales, myths, and real heroes."[65] Initiating a trend that became common practice during the next decade, Fox opened the film on May 25, before the usual onslaught of June openings. In certain engagements 70mm Dolby prints were used, and the initial release was limited to only forty-two theaters in thirty cities. The distributor hoped to establish positive word-of-mouth before widening the film's market in late June.

Breaking house records in many engagements, *Star Wars* proved to be even sturdier at the box office than its predecessor. By November 1977, six months after its release, the Lucas film replaced *Jaws* as the highest-grossing film ever. While its maintenance in the market obviously resulted from extremely enthusiastic word-of-mouth, the film also benefited from Fox's merchandising strategy. Fox executive Mark Pepvers commented, "George Lucas created *Star Wars* with the toy byproducts in mind. He was making much more than a movie."[66] (In fact, Lucas sought to control all merchandising rights for the film, but the final contracts specified an equal revenue split between Fox and Lucas after Fox's administrative costs were covered.)[67]

Part of the film's phenomenal success as a licensing property has been its diverse set of characters and its creative hardware. The film's completely novel environment and characters were so striking that Kenner Toys was able to go beyond the figures in the film and add new characters to their *Star Wars* line in keeping with the film's mythological world.

Superman, released for Christmas 1978, similarly exploited its merchandising potential. Producer Ilya Salkind was able to maximize the film's licensed products in large part because of the conglomerate structure of Warner Communications Inc. (WCI). Ten years earlier, the conglomerate purchased DC Comics, the publisher of the Superman adventures since 1939. This deal facilitated the licensed product developed in conjunction with the film released by Warner Bros. Another WCI subsidiary, the licensing Corporation of America, was assigned the task of allocating rights to different product companies; major companies involved with the promotion included Bristol Meyers, General Foods, Pepsico, Lever Bros., and Gillette. Warner Books issued eight separate *Superman*-related titles, and Warner Records released not only a soundtrack album but two singles.[68] Happy about the possibilities for cross-promotion of the film, Salkind enthused, "They're all part of the same conglomerate. That was a big advantage of going with them—besides their being a very good company. We had all the areas of merchandising and books and records and everything else with the same conglomerate. If we had dealt with another major we would have had a very difficult situation. . . ."[69]

By the end of the decade a number of other high—concept films were released—*The Deep* (1977), *Close Encounters of the Third Kind, Grease* (1978), *Jaws 2* (1978), and *Star Trek: The Motion*

Picture (1979)—all of them foregrounding marketing assets, wide distribution, and aggressive marketing. The shift toward these marketing-oriented projects has led industry analyst Lee Beaupre to designate the 1970s as "Hollywood's Marketing Decade."[70] The effects of these marketing changes were far-reaching. By 1976, data illustrated that box office was being generated from a wider base of theaters, reflecting the move toward saturation releases; from 1969 through 1975 the number of theaters accounting for the *Variety* key city box-office chart grew by 54 percent.[71] With increased television advertising, costs for marketing the average film increased dramatically in the second half of the 1970s; by 1980, print and advertising expenses averaged about $6 million per film (at a time when the average negative cost—all production expenses before prints, advertising, etc.—was more than $10 million). With advertising costs escalating even faster than increases in production costs, the breakeven level for films during this period became inflated. According to producer Salkind, a gross of less than $80 million for *Superman* would have been a "flat out disaster," while estimates before the release of *Close Encounters* placed the break-even point at a gross of close to $70 million.[72] With the higher box-office potential of breakthrough hits, a single film could make a studio the market share leader for the year. *Jaws* led Universal to a 25 percent market share in 1975 (the next highest studio had only 14 percent), *Star Wars* gave Fox a 20 percent market share in 1977, and the combination of *Saturday Night Fever* and *Grease* helped Paramount dominate with a 24 percent share in 1978.[73]

The pattern of wide releases, television advertising, and spiraling marketing costs continued into the 1980s, and, indeed, it still dictates the distribution plans of the major studios. These innovations can be traced back to the independent companies (including Tom Laughlin working as equal partners with Warner Bros.) and their aggressive advertising and seeking of new distribution arrangements from the mid-1960s through the mid-1970s. Through these independents working in art, adult, and family cinema, the studios were able to gauge the significance of new marketing techniques and novel forms of distribution. In turn, by adopting these innovations for their own product, the majors rebounded in the mid-1970s, experiencing greater box office for individual films than ever before. The era of the high-concept film also eventually limited the diversity of American filmmaking both within the studios and within the ranks of the independents. Focusing on marketing-oriented projects and searching for larger and larger hits, the studios looked to "tent-pole" films, a single one of which on its own could support a studio's yearly distribution schedule. Such efforts substantially limited the production of films that could not be described in a single sentence and that did not contain inherent marketing hooks. With their greater precision in targeting audience members through market research, studios were also able to exploit those markets, including the art cinema, that traditionally had been the domain of the independents. As with all aspects of the independent-mainstream relationship, this situation does not remain static. Indeed, by the end of the 1970s two of the most influential independents—Miramax and New Line Cinema—were in their infancy and would soon be ready to rejuvenate the world of commercial independent filmmaking.[74]

Notes

1. A saturation release pattern involves the widespread distribution of a film across North America at a single point in time rather than a tiered approach favoring a slow rollout concentrated at first in large cities.
2. "Click Roadshows," *Variety,* August 21, 1968, p. 17.
3. Ron Wise, "Fundraisers Miss Modest Film Ducats, An Easier Sell Compared to Legit," *Variety,* January 17, 1973, p. 24.
4. Lee Beaupre, "Dickstein's 'Star' Strategy," *Variety,* September 4, 1968, p. 2.
5. Lee Beaupre, "Third Roadshow Study: 'Funny Girl' Getting a Specialized Sell to Party Agents," *Variety,* August 23, 1968, p. 25.
6. As Beaupre describes it: "With the hindsight exception of *2001,* most roadshows cater to family audiences or, less frequently; 'serious' adults." *Variety,* August 14, 1968, p. 5.

7. "'Ethnic Roadshow' Policy Gives Marcus Epic Special N.Y. Dates," *Variety,* May 23, 1966, p. 21.
8. Lee Beaupre, "Clutch of Roadshows," *Variety,* August 14, 1968, p. 5.
9. Ibid.
10. John Gregory Dunne, *The Studio* (New York: Limelight Editions, 1968), p. 242.
11. Teresa Grimes, "BBS: Auspicious Beginnings, Open Endings," *Movie* 31-32 (1986): 57.
12. For a review of this transitional period, consult Jim Hillier, "Forty Years of Change," *The New Hollywood* (New York: Continuum, 1994), pp. 6–17.
13. "Foreign Pix Hope for More U.S. Dates with Curtailment of 'B' Productions," *Variety,* September 30, 1953, p. 3.
14. Todd McCarthy, "Exhib/Distrib Donald Rugoff Dies at 62," *Variety,* May 3, 1989, p. 7.
15. "Art-House Boom," *Newsweek,* May 28, 1962, p. 102.
16. McCarthy, "Exhib/Distrib Donald Rugoff," p. 7.
17. "Rugoff Cinema V Shakes Moribund Tone," *Variety,* October 5, 1966, p. 5.
18. Robert J. Landry, "Unsold in the Land of Sell," *Variety,* April 24, 1957, p. 5.
19. McCarthy, "Exhib/Distrib Donald Rugoff," p. 7.
20. In a move that reverses the usual protocol, Cinema V placed an industry ad thanking their agency (Diener, Hauser, Greenthal Co.) for their images; the ad was titled, "They make images to sell dreams." *Variety,* September 10, 1969, p. 47.
21. "Rugoff's N.Y. Times Ad for 'Organism' Chides Hub's Mixed-Reason," *Variety,* December 29, 1971, p. 1.
22. Stephen Farber and Estelle Changas, "Putting the Hex on 'R' and 'X,'" *New York Times,* April 9, 1972.
23. "From Nearly to Total Nude Pix," *Variety,* October 2, 1968, p. 1.
24. "'Curious': Sexy-Dull Shocker," *Variety,* March 19, 1969, p. 7.
25. Kent E. Carroll, "Some Fear to Be 'Curious,'" *Variety,* April 9, 1969, p. 5.
26. "Sex Dominates B'way First-Runs," *Variety,* March 19, 1969, p. 9.
27. "Dubious Yellow," *Time,* March 14, 1969, p. 98.
28. "Porno Study: 600 U.S. Film Sites Comprise Playoff For Sexploitation," *Variety,* October 7, 1970, p. 7.
29. Aubrey Tarbox, "High-Brow Novels to Screen," *Variety,* March 12, 1969, p.8.
30. For a history of the distribution innovations introduced by American National Enterprises, see Frederick Wasser, "Four Walling Exhibition: Regional Resistance to the Hollywood Film Industry," *Cinema Journal* 34 (Winter 1995): 51–65.
31. Lee Beaupre, "Utah Gospel of Four-Wall Sell," *Variety,* November 7, 1973, p.5.
32. For an industrial history of Sunn Classics, see Gary Edgerton, "Charles E. Sellier, Jr. and Sunn Classic Pictures: Success as a Commercial Independent in the 1970s," *Journal of Popular Film and Television,* October 1982, pp. 106–18.
33. Wasser, "Four Walling Exhibition," p. 55.
34. "'Four Wall' Sun International Reversing Distribution Field," *Independent Film Journal,* March 18, 1974, p. 7.
35. "'Billy Jack' as Labor of Love," *Variety,* November 10, 1971, p. 4.
36. "'Billy Jack': Happy Denouement of a Warners Courtroom Drama," *Variety,* November 7, 1973, p. 5.
37. Ibid.
38. Richard Moses, "The Rise, Fall and Second Coming of Four-Walling," *Variety,* January 8, 1975, p. 22.

39. Richard Albarino, "Billy Jack Hits Reissue Jackpot," *Variety,* November 7, 1973, p. 1.
40. Richard Kahn, "The Day Film Marketing Came of Age," *Variety,* October 30, 1979, p. 38.
41. Ibid.
42. Albarino, " 'Billy Jack.' Hits Reissue Jackpot," p. 1.
43. "Motivational Research in Promotion," *Variety,* June 26, 1974, p. 7.
44. "'Exorcist' Four-Walling Causes Trade Disruption," *Independent Film Journal,* March 4, 1974, p. 6.
45. See, for example, "Outsider Hits," *Variety,* November 6, 1974; "Hudson's Four Wall Deal," *Variety,* November 5, 1975, p. 3; Addison Verrill, "Amateurs Bring in Bonanza," *Variety,* February 2, 1972, p. 7.
46. Richard Albarino, " 'Billy' Sequel's Grand $11-Mil Preem," *Variety,* November 20, 1974, p. 61.
47. "Four-Walling, 'A Burgeoning Menace,' Stirs Exhib Wrath," *Independent Film Journal,* August 7, 1974, p. 12.
48. Frank Segers, "Pix Unions Scaling Up Four Walls," *Variety,* June 12, 1974, p. 1.
49. Kahn, "The Day Film Marketing Came of Age," p. 38.
50. "'Billy Jack' Sequel Four-Walls New York, Philly, Phoenix Areas," *Variety,* October 23, 1974, p. 76.
51. Ibid., p. 4.
52. Albarino, "'Billy' Sequel's Grand $11-Mil Preem," p. 61.
53. Larry Primak, "Jonas at the Pic Distributors Wall," *Variety,* February 5, 1975, p. 5.
54. Ibid.
55. "Col's Break Out Campaign to Launch Its Own Breakout," *Variety,* May 14, 1975, p. 6.
56. Ibid.
57. Jim Harwood, "Anticipated Success Mutes Squawks on Cost, Rental Terms," *Variety,* June 4, 1975, p. 7.
58. Harlan Jacobson, "U Introing Nat'l Coop Ads on 'Jaws,'" *Variety,* April 16, 1975, p. 3.
59. "CIC Shifts from Usual Foreign Marketing Pattern in 'Jaws' Bow," *Variety,* December 3, 1975, p. 3.
60. For an analysis of the economics and aesthetics of the high-concept film, see Justin Wyatt, *High Concept: Movies and Marketing in Hollywood* (Austin: University of Texas Press, 1994).
61. "Big Ballyhoo Gamble on 'Omen'; Fox Hopes Antichrist Is Saviour," *Variety,* June 30, 1976, p. 4.
62. Addison Verrill, "'Kong' Wants 'Jaws' Boxoffice Crown," *Variety,* December 22, 1976, p.1.
63. Stuart Byron considers several reasons for *King Kong's* ultimate commercial 'disappointment' (although he remarks that the film still earned a $40 million profit) in "Industry," *Film Comment,* March–April 1978, pp. 72–73.
64. Olen J. Earnest, "*Star Wars:* A Case Study of Motion Picture Marketing," *Current Research in Film: Audiences, Economics and Law,* ed. Bruce A. Austin (Norwood, N.J.: Ablex, 1983), p. 9.
65. Ibid p.11.
66. "E.T. and Friends Are Flying High," *Business Week,* January 10, 1983, p. 77.
67. Dale Pollock, *Skywalking: The Lift and Films of George Lucas* (New York: Harmony Books, 1983), p. 194.
68. "Merchandising New Abracadabra of Cinematic Showmanship," *Variety,* August 23, 1978, p. 6.
69. "Ilya Salkind Defines Disaster, *Variety,* August 30, 1978, p. 40.
70. Lee Beaupre, "Grosses Gloss: 'Breaking Away' at the Boxoffice," *Film Comment,* March–April 1980, p. 69.
71. "New Era of Custom-Fit Pix Releases," *Variety,* March 17, 1976, p. 48.

72. "How Close the Encounter to a Profit," *Variety,* November 9, 1977, p. 5.
73. A. D. Murphy; "North American Theatrical Film Rental Market Shares: 1970–1989," *Variety,* January 17, 1990, p. 15.
74. For an analysis of Miramax's and New Line's significance to the world of independent filmmaking of the last two decades, consult the section "The Outsider: The Era of the 'Major' Independent," in Justin Wyatt, "Economic Constraints/Economic Opportunities: Robert Altman as Auteur," *Velvet Light Trap* 38 (Fall 1996): 59–65.

Goldfinger

Albert R. Broccoli

The huge impact of *Dr No* was evident not just in its wide box-office appeal around the world, but also in the boost it gave to Fleming's books. Before the film took off, his spy adventures had done well, but his hero was not exactly a household name. Suddenly, after cinema-goers all came out for Bond, the sales of the paperbacks soared. James Bond was away and running. The world had got a new screen hero. The effect of all this success on Sean Connery was fascinating. We invested thousands of dollars in publicity campaigns to hammer home the message: Connery is James Bond.

Sean, at the beginning anyway, played along with it, enjoying all the door-opening, the flattery, the hero-worship that comes with the film-star package. Virtually overnight, *Dr No* had taken him out of the 'promising young actor' category and given him potential—if not actual—international status. The American movie director (quoted in the *Saturday Evening Post*) who said, 'Connery was on the garbage heap of acting until Bond' was strictly out of line. Sean, even in some of his very early films which flopped, was always interesting, often first-class. But in terms of recognition—what else matters to an actor?—007 was the career boost of a lifetime. Events will show to what extent Connery conceded that fact. Not that he hadn't earned all the kudos he received: he had taken a spoofy character and given it an exciting, appealing and very macho dimension.

In the euphoria that followed he began to flex his muscles not only as a screen performer, but also as a personality. No matter what he might have said in public, Sean could scarcely have objected to his sexy, cult-hero image. He knew that when he walked into a room, or was invited to parties, the women responded to his James Bond aura, not him as Sean Connery. I don't recall him issuing any public rebuttal when a newspaper described him as 'a walking aphrodisiac'. He could see there was a lot to be gained (he would eventually own shares in a bank) by keeping that game plan going. He enjoyed it, too—and why not? When you've been a truck driver and a labourer, it's great to wear Savile Row suits and be chauffeured around. And the fact that he is an excellent celebrity golfer today owes something to the golf lessons we arranged for him on *Goldfinger* for his scenes with the German actor Gert Frobe. We gave him time off to play, and be coached by professionals. Often we juggled with the shooting schedules so that he could slip away to hit a few balls on a nearby course. Nothing special about this. It was a fringe benefit—there were plenty of these—that we were glad to throw in for an actor of his calibre. And, to be fair, he had earned them.

With the next James Bond film still on the drawing-board, Harry and I, through our company Eon Productions, had time to make another picture outside Bond. But what kind of film? Thinking back over that episode and the decision we finally took—with our eyes open—reminds me of the answer Irving Thalberg often gave whenever he was asked the reason for his success: 'Two rules: never take one man's opinion as final. Never take your own opinion as final.' In the event, Harry shouldn't have listened to his own opinion, and I shouldn't have agreed with him! It resulted in both of us missing out on a minor bonanza to the considerable gratitude of certain characters who still can't believe their luck.

My partner, who had been a successful independent producer, never disguised the fact that he liked to spread himself over a variety of interests. He had a low boredom threshold, I guess. Once Bond was launched, he was restless for a diversion and keen to go ahead with an African safari spoof he had in hand. He had already gone a fair distance in persuading Bob Hope to come over to make the picture. (I heard whispers that as an inducement he promised Hope that he could deliver the Pope on one of the comedian's TV specials. Personally, I knew nothing about this and maybe His Holiness didn't, either.)

Anyway, Harry was eager to go ahead on the project when I walked in with an alternative suggestion. Donald Zec had written enthusiastically about a pop group then making quite a few waves up in a city called Liverpool. It was a major layout which was being plugged with the group's photos on billboards outside newsagent shops across the country. I had mentioned to Zec that Harry and I were looking for a non-Bond film to make. Donald thought about this for a while and then said, 'Look, this may not be your line of country, but there's something wild happening in the pop world which suggests a whole untapped goldmine to me. I wrote a spread in the paper today about a group called The Beatles. They're a zany foursome with long hair and Liverpool accents, and I wouldn't be telling you this except that apparently we sold more papers today than we did on the Queen's Coronation. Kids all over the country are crawling out of their beds just to steal The Beatles' pictures off the billboards. I don't see Oscars in this, but it seems to me you have the dream package: four certain stars and a whole new audience out there who might just kill to see them.'

Donald's logic convinced me, but persuading Harry proved to be a bit tougher. I remember looking over at my partner, who lay back in his leather desk chair, shoes off, his feet with the red socks on up on the desk. He is looking fixedly at Donald, who is looking fixedly back at him. Donald, in turn, is giving me that 'what-the-hell-am-I-doing-here-Cubby?' look. And the reason is, Mr Saltzman's round little black eyes are clouding over with disbelief. At which point Donald wrapped up his narrative as fast as he could and left. I turned to Harry and asked, 'Well, what do you think?'

He leaned forward—I recall this vividly—pounded the desk with the palms of his hands, then said, 'Listen, let me ask you something, Cubby. Would you rather make a picture with four long-haired shnooks from Liverpool—what's their name. . . ?'

'The Beatles,' I said.

'The Beatles, who nobody's ever heard of, when we've got Bob Hope—BOB HOPE!—all ready to go.'

Well, of course, when it was put like that, I wasn't sure I could give Harry an argument. By the normal rules of the game, Harry made sense. Bob Hope was a major star with acknowledged box-office appeal all over the world. Could we gamble on these four relatively unknown kids? The euphoria faded. Mr Broccoli and Mr Saltzman joined the ranks of those other geniuses who over the years made the wrong decisions for all the right reasons! One man's poison is another man's meat. We turned our backs on one of the biggest money-spinners in the world of entertainment.

A year later *A Hard Day's Night* is leaping towards a gross of $65 million; Walter Shenson, a publicity chief for United Artists, who made the film, is driving a Rolls or maybe a Cadillac; and the four 'long-haired shnooks' went on to reshape the styles and attitudes of an entire generation. While we went on to make *Call Me Bwana* with Bob Hope and a voluptuous Swede named Anita Ekberg.

In the event, the film did little more than cover its cost. (But it was a big break for Miss Ekberg, dubbed 'The Iceberg' by one newspaper and 'The Bore With the Bust' by another. Having Bob Hope as a co-star raised her professional status enormously. Socially, it brought her into contact with Sean Connery. There was considerable static generated between these two, which kept the gossips going for a while.)

I was glad to see *Bwana* out of the way, so that we could get down to making the second Bond film, *From Russia With Love*. We favored this film for several reasons. To many people, myself included, this was one of Fleming's best stories. The leading characters were well fleshed out. It was a tough, straightforward spy adventure. The public was familiar with the title, and it gave us an opportunity to shoot in one of the world's most exotic places, Istanbul. The story centers on an attempt to steal a vital decoding machine, the Lektor, and murder 007 in the process. The organization behind it, SPECTRE (Special Executive for Counterintelligence, Terrorism, Revenge and Extortion), dupes a beautiful Russian agent, Tatiana Romanova, into a plan to seduce, then execute, James Bond.

The popularity of the book, notably among women, was the strong love interest between the female agent and Bond. I liked the fact that it gave Bond an emotional, as well as physical, dimension. But there was an aspect to the story which led me and Harry into making a decision which was to be fundamental to all the Bond films. We decided to steer 007 and the scripts clear of politics. Bond would have no identifiable political affiliation. None of the protagonists would be the stereotyped Iron Curtain or 'inscrutable Oriental' villain. First, it's old-fashioned; second, it's calculated to induce pointless controversy, especially in these days of *glasnost,* with Mikhail Gorbachev (as of March 1988) the Flavour of the Month.

Fleming had made the Soviet Secret Service the 'heavies' in *From Russia With Love.* He called this murderous organization SMERSH, a name linking two Russian words, *'smyert shpionam',* which translate roughly as 'death to spies'. There was nothing fanciful about Fleming's plot. He'd based it on actual experiences in the 1930s, when he served in the Moscow bureau of Reuters News Agency. One of his assignments was to cover the trial of six British engineers working for the Metropolitan-Vickers Company. They were charged with spying and plotting against the Soviet state by sabotaging equipment at power stations and allegedly bribing Russian officials in exchange for secret information. Also charged with the six Britons was a dark, attractive Russian girl, Anna Kutusova, a secretary who worked for the company. She was supposed to have been the mistress of one of the accused men. It was a classic example of the 'beautiful spy' cliché, and Fleming clearly modelled Tatiana Romanova on her.

It was while he was reporting this case that Fleming built up his extensive knowledge of the way the secret police extracted information or confessions by torture or blackmail. We wanted to keep the motivation, but redefine the villains. Manipulating the seductive Tatiana is Rosa Klebb, a butch, crop-haired villainess, aided by Red Grant, a sadistic psycho drawn into the plan to kill Bond. It was Harry's idea to have the distinguished German actress Lotte Lenya play Rosa Klebb. It clicked with Fleming and me immediately. Ian had given this character—he'd seen the real McCoy in Moscow—evil overtones, with just a hint of lesbianism. (She lightly touches Tatiana on the knee, the girl recoiling in disgust.) The late Lotte Lenya, widow of the composer Kurt Weill, was a fine actress, and she made Rosa Klebb one of Bond's memorable adversaries. Her struggle with him as she attempts to kick-stab him with a switchblade in the toe of her shoe is real edge-of-the-seat action.

The casting of the girl to play Tatiana was not easy. Fleming describes her in the book as 'a young Greta Garbo'. There aren't many of those featured in the casting directories. Harry and I interviewed a couple of hundred girls of several nationalities. Some of these were already well known, including Magda Konopka, who is Polish, and Sylvia Koscina of Yugoslavia. We finally settled on Daniela Bianchi, a runner-up in a 1960 Miss Universe contest. She had fine features plus a touch of class, which brought her closer than anyone else to the Fleming prototype. She had to portray the discipline of a secret agent while also suggesting the vulnerability of a young woman with stirred emotions. (She seduces Bond, as ordered, wearing only a black velvet choker around her neck, but then defies the conventions of espionage by falling in love with him.) Daniela handled this character shift excellently.

Robert Shaw gave us terrific value, too, in his role as Red Grant. This character is a convicted murderer who escapes from a British jail to be recruited by SPECTRE as a top-grade killer. Shaw prepared for the role by putting himself through a ferocious bodybuilding course. He had to look as though he was built to take the vicious test punch to the midriff delivered by Rosa Klebb with a knuckleduster on her fist. Both he and Sean had lessons in Turko-Grecian wrestling in a Turkish gymnasium to prepare them for their confrontation on the Orient Express. The result is the most savage, heart-stopping duel you'll ever see in sixty seconds of screen time.

(Robert Shaw's death not long after was a great loss to me, and to the industry. He was not only a fine actor, especially in Shakespearean roles, but also a gifted writer. The film industry on both sides of the Atlantic could ill afford to lose this kind of talent.)

Dana loved Istanbul. She's always had the writer's curiosity about new places, different cultures. But she had other reasons for remembering the place. It was there that she really got to know Ian Fleming. In London he was mostly preoccupied with writing or his business affairs. At production meetings he'd sit there in his detached manner, occasionally, but always diffidently, suggesting an idea or two. He revealed very little of himself. But in Istanbul he was in his element. It was as though he were stepping back into the pages of his book. He loved the sounds, the spicy smells, the bazaars, the street merchants and the belly-dancers. Especially the belly-dancers. I can picture him now in one of Istanbul's exclusive restaurants, a quivering midriff an inch or two off the end of his Turkish cigarette, and his pale-blue eyes locked on the dancer's navel.

Here, away from the world of publishing and the hassle of agents, he could relax. He warmed towards Dana, and even—this was rare for him—discussed aspects of his writing with her. But then Ian always had a weakness for beautiful women! He loved talking about them. The way he describes the women in his books gives no clue as to whether he's seeing them through his own eyes or Bond's. One thing's for sure: Ian appreciated all types, hues and nationalities. His wife Anne, whom he adored, is on record as having written to him, claiming playfully that she seldom visited a capital city where she did not meet some woman with whom Ian had enjoyed carnal relations. But I suspect much of this was myth rather than fact, Fleming coming on with that suave lady-killing manner because he thought it was expected of him.

Dana and Ian went sightseeing together on a boat in the Bosporus. She found him a delightful, charming man and a great guide. He had been to Istanbul a year or so before, on assignment as a journalist covering an Interpol conference. He became very friendly with an Oxford-educated ship-owner, Nazim Kalkavan, who knew Istanbul's every treasure, every monument, every secret alleyway. All this information Fleming filed away in his mind, and it reappeared in his book *From Russia With Love*. He told me that the character Kerim, head of the Turkish Secret Service, was modeled on Kalkavan.

Kerim was a pivotal role in our script, and was played magnificently by the actor Pedro Armendariz. Pedro was a big attractive Mexican, a warm personality who'd been a star in his own country before having an even bigger success in Hollywood and Europe. He was not only a great actor but a fantastic human being. I thought he'd be terrific as Kerim, Bond's Secret Service contact in Istanbul. I met up with him in California and offered him the part. I didn't know until we were halfway through the picture that he had cancer. Apparently there were indications of it even before we started, but Pedro was determined to fight it. He had another reason, I was told. If he wasn't going to beat it, he wanted to leave money to his widow.

One of his big scenes involved a chase and a three-car pile-up featuring Bond, a moustached Bulgarian and Pedro. When Bond gets away, the Bulgarian shouts in fury at Armendariz, who reacts by casually flicking the ash off his cigar, saying, 'My friend, that is life.' When Terence shot that scene, we knew then, and so did Pedro, that he was a dying man. It was a delicate situation. We wanted to spare him any pain or discomfort. He was determined to finish the film. He had that kind of discipline, and he had the guts, too. He was desperate to prove that he could see the assignment through. The alternative was to recast the role, but none of us was prepared to do that.

So we figured out a solution which enabled us to shoot all Pedro's remaining sequences at Pinewood in one go. It was a very painful two weeks for the whole crew. To see this fine man, with that 'lovable bandit' smile of his, going rapidly downhill was hard to take. I don't know how, what inner strength he grabbed hold of, but he performed right through to the last shot.

Ironically, when Terence afterwards went to have a drink with Pedro there was an echo of that scene in Istanbul. Terence was sad, and it showed. The Mexican flashed his famous teeth in a smile. He had a cigar in his hand. He remembered the scene. Tapping the ash off, he repeated, 'My friend, that is life.' We had a dinner party before he left to return home to Mexico. It was June 1963.

A couple of years earlier his close friend, Ernest Hemingway, also faced with a crippling illness, had shot himself. While Pedro was at UCLA Medical Center in Los Angeles for special treatment, he asked his wife to bring him his antique pistol so that he could have it repaired in California. Not long after, in his bed, he took the gun from under his pillow and killed himself. It was tragic, of course. But to many of us it was also brave and typical of the man.

The second-unit work on *From Russia With Love* hit quite a few problems. There was sickness among the cast; some of the motorboat sequences had to be aborted and re-staged in Scotland. An important scene in the film has Bond, Tatiana and Kerim escaping through an underground sewer, chased by an army of brown rats. Under British regulations, we weren't allowed to use wild rats in British films. Syd Cain hit on the idea of coating tame white rats with cocoa, but by the time we got around to shooting the scene they were tired. They wouldn't budge; instead they started licking the chocolate off one another's backs. We now had piebald rats and a lot of spare cocoa. It was a key sequence, so we took a small unit to Madrid, where we'd heard there was a Spanish rat-catcher who could lay his hands on two hundred brown rats. Or two thousand, if we'd needed them. We shot the whole scene in a garage with a sheet of plate glass between us and them. The ratcatcher thought we were being unduly hesitant. But then so did the tarantula handler in *Dr No*.

The final scenes of *From Russia With Love* were shot in the last week of August 1963. There were some brilliant back-up features to the film. It was our first effective use of what became known as the 'Bond gadgets': specifically, the special black attaché case handed to Bond by the head of Q branch, Boothroyd, played by Desmond Llewelyn. Based on Fleming's description, it was created by the special-effects genius John Stears and the art director Syd Cain. The case contained gold sovereigns, a throwing knife, .25-calibre ammunition and a folding Armalite Survival Gun with a telescopic infrared lens. There was also a harmless-looking tin of talcum powder which, in fact, was a trick canister of tear-gas.

Dick Maibaum wrote some great dialogue for the scene where the boffin instructs Bond, in the tones of a headmaster, 'Normally, to open a case like that you move the catches to the side. If you do, the cartridge will explode in your face. Now, to stop the cartridge exploding . . .' It's a great scene, played for humour, but at the same time it offers an intriguing insight into the hardware of deadly espionage. Which is what Fleming's popularity was all about. Another clever idea, superimposing the titles on the sinuous body of a Turkish belly-dancer, was masterminded by Robert Brownjohn and Trevor Bond.

The film opened in London to an enthusiastic reception, with considerable praise for Sean. It became the top money-maker of the year worldwide. Bosley Crowther in the *New York Times* was totally enraptured by Daniela Bianchi, and as for the film, he begged: 'Don't miss it . . . just go and see it and have yourself a good time.' The influential *Variety,* predicting 'big box office', declared unequivocally: 'Ian Fleming's British Secret Service Agent James Bond cannot miss. *From Russia With Love* is a preposterous, skillful slab of hard-hitting sexy hokum . . . directed by Terence Young at a zingy pace . . . the cast perform with an amusing combo of tongue-in-cheek and seriousness and the Istanbul location is a bonus. Connery . . . is well served, not only actionwise, but by some crisp wise-cracking dialogue by Richard Maibaum. Robert Shaw is an impressive, icy, implacable killer and the late Pedro Armendariz weighs in with a formidable, yet lightly-played performance.'

Entertainment Today was just as enthusiastic, commenting: ' . . . the film proved to countless skeptics that the James Bond films were being made by people who knew what they were doing . . .' This was true, although I could not pretend that the successful partnership between Harry Saltzman and myself looked set to last for ever. We were different in style, temperament, and in our attitude to film-making. To me, sustaining Bond as a top international box-office attraction meant staying with it, living with it, without hankering after other things. It had achieved a unique success, but there was always the temptation to believe that it had a kind of built-in momentum of its own. It didn't. Each James Bond film is as demanding creatively as the first. The pictures must never have the flavour of tired thinking or recycled scenarios. To me, that meant then—and means now—that Bond is a full-time occupation.

And here I'm exceedingly fortunate, since Dana is just as involved with the Bond pictures as I am. Her name isn't among the credits, but her input has always been valuable, often crucial. There's always been a lot of love in our household, and Dana is at the heart of it. She somehow manages to keep that generating current going wherever any of us might be in the world. Her son Michael, and Tina, Tony and Barbara are all devoted to her. And I'm not exactly at the back of the queue.

While our first two films and the James Bond books swept the world, Ian Fleming, who began it all, was having a tough time. In his early film negotiations with Kevin McClory, which were finally aborted, one controversy remained. It hinged on whether McClory and his associate Jack Whittingham should be acknowledged as having contributed material for his book *Thunderball*.

In November 1963 Kevin brought the case to the High Court in London. It would lead to two years of contentious argument, over which time Fleming became increasingly weary. He was a creative writer, not a showbiz litigant. And even before all that began, his heart condition was worsening—a fact he concealed from most of us. As the case dragged on, our own interest in *Thunderball* had to be shelved again. We turned instead to *Goldfinger*.

This was a strong story with a fascinating villain. Auric Goldfinger's master plan is to detonate a small atomic bomb in Fort Knox, which would hugely increase the value of his own hoard of $60 million worth of gold bullion. Terence Young wasn't sure he wanted to make another Bond picture, and went off to direct *The Amorous Adventures of Moll Flanders*. We approached Guy Hamilton, who had originally turned Bond down but was eager to do this one. I've always liked Guy Hamilton's work. He shoots with a lot of pace and style, and also has a flair for comedy: all the elements intrinsic to Bond. Guy was also a low-handicap golfer, which immediately gave him points with Sean. Before he came to us, Guy had made some impressive films, including *The Colditz Story, An Inspector Calls, The Devil's Disciple* and *The Best of Enemies*.

The moment we began casting, we hit a problem. Obviously, choosing the actor to play Goldfinger was crucial. There was initial disagreement over who that actor should be. Harry was all for the American actor Theodore Bikel, who played the adventurous Hungarian in *My Fair Lady*. I was just as insistent that we use the German Gert Frobe. He was a bulky, bullet-headed character who was not only well known in Germany, but had also played a role in *The Longest Day*. What impressed me was that he could be menacing, yet had a great sense of humour. But Harry kept pushing Theodore Bikel until finally I said, 'All right, let's get him over here and make a test.' There was always the chance Harry could be right. We flew this actor from New York to London and made the test. He was no Goldfinger.

Even so, Guy and Harry remained unsure about Frobe. They protested he didn't speak English too well and was not a star, merely a character actor. I said we were not looking for stars. We were looking for the ideal Goldfinger. There was only one way to find out. I flew to Munich to speak to his manager, a German woman. Frobe's hair was sand-coloured, but not as red as the script called for. I told her I'd like to have Gert redden his hair and then come and see us in London. When Guy saw him, his eyes lit up.

'Gee! Who's that?'

'That's Gert Frobe,' I told him.

'We have to test him. He looks the right man to me,' said Guy.

It's true Frobe's English was sketchy. But that was never going to be a problem. We could always dub another voice over his. What mattered was he made a great Goldfinger.

To bring in some fresh thinking to the screenplay, we engaged the late Paul Dehn, a fine writer and distinguished film critic. He and Dick Maibaum sparked ideas off each other in what turned out to be a very productive and highly professional collaboration.

Two important pieces of casting remained: an actor to play Oddjob, and an actress for Flemings butch but sexually free wheeling female, Pussy Galore. Casting the Japanese wrestler Harold Sakata as Oddjob was, like Frobe, a spot-on choice. He was not an actor, but I didn't see that as a particular handicap. That square head, the quizzical Oriental eyes, and the sheer tonnage of the man made him the perfect henchman to the master criminal Goldfinger. Instinctively, he managed to convey a hint of icy humour, which made audiences shudder in their seats. If you guessed that offscreen Sakata (known as Tosh Togo in his wrestling days) was probably a bit of a pussycat, you'd be right. He was a friendly, gentle giant who, though he had no dialogue in the film, grunted his way to international recognition. He died some time back, but he'll long be remembered. He created a whole new role model for the screen heavy.

It was Guy Hamilton who suggested Honor Blackman to play Pussy Galore. All her crinkly leather action and shoulder-throws she did so effectively in *The Avengers* virtually clinched it for her to tussle with James Bond. The casting complete, I drove to London Airport with Guy Hamilton and Dana *en route* to the States for the Fort Knox sequences. Also with us just for the ride to Heathrow was Dana's son Michael. He'd been in London only a couple of days.

I began turning over in my mind all the complex problems we were going to have to face on the location. There were intricate flying sequences, ground shots near the Fort, and we'd have to move carefully in a sensitive area guarded by crack units of the US Army.

Michael, before going to law school, had spent two years at a military school, then graduated from Harvey Mudd University in Claremont, California, with an engineering degree. He was on summer vacation and had been accepted at Stanford Law School. I could see that experience being valuable back-up in our contact with the military and also with the technical stuff around Fort Knox. Moreover, we had only a handful of crew on that location and could use a versatile character like Michael. So it was not nepotism or an idle whim which made me say to him as he stood there in just a shirt and pair of trousers: 'Too bad you don't have your passport. You could be of some help on this trip.'

'As a matter of fact, I do have it with me in my pocket,' he said (looking questioningly at his mother—Dana had waited for months for him to come to England to visit us).

I looked at Dana. 'I could use him.'

Michael said, 'Mom?'

Dana smiled. 'Go, if that's what you want.'

'Then consider yourself hired!' I said, and bought an extra ticket to New York. A day later Michael was with us in Kentucky, a hard worker and a very fast learner.

We went through the motions of seeking permission from the US Treasury Department to shoot inside Fort Knox. Firmly but courteously, they refused. Their interest in movies in general, and James Bond in particular, didn't extend to giving us an insider's view of how the greatest concentration of bullion in the world is guarded. But Ken Adam's ingenuity and research produced a spectacular substitute. His concept of what the inside of the depository looked like was close to genius. Built on several levels of chrome and steel, behind which the gold bars were stacked, it was a breathtaking arena in which Oddjob is finally eliminated.

Outside of the Pinewood stages, we constructed the Fort Knox exterior, complete with big electric gates, concrete drive and long stretches of wire barricades. While the engineers were preparing all this, we were within shouting distance of the real thing, under the alert scrutiny of armed elements of the US military.

Permission to use troops was hard to obtain. We were not allowed to pay them, so remuneration had to come in the form of an allowance for cleaning uniforms or whatever. In the event, we received all the permissions we required, and much of that was due to Charles Rushon, a friend of mine and former Army colonel. Ted Moore's photography, together with all the stunt work, created a landmark in spy adventure films. The imitators would soon be climbing on to the bandwagon. (We had to stretch a point with Pussy Galore's flying circus. Flying females were thin in the air over North Kentucky, so I hired some male pilots from a nearby flying school, rigged them out in black jump suits and blonde wigs. They looked pretty good, too, but couldn't wait to get rid of the gear.)

There was now the problem over Pussy Galore. Not the character, but the name. Fleming was no shrinking violet. He'd been around and was familiar with the vernacular of Vegas bachelors and men's locker-room conversation. My mischievous friend knew only too well the double entendre behind the name Pussy Galore. So, apparently, did his American publisher, who read the manuscript of *Goldfinger* and laid it on the line: 'You just can't use this name, Ian.'

Fleming, who'd been to Sandhurst, Britain's equivalent of West Point, was not used to being told what he couldn't do. 'Oh yes I will,' he said, 'and not only that, we're going to get away with it!' Well, that was fine for Ian Lancaster Fleming. He only had the publisher to contend with.

We were also advised against using the name. But our view was quite simple: we were filming the book; Pussy Galore was a pivotal character in the story; that's what Fleming named her; there seemed no reason to call her anything else. Dick Maibaum was prepared to change it to Kitty Galore, but Fleming, rightly, thought that would be nonsense, since millions who'd read the book would be mystified. In those days we didn't submit scripts beforehand to so-called censors.

Geoffrey Shurlock was the man behind the then influential Production Code of the MPEA (the same sort of character who had come out against *The Trials of Oscar Wilde*). We saw no reason to clear the script with him, and used the dialogue as written. At a Royal Premiere, Honor Blackman was presented to Prince Philip. The following morning one newspaper gave it front-page treatment under the heading 'Pussy and the Prince', It was an irresistible heading which amused everybody, including the Palace. Another newspaper had a similar headline.

By then Geoffrey Shurlock had been told that *Goldfinger* had been premiered in London without him having read or approved script. This upset him. He was even more miffed when he heard there was an actress featured in the picture named Pussy Galore. He began to make waves, and I had to drop everything in London and fly over to the States to talk to him. He said flatly that he was not going to permit me to release the picture.

'How can you do that?' I said. 'We've spent millions of dollars—you can't just censor it because of a name.' (I was never for censorship anyway; the public are the best judges.)

'I know what you're saying, but I can ban this picture,' was his answer.

I then played the ace. I had brought with me all the tear sheets of the British papers which carried pictures of Prince Philip meeting Honor Blackman. Some said, 'The Prince meets Pussy'; others, 'Pussy and the Prince'. I showed them to Shurlock, 'Look these. If the picture is good enough for Prince Philip and the people of London to see, that ought to be all right over here. Second, look at those headlines. There's obviously nothing wrong with the word 'Pussy' . . . that's her name! It's been accepted in England, and dammit, if it's OK with them what are you worried about?!'

He looked again at the tear sheets, then at me, paused a while and laughed. 'Ah, OK, Cubby, you win.'

LESSON ELEVEN

The Rating System

CARA and the Emergence of Responsible Entertainment

Kevin S. Sandler

> *When Al Van Schmus—the last of the Breen Boys—retired, the Classification and Rating Administration lost all resemblance to the Production Code Administration. Or did it?*
> —Leonard J. Leff and Jerold L. Simmons, The Dame in the Kimono

A regulatory facelift could not have come at a better time when the MPAA established the Code and Rating Administration (CARA—changed to Classification and Rating Administration in 1977) on November 1, 1968; the motion picture business in the United States was in shambles. Declining attendance, shifting cultural mores, cinematic free expression, and independent and foreign film competition led producers, distributors, and exhibitors to discard long-standing codes of industry conduct and cooperation for short-term personal gain. These abandoned "gentleman rules," as Jon Lewis calls them, dissolved a business arrangement between the three branches of the motion picture business that guaranteed the appearance of harmless entertainment to Hollywood's various audiences and detractors.[1] The standards and practices of the industry's centralized process of self-regulation were impotent amidst this undoing, unable to endow Hollywood entertainment with an affirmative cultural function so systematically accomplished in the past. The MPAA had to reconceptualize its products whether it wanted to or not.

Despite these obstacles, the rating system prevailed, surpassing the tenure of the Production Code Administration (1930–1966) as it celebrated its thirty-ninth year in 2007. Instead of a uniform PCA seal, CARA currently assigns one of five age-based rating categories to a film: G (suggested for general audiences); PG (parental guidance suggested); PG-13 (parents strongly cautioned); R (persons under 17 not admitted, unless accompanied by parent or adult guardian); and NC-17 (no one 17 and under admitted). Since the inception of a rating system, the MPAA and its longtime president, Jack Valenti (who retired in 2004 and was replaced by Dan Glickman, who served as secretary of agriculture under Bill Clinton), have repeatedly differentiated the self-regulatory policies and procedures of CARA from its predecessors: "a voluntary rating plan" that "assures freedom of the screen," announced a 1968 press release; "a totally new approach," declared Valenti for *Daily Variety* in 1975, that "would no longer 'approve or disapprove' the content of a film": a replacement for "a stern, forbidding catalogue of 'Dos and Don'ts' [that had] the odious smell of censorship," wrote Valenti in a 1991 industry pamphlet. And in 1998 an MPAA press release proclaimed that the voluntary rating system replaced "an absurd manifesto called the Hays Code,"[2] These accounts indicate that the MPAA always wanted consumers to believe that CARA and the PCA were entirely separate regimes, distinctive markers of censorious "Classical Hollywood" and liberated "New Hollywood." Valenti frequently expressed this sentiment of CARA being a more modernized system, one that allowed the filmmaker "to tell his story in his way without anyone thwarting him,"[3]

Valenti's words seem initially plausible. First, different age categories gave filmmakers greater creative leeway than a single-seal-for-all-audiences approach. Content and themes previously forbidden by the PCA were now more permissible under a classification system. Second, moral absolutism, once the backbone of the Production Code, gave way to a world of moral relativism under classification. Film ratings were a determination of the possible suitability of a film for children and were not grounded in Catholic doctrine. Last, CARA regulated films only after their completion. Unlike the PCA, CARA did not actively shape film narrative and form during the production process in order to ensure mass distribution and exhibition of Hollywood's products. Classification, it would appear then, enabled and permitted freer expression in Hollywood films than self-regulation under the Production Code.

Freer expression? Indeed. Free expression? Definitely not. This chapter will demonstrate that CARA functioned similarly to the PCA in one key respect: to control entryway and participation into the legitimate theatrical marketplace. I will first argue that classification reestablished a system by which the MPAA could govern the flow of product through the production, distribution, and exhibition sectors of the Hollywood film industry. Together with the full cooperation of the National Association of Theatre Owners (NATO) by 1973, the MPAA, through CARA, was able to construct a new model of entertainment, what I call "responsible entertainment," an industry standard that functioned much like "harmless entertainment" during the Production Code. Responsible entertainment required, above all, a collective adherence and commitment by the major distributors and exhibitors to completely abandon the use of the X/NC-17-rating product line. By regulating all Hollywood films into R categories or lower—what I call the Incontestable R—the industry could ensure the suitability and respectability of Hollywood's products in the eyes of audiences. Hollywood, in other words, updated its business practices (a rating system enabling free expression) without changing its business model (entertainment for all ages). The remainder of the chapter will focus on the mid-1970s to 1990, a period of notable rating cases when filmmakers and opportunistic distributors challenged the boundaries of the Incontestable R, causing a momentary rupture in the guise of responsible entertainment. Moments like these were few, I argue, but they highlighted the fact that the rating system, while enabling greater creative freedom than the Production Code, still is a virtual synonym, in the words of Bruce A. Austin, for both "self-preservation" and "self-interest," the same ideals that have motivated the MPAA for more than eighty years.[4]

Responsible Entertainment and a New Code of Self-Regulation

In his 1990 *American Film* article "What Will H. Hays Begat: Fifty Years of the Production Code," film critic and historian Charles Champlin correctly asserts that the Production Code never truly ended; it was momentarily sidetracked, then gradually transformed into a classification system, another "voluntary and self-regulating way of heading off more imposed censorship,"[5] This new "way" of self-regulation not only served once again as a buttress against federal legislation, but it also helped to reestablish the commercial efficiency of the Hollywood film industry under the guise of responsible entertainment.

In beginning to understand CARA as a reformulation of the MPAA's business practices rather than an overhaul of its operations, it is important to realize that the rating system was actually always intended to be a "production code" for the major Hollywood distributors just like its predecessor. On the surface there were many points of continuity between the two administrations. CARA originally stood for the Code and Rating Administration, and many PCA administrators moved over to CARA (which also occupied the same Hollywood offices for a time). Eugene Dougherty, the senior member of the Production Code staff who served under Joseph Breen and Geoffrey Shurlock, became CARA's first chairperson. Shurlock himself remained as a consultant. Also retained was Richard R. Mathison, a PCA staff member since 1965, and longtime examiner Albert E. Van Schmus, who continued in his role as a senior examiner until his retirement in 1982.[6] The CARA seals maintained the numerical sequence set by the PCA seals.

To be sure, the Production Code was definitely a more determining and constrictive force in the constitution of Hollywood-produced films from 1930 to 1966. Van Schmus admits that its single-seal-for-all-audiences standard was undoubtedly censorship of free expression: "I always looked upon myself as a censor. I admit it. That's what I was there for, to try to talk somebody out of doing something in their script."[7] The rating system liberalized the Code, allowing filmmakers to theoretically address any and all subjects across various age categories. CARA examiners looked at a film's theme, content, and treatment of subject matter to determine its appropriateness for children. In the early years a rating of G, M (later GP then PG), or R was then assigned to those films that all or some parents may find acceptable viewing for their children. An X rating was awarded to films off-limits to children under sixteen (later under eighteen). In any case CARA, unlike the PCA, guaranteed a rating "category" to each applicant and nearly unlimited cinematic expression to all.

Yet an examination of the official 1968 Code of Self-Regulation reveals a less altruistic side to the MPAA, one that supports a claim made by outgoing PCA head Geoffrey Shurlock at the time of CARA's creation: "We'll use the same standards that we've used for 30 years in applying the code."[8] In fact, the 1968 Code was practically a carbon copy of the 1966 Code (which itself was based on the 1930 Production Code), with one key difference: a four-tiered rating system replaced the Suggested for Mature Audiences tag. Even the "Declaration of Principles" and "Standards of Production" were lifted directly from the 1966 Code of Self-Regulation to guide administrators about matters of sex, violence, and other wrongdoings in considering motion pictures for ratings approval. These replications confirm Van Schmus's pronouncement that the 1966 Code of Self-Regulation was merely an "advertising effort" in preparation for classification.

Even so, contained in the language of the 1966 and 1968 Code documents lies the foundation of boundary maintenance under CARA, what I have previously referred to as "responsible entertainment." The word *responsible* is stated four times throughout both Codes, and none of these four is more important than the one employed in the "Declaration of Principles": "To encourage artistic expression by expanding creative freedom," and "To assure that the freedom which encourages the artist remains *responsible* and sensitive to the standards of the larger society."[9] Valenti elaborated more on these tenets in a section entitled "Censorship and Classification-by-Law Are Wrong" from a "Personal Statement" released in connection with the announcement of CARA and the 1968 Code:

> *We will oppose these intrusions into a communications art-form shielded and protected by the First Amendment. We believe the screen should be as free for filmmakers as it is for those who write books, produce television material, publish newspapers and magazines, compose music and create paintings and sculptures.*
>
> *At the same time I have urged film creators to remember that freedom without discipline is license, and that's wrong, too. I have, in the many meetings I have had with creative people in film, suggested that the freedom which is rightly theirs ought to be a* responsible *freedom and each individual film-maker must judge his work in that sensible light. I'm cheered by the response to my suggestions.*[10]

The balance between artistic expression and cultural sensitivity, what Valenti delineated here as "responsible freedom," is essentially the philosophy behind "responsible entertainment" in the classification era. A process for determining the upper threshold of responsible entertainment and CARA's strategies for effectively enforcing this boundary was never outlined in the 1968 Code. At CARA's inception, though, a policy to negotiate these concerns can be found in the new Code's proclamation, "Freedom of expression does not mean toleration of license." Often repeated by Valenti throughout his tenure, this phrase points to the strategies the MPAA envisioned for responsible entertainment at that time and the ones it currently upholds now.

How, then, did the MPAA reconcile two contradictory objectives in the Code of Self-Regulation, one in which creative freedom could flourish as long as it was balanced by a sense of self-restraint and social responsibility? Or as Valenti succinctly put it again: "Every filmmaker ought to be able to tell a story the way he wants to. But that kind of freedom ought to be harnessed."[11] The MPAA did so by having it both ways, by perpetuating the belief that CARA supports free expression of filmmakers while at the same time actively discouraging the use of the X rating among its membership. In this manner the MPAA could subscribe to a framework of creative license but still function according to an affirmative cultural model of entertainment. As a result, the MPAA could manage the flow of product through every sector of the film industry under its own terms of boundary maintenance—responsible entertainment—while also publicly denying its role as a censor.

Before this could happen, Valenti needed the industry to adhere to the standards of responsible entertainment not only in theory but in practice. The success of CARA depended on the collusive support of its judgments by the members of the MPAA and NATO. What responsible entertainment might look like or feel like or taste like was anybody's guess at the time. But Valenti knew early on that the menu did not include the X rating.

The MPAA and the X Rating

In a 1977 hearing on Capitol Hill Jack Valenti outlined the principles that led to the success of the MPAA rating system:

> *Let me tell you that the linchpin of this rating system was the interlinking of essential ingredients. First, the system must have integrity, must have probity. It must be proof against pressure from all sides, majors and independents, from anyone who has a personal economic stake, or anyone who may assume they have an economic stake, in the outcome of the ratings. . . . Second, we had to have a partnership of everybody involved in films, the retailer, the theater owner who exhibits the film, the independent director and producer, and the major director and producer. . . . Third, a policy mechanism had to be created so that if someone felt aggrieved by a rating, he had a place to go. You can't have a czar or a dictator saying, "That is it, and no more." Four, and this is the crux of the system, it really had to perform a service for parents. Otherwise, the ratings had no meaning. Those were the four indispensable elements that formed the recipe for the rating system.*[12]

When the MPAA established CARA in 1968, these four elements were effectively set in place. Lending initial integrity to the system was the creation of the X rating, which barred those under sixteen and quieted concerns about children's access to sexually explicit material. I will examine the advent of the X in terms of two of the three major partners in CARA: the MPAA (the seven "majors" minus RKO, which had its assets stripped by Howard Hughes in 1955, plus two new independent distributors: Allied Artists and Avco Embassy) and NATO (which represented most of the major exhibition chains). The third partner in CARA was the International Film Importers and Distributors of America (IFIDA), a trade organization representing a mass of independent companies, which played little role in the rating system.[13] If any distributor disagreed with an assigned rating from CARA's Rating Board, one had the opportunity to appeal the original rating to CARA's Appeals Board. And written into the principles of the Code of Self-Regulation was a commitment to parents to help them "determine whether a particular picture is one which children should see at the discretion of the parent; or only when accompanied by a parent; or should not see."[14]

An industry-wide commitment to these goals was necessary to lay the foundation of responsible entertainment. The MPAA needed protection from moral reformers and politicians. NATO was bound by the courts to keep sexually explicit material away from children. And Valenti, wanting no part of any of them, wished to keep the industry, in the words of Jon Lewis, "out of the dirty movie business."[15] It was not until 1973, however, that the members of the MPAA and NATO collectively abandoned the use of the X rating, a category that had quickly become anonymous with "the dirty movie business" shortly after the inception of CARA.

"The stigma of the X," Justin Wyatt explains, was the result of the rating's widespread and pronounced use as a marketing tool in the late 1960s and early 1970s to tap into a market segment of adult viewers previously ignored by Hollywood. Mainstream filmmakers, distributors, and exhibitors took advantage of the creative freedom and notoriety provided by an adults-only category, as did exploitation, filmmakers and pornographers. This inter industry practice, Wyatt notes, created initial confusion over the meaning of the X rating, dividing the adult-film marketplace into three distinct areas: serious "adult dramas," like *A Clockwork Orange* (1971), primarily distributed by the MPAA signatories and incorporating graphic, though simulated, sex scenes and/or adult subject matter; "soft-core" exploitation *(Cherry, Harry & Raquel* [1969]); and "hard-core" pornography *(Deep Throat* [1972]), the domain of the independents and marked by differences in sexual content, exhibition, and pricing.[16] As a result of the category's appropriation by members of the legitimate and the non-legitimate film industry for exploitative purposes, the X quickly became associated with pornography, providing little chance for serious artistic filmmakers to adopt the rating. It became clear that if filmmakers wanted to make responsible Hollywood entertainment in the classification era, they had to make it with an R rating or go outside the legitimate theatrical marketplace.

The fact that independent distributors could self-impose the X was the result of the MPAA's never copyrighting the category, unlike the other ratings. I am uncertain, though, if this omission was a legal maneuver on the part of Valenti or a Machiavellian scheme of his to force filmmakers to use their creative freedom "responsibly." In the case of the former, Valenti stated in a 1975 MPAA press release that his original intent was to have only three ratings—G, M, and R—because it was his view that parents should have the right to take their children to any film they choose. He said, however, that NATO urged him to create the X category out of fear of legal redress under *Ginsberg*, the 1968 Supreme Court case that ruled that material could be considered obscene for children but not for adults.[17] He supplements this legal explanation in a 1990 interview, claiming that the X rating was not copyrighted because the MPAA charged a fee for its rating service. The X "had to be open-ended," he said, "so that if somebody doesn't want to submit a picture [to the MPAA], they can use the X. Otherwise, we could be challenged on First Amendment grounds."[18] As for the Machiavellian rationale, it is hard to believe that Valenti did not anticipate the appropriation of the uncopyrighted X by soft- and hard-core pornographers. The X permitted any and all representations of sex and violence to be subsumed under its category. The basic principle of responsible entertainment—"freedom of expression does not mean toleration of license"—could never be contained within a no-limits classification. Even if there is some truth to Valenti's legal justifications for not copyrighting the X, the excuses peculiarly support a system of boundary maintenance dependent on that rating's stigmatization and abandonment.

Whatever the reason(s) may be for failing to copyright the X, the MPAA pretty much avoided the "dirty movie business" for both serious adult works and soft-core features from the very beginning of CARA. The number of X-rated films released by the MPAA signatories (Columbia, MGM, Paramount, 20th Century-Fox, United Artists, Universal, and Warner Bros.) between November 1, 1968, and October 8, 1973, totaled only twenty-five pictures (1968: 4; 1969: 8; 1970: 7; 1971: 5; 1972: 0; and 1973: 1).[19] Many of these films were foreign produced, including adult dramas *(The Damned* [1969]; *The Devils* [1971]), soft-core sexual comedies *(The Best House in London* [1969]), and a documentary *(The Body* [1971]). Only a small proportion was U.S. produced, including serious-minded films like *Medium Cool* (1969),[20] *Midnight Cowboy* (1969), and *Last of the Mobile Hot-shots* (1971), as well as sexual farces like *Can Hieronymus Merkin Ever Forget Mercy Humppe and Find True Happiness?* (1969) and *Beyond the Valley of the Dolls* (1970). The shrinking year-to-year number of legitimate X pictures produced stateside and released by the majors reflected the rating's instant cultural stigma and especially its economic liabilities: the category's age restrictions prevented a large portion of the potential audience from ever purchasing tickets.

When some MPAA signatories did exploit the notoriety provided by the X rating and its suggestion of "uncensored spectacle," as did Warner Bros. with *Girl on a Motorcycle* (1968), for example, they met with a harsh reception. One unnamed Warner Bros. executive said, "[The Code staff] asked us to make some cuts, but we decided to go ahead and take the X rating and make some money."[21] But after *Girl on a Motorcycle*'s disastrous performance at the box office, Warner Bros. rereleased the film with an R rating and a new name *(Naked under Leather)* after removing an erotic lovemaking scene and Marianne Faithfull's masturbation scene. Paramount's *if . . .* (1968) and the independent Sigma III film *Greetings* (1968) were also released in edited R versions after their initial X runs.[22]

The rereleasing of *Girl on a Motorcycle, Greetings,* and *if . . .* with R ratings in 1969 suggests that both MPAA and independent distributors became quickly disenchanted with the box-office potential of serious-minded X-rated pictures. Their initial eagerness to take advantage of the adults-only rating gave way almost immediately to its cultural stigmatization. By July 1969 certain newspapers had begun to reject advertisements for X-rated films, and many TV and radio stations established policies refusing to run trailers for them. Some stations would not even run ads for M-rated films before 10 p.m.[23] Moreover, difficulties in promoting X-rated films exposed the rating's inherent economic limitations to the MPAA signatories: the age restrictions simply made them a poor financial investment. If an R could play to a mass audience, so the executives thought—albeit one that required adult supervision for children—why not cut a film to fit the lower category's requirements? In fact, the *New York Times,* on the very day of CARA's formation, reported that MPAA members were already editing their films down from an X rating before they were even officially rated. The newspaper stated that Paramount had removed some obscene dialogue from a prison film, *Riot* (1969), to get an R;[24] the *Times* also reported that Michelangelo Antonioni would excise a four-letter word for copulation in the script for MGM's *Zabriskie Point* (1970) if its inclusion meant an X. "The general view" in the industry, wrote *Newsweek* four months later, in February 1969, was "that, while nobody quite knows what draws an X rating, it is something to avoid."[25]

Even the commercial and artistic success of *Midnight Cowboy* (1969) failed to establish a trend in X-rated film production. *Midnight Cowboy*'s triumph, suggests Jon Lewis, had more to do with its kinship with prestige adults-only pictures like *Bonnie and Clyde* (1967) rather than with soft- or hard-core features like *I Am Curious (Yellow)* (1967) and *3 in the Attic* (1968), two other X-rated films in the top-twenty box office for 1969.[26] By the end of the decade, too many "dirty" movies had already damaged beyond repair the adults-only rating's commercial viability. In his 1972 book, *The Movie Rating Game,* former CARA intern Stephen Farber confirms the widespread avoidance of the X by 1970: "By now the X has lost whatever chance it might have had to achieve respectability," he said. "Several studios have made it a policy to produce *no* X films, and most studio contracts with directors stipulate that the director must win an R or less restrictive rating on the finished film." The X may even keep some films from being made at all. Farber identifies already completed films like *Joe* (1970), *Hi, Mom!* (1970), and *Straw Dogs* (1971) as being cut by their distributors so they could be awarded an R.[27]

At the same time that the MPAA signatories put policies in place to abolish the X rating as a business strategy, CARA further protected MPAA interests by instituting a new policy of its own to assure that more films could be awarded R ratings. In 1970 CARA raised the R and X age limits from sixteen to seventeen in order to absorb previous X-rated content into the R category. This bump, in the words of CARA chairperson Eugene Dougherty, was intended so that "no serious film-makers would want to go beyond the limits of the R."[28] The term *serious* appears to be CARA's (or, at the very least, Dougherty's) synonym for self-restraint, the responsible kind of entertainment Valenti envisioned for the Hollywood film industry. Indeed, no U.S.-produced, MPAA-distributed films actually did go beyond the boundaries of the R for a long time after 1970. Only auteur-driven foreign productions distributed by the majors carried the badge—Stanley Kubrick's *A Clockwork Orange,* Pier Paolo Pasolini's *Decameron* (1971), Ken Russell's *The Devils* (1971), Bernardo Bertolucci's *Last Tango in Paris* (1973)—as did a few soft-core features: *Emmanuelle* (1974) and *Inserts* (1976).

The near-abandonment of the X rating and the expansion of the age range for R pictures in 1970 also caught the attention of *Variety* at the time. The trade paper described 1970 as the year of the "wandering X and R," because of the number of films seemingly of X caliber that drifted over into R and, strangely, even into GP territory.[29] Films like *Women in Love* (male frontal nudity) and *The Boys in the Band* (homosexuality) earned R ratings, whereas a year earlier they may have been given X ratings. Statistics support these claims. R ratings accounted for only 23 percent of films from 1968 to 1969 but rose to 37 percent from 1969 to 1970 and gradually increased through the early part of the decade, reaching a plateau of 48 percent from 1974 to 1975.[30] As a result of these changes to MPAA and CARA policies, Valenti redesigned a system that was more inclusive of MPAA product while simultaneously promoting Hollywood as a responsible industry committed to making mass audience films. The R rating became the tag that signified Hollywood, and the X became associated with U.S. independent and foreign art fare, as well as soft- and hard-core pornographic films. Writing in the *Journal of the University Film Association* in 1971, Julian C. Burroughs Jr. foresaw this strategy by the MPAA as a means of reducing criticism of its projects and staving off federal legislation. "The major motion picture companies which are represented by the MPAA," he said, "will have to decide how far they are willing to follow the 'anything/everything goes' trend. To put it another way, as long as the majors—and others who would aspire to general public favor—allow good taste to play a significant role in their productions and promotions, they are not likely to lose the support of the majority of Americans."[31]

The following year, the Associated Press reported in April 1971 that "the day of the X rated film appears to be over" for the MPAA signatories. In this story Columbia Pictures reiterated its stance against releasing X-rated pictures, and James Aubrey, president of MGM, explained why his company no longer was in the business of making X films: "Everybody was caught in the newfound freedom. The industry wallowed in it. But while permissive films might have been successful six months ago, they aren't now." 20th Century-Fox also abandoned X-film production after the back-to-back box-office bombs of the soft-core *Myra Breckenridge* and *Beyond the Valley of the Dolls* in 1970. "The board of directors decided then never again," said a Fox studio source, "not for all the money in the world." Even smaller, semilegitimate, independent distributors were abandoning the rating. Samuel Z. Arkoff, chairman of American International Pictures, remarked in May 1971: "It's good business sense today to make only Gs and GPs," and independent distributor Donald S. Rugoff admitted, "I never bought a film before with ratings in mind but I do now. The hassle just isn't worth it."[32] How quickly the X became an oddity for MPAA signatories is summed up by a *Variety* headline in July 1971: "WB acceptance of X for 'The Devils' a Rarity Nowadays for Major Film."

Even with MPAA-member unity over the branding of the X, Hollywood's new form of boundary maintenance could only succeed with the joint cooperation of NATO. Exhibiting adults-only pictures in legitimate first-run houses still gave the public impression that the MPAA sanctioned all these films, even if they were not reviewed and awarded an "official" X by CARA. The infiltration of adult-themed films, however, came at an inopportune time for the industry. As Justin Wyatt notes, in 1969 the majors suffered more than $200 million in losses, weekly attendance was almost one-sixth of its 1946 high, and "the youth 'revolution' served to feed the increasing freedom in terms of subject matter, further enhancing the marketability of the adult/porno feature."[33] Abandoning the X might have been the last thing on the minds of NATO exhibitors at a time of floundering box-office receipts.

NATO and the X

On the day of the inauguration of CARA in 1968, *New York Times* film critic Vincent Canby reported that proponents of the rating system saw two possible reasons why it could fail, both related to the X: first, X-rated films would prove so successful that they would stimulate more production; and second, as a result, exhibitors might loosen their enforcement of the rating, inviting new calls for governmental censorship and putting pressure on the Rating Board to place limits on the number of X films released.[34] He was right on both accounts. The X rating did prove to be a successful marketing category for distributors in the early years of CARA, and exhibitors were negligent in their handling of the adults-only category, igniting criticism and calls for reform of the rating system. To give rise to the era of responsible entertainment, the MPAA abandoned the product line altogether. NATO needed to recalibrate its box-office policy as well.

A new working relationship between the MPAA and NATO was absolutely mandatory after the Production Code since enforcement of the Code of Self-Regulation no longer fell on the shoulders of the distributors but on the theater owners themselves. In 1968 NATO made clear in the *NATO News*, a monthly bulletin available only to its members, that it shared responsibility with the MPAA for the system's success: "The local box office is the crucial point at which the rating system will succeed or fail. No amount of publicity or church support can guarantee the plan unless exhibitors themselves understand it, enforce it at their theatres, and work to create favorable public opinion in their communities. A lack of support on the part of theatre owners can only serve to create the circumstances which encourage hard feelings and, ultimately, censorship."[35] Enforcement would include checking IDs for X-rated films, ensuring that children were accompanied by a parent for R-rated films, patrolling theaters for children jumping screens, refraining from playing an R- or X-rated trailer in front of a G- or M-rated feature, being aware that the severest rating prevailed on a double feature, running the rating trailer before each film, and educating theater staff on the differences between the ratings.

Some of the criticism of the rating system in its first few years can be attributed to NATO's failure to carefully implement these obligations, many of which unsurprisingly centered on the X rating. Newspapers reported that neighborhood theaters neglected to police the box office. For example, the *New York Sunday News* found in July 1969 that underage children were being admitted to X-rated films and that exhibition policies sometimes allowed X trailers to accompany R films. The article reported the horror of one woman who took her fourteen-year-old son to see the R-rated *Goodbye Columbus* only to view the coming attraction of the X-rated *I, a Woman II*. [36] In other instances inattentive exhibitors showed X-rated trailers with G-rated films. It certainly did not help that 'opportunistic distributors took advantage of the new system at NATO's expense by releasing films with two ratings—with and without restrictive footage—to play for different audiences and theaters across the country.[37] The problems the X rating immediately posed to local theater owners led to a plea in July 1969 by the *Motion Picture Herald*'s Charlie Poorman to exhibitors to forgo X-rated features altogether. "While it is true that a powerful segment of the populace will patronize the maximum in perversion," he said, "there is no industrial future in this." He believed that the X rating "doesn't represent our best cinematic efforts" and suggested that theater owners replay older films in lieu of "unsuitable" ones.[38]

Two months later, a survey conducted by Young NATO, a committee of second- and third-generation exhibitors in the organization, reported that 47 percent of its respondents—who accounted for 89 percent of the nation's thirteen thousand theaters—automatically excluded X-rated films already from potential engagements for their theaters. The survey also supported claims that theaters carelessly enforced rating restrictions, with 30 percent of those NATO theaters playing X pictures to underage patrons.[39] For at least half of NATO's members, banning X films avoided the expense of modifying prints and trailers for local censor boards (most of which would cease their operations by the mid-1970s). These costs, partially if not entirely, would fall on the individual theaters. It also helped exhibitors to avoid community pressure, especially if they could not properly promote an X film in the local newspaper. Justin Wyatt viewed this split reaction to the economic opportunity of adult film in NATO's membership as reflecting a division along urban and rural lines. Ever since the *Miracle* decision forced the MPAA to divorce itself from exhibition and created numerous independent theater owners and chains, small-town exhibitors were more reluctant to play adult pictures than their big-city counterparts because of a lack of support from their communities.[40] These policies corresponded with the growing number of newspapers in small cities that refused to accept advertising for X films. While the newspaper chains in urban centers (New York, Philadelphia, Chicago, Los Angeles, and San Francisco) did not turn away advertisements, dailies in smaller cities (Birmingham, Chattanooga, Miami, Milwaukee, San Diego, Wichita) banned X-rated ads to conform to the standards of their respective communities.[41] In November 1969 the MPAA listed twenty-three such newspapers that would not take ads for X-rated films, a number that jumped to thirty-four newspapers by July 1972 and included major metropolitan city newspapers such as the *Detroit News, Cleveland Plain-Dealer, Cincinnati Enquirer,* and the *Boston Herald-Traveler*.[42]

Community grievances, inconsistent exhibitor policies, and media bans such as these fueled public concerns over the availability of obscenity to minors and renewed calls for federal censorship of motion pictures. On January 28, 1970, just prior to the release of the report of the President's Commission on Obscenity and Pornography, Valenti appeared before a subcommittee of the Committee on the Judiciary in the House of Representatives to oppose an impending bill to regulate local exhibition of theatrical motion pictures. He reassured Congress that NATO overwhelmingly supported the rating system and that voluntary self-regulation on the part of the film industry was the best course of action. Drawing from results of the Young NATO survey, as well as the MPAA's own recent study conducted by the Opinion Research Corporation (a survey of CARA's awareness and usefulness to parents that has been conducted every year since), Valenti announced two principal revisions to the Code of self-regulation to clarify the rating system to politicians, parents, and patrons at the box office. Mentioned earlier in this chapter, these revisions included the replacement of the M, supposedly the least understood of the four categories, with the GP (all ages admitted but parental guidance suggested) and the raising of the age limit for the R and X categories from sixteen to seventeen.

Throughout his tenure Valenti would often make such cosmetic adjustments to the system of boundary maintenance, changes that were honest enough to placate Hollywood's detractors but inconsequential enough not to endanger the economic and political interests of the MPAA. At this crossroads Valenti's diversionary tactics obfuscated the MPAA's overwhelming reliance on NATO for CARA's success and effectiveness. He used the occasion not to criticize exhibitors, who were the linchpins of the rating system, but to lend his unwavering support for the medium's First Amendment protection while also criticizing those "smut pushers," "salacious pornographers," and "fastbuck peddlers of garbage" who infringed on the privilege of creative freedom for others. The fact that these "fastbuck peddlers of garbage" found homes for their films at NATO theaters went unmentioned as Valenti's closing remark at this hearing reified the rating system's main objectives and its blueprint of responsible entertainment—"freedom of expression does not mean toleration of license":

> *Too often, it appears to me, the public does not differentiate between the responsible filmmaker and the irresponsible. There is a difference, a decisively important one. . . .*
>
> *The responsible leaders in the motion picture industry will not permit this medium to be tarnished. Personally I shall never cease, whatever the cost, to fight for self-regulation and self-restraint. I shall condemn obvious and gratuitous trash no matter where it comes from or who cashes in on it.[43]*

While Valenti could ensure that the MPAA carried out this responsibility through the self-regulatory operations of CARA, he still needed NATO theater owners to abandon any and all exhibition of X-rated pictures, many of which made more money than some legitimate Hollywood releases at the time.

That very same day, in the pages of a safer, less-public form—*Variety*—Valenti attacked Loews for eroding faith in the rating system. In this unprecedented criticism of a major theater circuit, he chastised the exhibition chain for booking the Danish sex film *Without a Stitch* (1970) in State I and Cine, two Manhattan first-run theaters. In no uncertain terms he made it clear to NATO that its members could not simultaneously be serving the needs of both sex voyeurs and a responsible community enterprise:

> *I told the chief executive of [Loews] that if other large, responsible theater operators decide to play this kind of film, then we are going to be witness to the death of quality exhibition in this country. The theater cannot have it both ways. The theater cannot be half quality and half smut. . . .*
>
> *If there is a proliferation of the quasi-porn film playing in first-class houses to the exclusion of product of wider appeal, we are in trouble.[44]*

Following Valenti's tirade, Tonlyn Productions, the independent distributor of *Without a Stitch*, filed a $30-million damage suit against the MPAA. The company claimed that Paramount head, Charles G. Bludhorn, told Loews that it would withhold its products from the chain if it continued to book X films from non-MPAA members. At the same time these bullying and perhaps illegal anticompetitive practices took place, 175 bills calling for film censorship or punitive actions against exhibitors were pending in state legislatures. Proposals ranged, for example, from official state film classification and bans on R and X trailers to taxes of five cents per G admission up to fifty cents per

X admission.[45] Although many of these bills were later found to be unconstitutional, they pointed to the X rating's growing association with bawdiness and pornography by many legislators around the country. This, in effect, convinced more NATO members to abandon its use.

Valenti's remarks to the U.S. House of Representatives and in *Variety* spelled out the MPAA's commercial strategy in the age of classification: only CARA-certified films rated R or lower should play in NATO theaters. Films officially rated X (with or without serious artistic pretensions) and especially those without an MPAA rating ("unrated") were greatly discouraged, since the outermost rating category and its unrated stepchild would always imply a violation of CARA's responsibility to the "standards of the larger society." The wedge driven between "quality" adults-only films and pornography, be they X or unrated, would forever distort the rating system, particularly for independent distributors. If they wanted access to the legitimate marketplace, they would have to play by the MPAA's rules under the MPAA's rating system in mainly NATO-owned theaters. In CARA's first few years many independents had rated their films X for surefire booking. But rapid changes in public acceptance and taste toward the adults-only rating and "soft-core" compelled them to work with, rather than against, the rating system. As a result, more and more independent distributors started to comply with CARA, submitting their products for classification so they could secure bookings in better, more lucrative, houses.

Like the Production Code, the rating system eventually became a gateway to the legitimate film marketplace: a code of production, distribution, and exhibition serving the major players in the industry. In 1972 domestic theater admissions rose roughly 20 percent over the previous year, primarily because of *The Godfather,* halting a seven-year slide, while total box-office revenues surged from $1 billion to $1.64 billion.[46] At the same time that Hollywood rediscovered how to make money, the R rating solidified itself as a marker of responsible entertainment in the New Hollywood.

The Incontestable R

In 1972 Valenti's repeated warnings to the MPAA signatories against producing and distributing soft-core films or irresponsible entertainment finally had an effect: Hollywood did not release any X-rated pictures that year.[47] The abandonment of the adults-only product line certainly had an effect on the industry's image. *Variety,* in its annual overview of CARA, noted that Hollywood's sudden shift away from X-rated material effectively helped to reduce public criticism of the standards for its other categories.[48] Obviously, the MPAA could never totally eliminate criticism of its members' practices, but acceding to CARA the authority to excise potentially problematic material from "serious" adults-only films to accommodate an R rating accomplished two important things: it gave the appearance that the film industry was responsible and ensured that Hollywood's products were available to audiences of all ages, R-rated guardian or no guardian. The development and maintenance of this practice created what I call the "Incontestable R," an aesthetic and discursive framework that guaranteed all R-rated films to Hollywood's audience as responsible entertainment.

Exhibitor cooperation was essential to the R's incontestability, and many NATO members, particularly small-city exhibitors, pledged their allegiance to the rating system and the abandonment of the X. Still, certain NATO members continued to exhibit soft- and hard-core films with MPAA X ratings or self-applied X ratings until the middle of 1973. During that time hard-core films like *Deep Throat, The Devil in Miss Jones,* and *Behind the Green Door* were quite successful in the marketplace, outgrossing many Hollywood films. What finally secured an industry-wide commitment to responsible entertainment were a series of obscenity rulings handed down on June 21, 1973, by the U.S. Supreme Court under the leadership of conservative chief justice Warren Burger, appointed by Richard Nixon in 1969.

In the two cases most relevant to the film industry—*Miller v. California* and *Paris Adult Theater I v. Slaton*—the Court reaffirmed that obscene material—defined as the depiction or description of hard-core sexual content—had no protection under the First Amendment. In the five-to-four *Miller v. California* opinion the Court rejected the idea of the Warren Court's national standard for defining obscenity, as well as its test for obscenity: "utterly without redeeming social value." Instead, it gave power to the states to determine what constitutes obscene material under local, rather than national, community standards. A specifically defined state offense, wrote the Court, would be "limited to works which taken as a whole, appeal to the prurient interest in sex, which portray sexual conduct in a patently offensive way, and which, taken as a whole, do not have serious literary, artistic, or political value."[49]

In *Paris Adult Theater I v. Slaton* the Court upheld (again five to four) the rights of states to regulate exhibition of obscene material to consenting adults, even those theaters with restrictive admission policies for minors. It also ruled that constitutional doctrines of privacy in the home did not protect obscene matter in public places like adult theaters. These reinterpretations of obscenity law in relation to the First Amendment elaborated on the standards given back to the states in *Miller v. California,* leaving content regulation open to prosecutors in individual communities.

Local and state authorities quickly took advantage of these rulings, seeing them as an opportunity to legally attack serious, artistic pictures given *Miller*'s vague guidelines of what constituted obscenity. Most notorious was a ruling by the Georgia Supreme Court declaring the R-rated *Carnal Knowledge* (1973) to be obscene, even though it only contained brief nudity, some salty language, and no hardcore—real or simulated—sexual conduct. The U.S. Supreme Court, however, in a unanimous decision in *Jenkins v. Georgia* in June 1974, argued that the film "did not depict sexual conduct in a patently offensive way" and made it clear that under the *Miller* standards obscene material had to be "hardcore" sexual conduct.[50] Despite this clarification, local district attorneys were already and would continue to be quite successful in winning legal injunctions against screenings of *Deep Throat* in various cities, such as Atlanta, Baltimore, and Memphis.[51] Injunctions such as these effectively sealed the fate for hard-core film exhibition and the X rating in all but a few selected urban markets.

Thanks to the U.S. Supreme Court, the MPAA had almost exclusive control over the legitimate theatrical marketplace. Previously uncooperative NATO exhibitors, now completely vulnerable to this new obscenity standard, had no choice but to acquiesce completely to the rating system, whose MPAA-member distributors by this time had given up on the X rating. For both the MPAA and NATO the R rating would prove to be an incontestable bulwark in the absence of the X, serving as a seal of approval for responsible entertainment in the classification era. The birth of the Incontestable R, in effect, was the death of the Hollywood X.

Despite the *Carnal Knowledge* victory, proponents of free expression—especially critics and filmmakers—were not happy with the results of the *Miller* ruling or the MPAA's response to it. A *New York Times* story in December 1973 echoed many disparagements directed at the MPAA during this time. Stephen Farber (who at that time regularly wrote articles about the rating system) and Estelle Changas (who interned with him at CARA) criticized the MPAA for its reluctance to openly challenge *Miller*'s supposed infringement of the First Amendment, its readiness to avoid adult material, and its willingness to trim films down from an X to an R rating. They described a series of projects that either had been cancelled or altered in light of the Court's decision. For example, a major distributor backed out of financing Arthur Hiller's film of Hubert Selby Jr's violent street novel *Last Exit to Brooklyn* (later made in 1989) because of its financial risk factor. Additionally, Universal vice president Ned Tanen, Columbia producer Larry Gordon, and director Robert Altman all had rejected or considered rejecting scripts containing potentially controversial elements. "I was just reading a script that has a sexual scene with a young man and a prostitute—a comic scene," Altman recounts. "And without *even* wanting to, I found myself thinking, 'This is going to be a problem. How am I going to do it? Is it really necessary, and should it be done in a very explicit, funny way? But if I do it that way, I don't know if it can be shown.'" For *Alice Doesn't Live Here Anymore* (1974) Martin Scorsese received a five page memo from Warner Bros. detailing strategies for rewriting dialogue and for protection shots in case of objection by CARA, local communities, or television stations. One admonition read: "Love scenes must show 'taste' and not show lovers." Such aesthetic and economic concessions to obscenity regulation, stated Farber and Changas, were "incompatible" with artistic freedom and according to Altman "actually spawned the acceptance of censorship" by the Hollywood community.[52]

Valenti's series of editorials and articles after the *Miller* decision clearly demonstrate the MPAA's position regarding accusations of censorship in the rating era. Valenti would articulate a realistic stance condemning governmental infringement on the First Amendment, except in cases of hardcore pornography, while categorically denying that classification was a form of censorship. In a same-day response to the Farber and Changas piece Valenti lamented the Court's decision on obscenity law ("We may curse it, defy, theorize it, but there it is. It won't go away."), but he called for action to assure that "serious, entertaining works of drama and comedy are not hauled into court" under an overly broad obscenity statute. He also assertively pronounced that the "MPAA rating board is not a censor," that "[it] does not command (nor could it if it tried) any filmmaker to edit one millimeter of film." Any decision to take a lesser rating to reach a larger audience, he believed, lies with the individual filmmaker, not with CARA, whose "sole objective is to give information to parents about the content of films so that parents can make decisions about their children's movie going." To Valenti industry self-regulation enabled creative expression, whereas the alternative—governmental classification—would quash it.[53]

If critics like Farber and Changas overestimate the power that CARA wielded in regulating X-rated MPAA films almost out of existence in 1973. Valenti underemphasized the role that he, the MPAA, and CARA play in shaping the Incontestable R practice. In the eyes of Valenti, and there is no reason to doubt this, the X rating was a legitimate category. "[It] does not mean 'obscene' or 'dirty,'" he frequently said. "X simply means unsuitable for viewing by children."[54] Valenti, though, never publicly condemned the industry's avoidance of the X rating or endorsed its practice of the Incontestable R. The fact remains that he, as the president of the MPAA and overseer of CARA, was paid by the major film distributors to protect their economic and political interests. If responsible entertainment is the standard by which this is safeguarded, and if it is not inclusive of the X rating, so be it.

The MPAA was never a trade organization to defend artists' rights or to ensure competitive markets anyway. The MPAA staved off classification for many years with an ineffective Production Code despite the awarding of First Amendment protection to motion pictures in the *Miracle* case. In addition, the MPAA also reintegrated distribution and exhibition through a collusive arrangement with NATO in the rating system twenty years after the *Paramount* decree. The abandonment of the X rating preserves this arrangement with CARA, its trusty knave of responsible entertainment. When Ralph Bakshi, director of the animated X-rated (though independently released) *Fritz the Cat* (1972) and *Human Traffic* (1973), claims he doesn't "know of a single director who hasn't been told not to make an X film," he expresses the view that it is not necessarily the muscle of CARA that dictates the rules but rather the might of the MPAA signatories.

With the MPAA's and NATO's virtual abandonment of the X by 1973, it became the primary responsibility of CARA's Rating Board to guarantee that all R-rated products—be they MPAA or independently distributed films—were free of X-rated residue before getting released in theaters. Some of the criticisms aimed at CARA during this time, however, were due to its inconsistent and unreliable policies for the X rating, as well as its other categories. Much blame has been assigned to chairperson Aaron Stern, a former rating consultant and psychiatrist on the faculty of Columbia University's College of Physicians and Surgeons, who replaced Eugene Dougherty as head of CARA in July 1970. In *Freedom and Entertainment* Stephen Vaughn characterized Stern as "too judgmental, intolerant of dissent, and eager to please the Catholic Church." Farber and Changas found him to be a "psychological crusader" against the "youth culture" of the time, handing out harsher ratings to movies if they contained "immaturity," "rebelliousness," or "liberal attitudes toward sex," Stern also seemed mesmerized by his power as chair, helping to edit films after their submission to CARA and frequently talking to the press about the rating system. It was this last point that particularly incensed Valenti, who wanted CARA to have only one voice: his own.[55]

Stern's interest in the educative potential of the cinematic form, however, did not translate into a similar protection of the economic and political interests of the MPAA, the rationale for CARA's existence in the first place. His public assaults against the X rating—against responsible entertainment—during his time in office must have been a major reason for his dismissal by Valenti at the end of 1973. In 1972, Stern told the *Los Angeles Herald Examiner* that "My strategy is to design a rating system in such a way that the only way you can have a more intrusive system is by defeating not only the constitutionality of the United States but the spirit of the government. If the rating system were called upon to defend itself as a noncensoring action, it could not defend itself. The fact that we keep somebody out of the theater is literally not defendable. I'm absolutely opposed to the X rating."[56] Unlike the U.S. Supreme Court, Stern believed children should not be denied access to films intended for adults, and unlike the MPAA signatories, Stern deplored the bargaining of shots or line of dialogue between producers and the Rating Board to get a particular rating. Given such comments, it is not surprising that Valenti later admitted he made a mistake in putting a behavioral psychiatrist in charge of CARA. "There were a lot of things we didn't agree on," Valenti said. "Nothing personal. It was his views on movies in general, demeanor, the ratings system, how he viewed certain things, the stance he was taking in the press, which was not consonant with the motives of the ratings system."[57]

To restore harmony in the rating system, Valenti replaced Stern with Rutgers University communication professor Richard Heffner in July 1974, who remained the chair of CARA until the end of June 1994. Heffner's personal disposition and approach to rating films could not be more different from his predecessor's. Under his administration ratings were assigned to films by a majority vote of the Rating Board, who based their decisions not on moral or psychological precepts but on contemporary parental attitudes toward film content. And unlike the PCA or CARA before it, Heffner's Rating Board did not assist in the editing of the films themselves; that task fell on the shoulders of filmmakers and distributors. It would appear that Valenti had found in Heffner a loyal and obedient chairperson, especially since the two lasted twenty years together. Their relationship, however, was often marked by disagreement and animosity, particularly involving the appeals process. The history of the Incontestable R through 1994 can be viewed, I believe, as a history of Rating Board decisions and Appeals Board reversals, of parental surrogacy and studio favoritism, of Heffner and Valenti. When the X was at stake, these contentions sometimes damaged, but never fully toppled, the bastion of responsible entertainment.

Notes

1. Jon Lewis, *Hollywood v. Hard Core: How the Struggle over Censorship Saved the Modern Film Industry* (New York: NYU Press, 2000), 135.
2. MPAA, Personal Statement of Jack Valenti, President, Motion Picture Association of America, in Connection with Announcement of New National Voluntary Film Rating System, Oct. 7, 1968; Jack Valenti, "The Movie Rating System," *Daily Variety*, 42nd Anniversary Issue, Oct. 28, 1975; MPAA, The Voluntary Movie Rating System: How It Began, Its Purpose, the Public Reaction, 1991; MPAA, Voluntary Movie Rating System Celebrates 30 Years of Providing Information to America's Parents, press release, Oct. 27, 1998.
3. Valenti, "The Movie Rating System."
4. Bruce A. Austin, "Making Sense of Movie Rating Statistics," *Box Office*, Oct. 1991, 45.
5. Charles Champlin, "What Will H. Hays Begat: Fifty Years of the Production Code," *American Film* 6, no. 1 (Oct. 1990): 42–46, 86, 88.
6. Stephen Vaughn, *Freedom and Entertainment: Rating the Movies in an Age of New Media* (Cambridge, UK: Cambridge University Press, 2006), 29.
7. Albert E. Van Schmus, interview by Barbara Hall, Academy of Motion Picture Arts and Sciences Oral History Program (1992), 102.
8. Quoted in "Movies—G, M, R, X," *Newsweek*, Oct. 21, 1968, 98.
9. MPAA, *Motion Picture Production Code and Rating Program: A System of Self-Regulation*, Motion Picture Association of America, 1968 (my emphasis).
10. MPAA, Personal Statement of Jack Valenti (my emphasis).
11. Quoted in Kim Masters, "Rating Game," *Premiere* (U.S.), Sep. 1988, 64.

12. *Movie Ratings and the Independent Producer: Hearings before the Subcommittee on Special Small Business Problems of the Committee on Small Business*, 95th Cong., 1st sess. March 24, April 14, May 12, June 15, and July 21, 1977. H. Rep. 90–916, 3–4.
13. The International Film Importers and Distributors of America was a less-powerful and now defunct trade organization, going out of service in 1978. According to the IFIDA Film Directory, 1968–1969, its members included Adelphia Pictures, Allied Artists, American International Pictures, Avco Embassy, Cinemation, Distribix, Grove Press, Janus, Joseph Burstyn, Sherpix, and Silverstein International, to name a few.
14. MPAA, *Motion Picture Production Code and Rating Program* (my emphasis).
15. Lewis, *Hollywood v. Hard Core*, 153.
16. Justin Wyatt, "The Stigma of the X: Adult Cinema and the Institution of the MPAA Ratings System." in *Controlling Hollywood: Censorship and Regulation in the Studio Era*, ed. Matthew Bernstein (New Brunswick, NJ: Rutgers University Press, 1999), 250–251.
17. Jack Valenti, "The Movie Rating System."
18. Wyatt, "The Stigma of the X," 241, quoting from Glenn Collins, "Film Ratings: Guidance or Censorship?" *New York Times,* April 9, 1990.
19. These statistics are not based on *Variety*'s rating tabulation that charts a year from November to October. These numbers are based on the actual year and come from "X-Rated Films, 1968–1973," *Hollywood Reporter,* 43rd Anniversary Edition, Nov. 1973. If we include Allied Artists and Avco Embassy, the smallest and short-lived of the MPAA signatories, who released a slate of legitimate and soft-core products, domestic and foreign, X-rated and otherwise, these statistics would look as follows: 1968: 4; 1969: 10; 1970: 11; 1971: 7; 1972: 1; and 1973: 2.
20. In 1970, only a year later, Paramount won an appeal against the X rating for *Medium Cool,* obtaining an R rating for the film.
21. Quoted in Vincent Canby, "For Better or Worse, Film Industry Begins Ratings," *New York Times,* Nov. 1, 1968.
22. "X Marks the Spot." *Newsweek,* Feb. 24, 1969, 101.
23. Bob Lardine, "Movie Industry Is on a Spot Marked X," *New York Sunday News,* July 20, 1969.
24. *Riot* eventually was awarded an M and was criticized for its mindless violence and homosexual candor.
25. "X Marks the Spot," 101.
26. Lewis, *Hollywood v. Hard Core,* 153. United Artists self-imposed the X on *Midnight Cowboy* rather than officially being awarded the rating from CARA.
27. Quotation ("By now"), in Stephen Farber, The *Movie Rating Game* (Washington, D.C.: Public Affairs Press, 1972), 49, 50–51, 66–67. At this time scripts were still vetted by CARA, just as in the days of the PCA, but only in regard to the rating that it may receive on completion of the film.
28. Quoted in Farber, *The Movie Rating Game,* 51.
29. A. D. Murphy, "$-Sign over MPAA Alphabet, Distribs Wanna Shun Risky 'R,'" *Variety,* Nov. 25, 1970, 5. Even though the M (later the GP then PG) category was frequently a site of contestation in the early years of CARA, I hardly believe that films of X caliber found their way into this rating. *Variety* does not provide any evidence for this assertion.
30. Wyatt, "The Stigma of the X," 244; Lewis, *Hollywood* v. *Hard Core,* 188. These statistics are drawn from data in *Variety,* which counts the MPAA calendar year as November to October since CARA was established on November 1, 1968.
31. See Julian C. Burroughs Jr., "X Plus 2: The MPAA Classification System during Its First Two Years," *Journal of the University Film Association* 23, no. 2 (1971): 53.
32. Aubrey quoted in Associated Press, "X-Rated Films Shunned," *Christian Science Monitor,* April 13, 1971; Fox source quoted in Jack Langguth, "Doctor X," *Saturday Review,* Dec. 2, 1972; Arkoff and Rugoff quoted in "Rating the Rating System," *Time,* May 31, 1971, 73.

33. Wyatt, "The Stigma of the X," 239.
34. Canby, "For Better or Worse."
35. "Film Rating System Announced: Four Ratings Geared to Protect Children," *NATO News*, Oct. 1968, 1, 4.
36. See Lardine, "Movie Industry Is on a Spot Marked X," 10.
37. See Vincent Canby, "Why Do They Laugh at 'G' Movies," *New York Times*, Nov. 2, 1969.
38. Charlie Poorman, "Survival Booking . . . in the Days of G, M, R, and X," *Motion Picture Herald*, July 16, 1969.
39. See "Young NATO Polls Theatres," *NATO News,* Dec. 1969, 8–9. Young NATO suspected that the percentage of theater owners avoiding X-rated films decreased since the time of survey.
40. Wyatt, "The Stigma of the X," 249–250.
41. " 'Protecting Public' vs. 'Censorship,' " *Variety,* Feb. 25, 1970, 7; "Newspaper Rating Problems Grow," *NATO News,* Sep. 1969, 13.
42. Burroughs, "X Plus 2," 48. Cited from *New York Times,* Nov. 28, 1969; Leonard Gross, "What's Blue at the Movies?" *Los Angeles Times West Magazine,* July 16, 1972, 20; Vincent Canby, "The Ratings Are Wrong," *New York Times,* June 4, 1972.
43. MPAA, *Statement by Jack Valenti, President, MPAA, before Subcommittee NO. 3 of the Committee on the Judiciary House of Representatives,* Jan. 28, 1970.
44. Quoted in Gene Arneel, "Valenti Raps Loew's 'Stitch' Booking; Can't Be Voyeur & Respectable Biz," *Variety,* Jan. 28, 1970, 4.
45. "Harris Sues MPAA, TOA, Par Alleging Conspiracy and 'Trade Libel' *vs.* 'Stitch,' " *Variety,* Feb. 11, 1970, 4. The suit also states that Paramount was upset that the $15-million *Paint Your Wagon* playing at Loew's State II was making much less money than the $1-million *Without a Stitch,* which shared the same building; "Clagett Tidying MPAA's New Bills; 39 Wanna Tax X," *Variety,* March 25, 1970, 5; Gene Arneel, "Censor Threats Haunt MPAA; Just Too Much, if Mostly Silly," *Variety,* March 18, 1970, 5.
46. Thomas Schatz, "The New Hollywood," in *Film Theory Goes to the Movies,* ed. Jim Collins, Hilary Radner, and Ava Preacher Collins (New York: Routledge, 1993), 16.
47. Again, I am not counting the smaller distributor, Avco Embassy, which released the relatively unknown exploitation film *A Place Called Today* with an X in 1972.
48. A. D. Murphy, "Code in Perspective over 4 Yrs.: Measure Indie Production Flood; U.S. Makers Seek G and PG Ratings," *Variety,* Nov. 8, 1972, 19. The trade paper also added that the possibility of a new adults-only rating to cover "quality" films had been severely undermined after Stanley Kubrick pulled *A Clockwork Orange* out of release in August for sixty days in order to qualify for a lower rating after cutting two scenes.
49. *Miller* v. *California,* 423 U.S. 15 (1973); *Paris Adult Theater I* v. *Slaton,* 423 U.S. 49 (1973). In *Miller* the Court did offer some examples of what a statute could regulate as obscenity: (a) patently offensive representations or descriptions of ultimate sexual acts, normal or perverted, actual or simulated; and (b) patently offensive representations or descriptions of masturbation, excretory functions, and lewd exhibition of the genitals.
50. *Jenkins v. Georgia,* 418 U.S. 153 (1973).
51. Lewis, *Hollywood v. Hard Core,* 262.
52. Stephen Farber and Estelle Changas, "What Has the Court Saved Us From?" *New York Times,* Dec. 9, 1973. See also, "Has the Supreme Court Saved Us from Obscenity?" *New York Times,* Aug. 5, 1973.
53. Jack Valenti, "To Rate a Film Is Not to Censor It," *New York Times,* Dec. 9, 1973. See also Jack Valenti, " 'Censorship Is Deadly,' " *New York Times,* Aug. 5, 1973; Jack Valenti, "Editorial," *New York Times,* Feb. 24, 1974.

54. Jack Valenti, "Ratings Are for Parents, Not Critics," *New York Times,* June 18, 1972.
55. Vaughn, *Freedom and Entertainment,* 32. Vaughn quotes from Farber and Changas, "Insiders Rate Film Code Board as 'Unreformed,'" *Los Angeles Times,* Aug. 8, 1971, Calendar sec.
56. Stern quoted in "The War between 'Censors' and Producers (Rated R)," *Los Angeles Herald Examiner,* July 16, 1972. Also see "Stern Quitting as Code Chief," *Daily Variety,* Dec. 3, 1973; Will Tusher, "Stern to C.P.I.; Hunter Tops Brut; Netter Out," *Hollywood Reporter,* Dec. 3, 1973.
57. Robert Landry, "If You Make an X, Take an X," *Variety,* Sep. 9, 1970, 1, 24; Valenti quoted in Moira Hodgson, "Movie Ratings—Do They Serve Hollywood or the Public?" *New York Times,* May 24, 1981.

LESSON TWELVE

Auteur Renaissance

"*The Last Good Time We Ever Had*": Remembering the New Hollywood Cinema

Noel King

That an aesthetically experimental socially conscious cinema d'auteur *could exist simultaneously with a burgeoning and rapacious blockbuster mentality was extraordinary, but it became the defining mark of 1970s cinema. That the two could co-exist for long, however, was an illusion as ephemeral as the notion of liberal ideological consensus.*[1]

Who the hell is talking to you like this? How OLD is he? The author is 52 and he loved the decade of the 1970s and its movies. We had movies then that you had to watch. *Many of them had unfamiliar shapes, new narrative structures or strategies. They began late. They switched course. And they did not end well or happily or comfortably. Sometimes they broke off in your hands, or your mind.*[2]

The economic disaster of 1970 produced a lot of official proclamations of change, but in the final analysis things didn't change very much. For all the successes of a few small films, it was finally the more predictable successes of big films and big stars that carried Hollywood bookkeeping back into the black. Now, more than ever before, Hollywood is on the lookout for the "presold" project, the films that come with a formula for guaranteed success: films based on runaway best-sellers and hit plays, or films with stars who in themselves are so big that they generate their own publicity.[3]

I

In *A Confederate General at Big Sur,* Richard Brautigan refers to "the last good time this country ever had."[4] As we move into the twenty-first century, that phrase also captures the way we are invited to remember the period of New Hollywood Cinema, as a brief moment of cinematic aesthetic adventure that happened between the mid-1960s and the mid to late 1970s and then vanished. In his recent history of this period, *Lost Illusions,* David Cook sees the years from 1969 to 1975 as an "aberration" (pxvii), a "richly fruitful detour in the American cinema's march towards gigantism and global domination," (p. xvii) as the franchise triumphs over the notion of the individual film. And in his review of the most recent edition of Robert Kolker's *A Cinema of Loneliness,* Jon Lewis, one of the most prominent of contemporary historians of contemporary Hollywood, refers to "this wonderful and brief moment" of New Hollywood.[5]

Of course any notion of a "New Hollywood" will always be a discursive construction of a particular kind. Different critical accounts seek to describe changes in Hollywood filmmaking in the period from the 1960s to the present, and although these acts of criticism target an agreed period of Hollywood film history they make different claims for what is significant about that period. The result is that "New Hollywood" does not remain the same object across its different critical descriptions. We encounter a series of competing accounts of "the new" in relation to "New Hollywood".[6]

But one strong strand of criticism sees "New Hollywood" as a brief window of opportunity running from the late 1960s to the early 1970s, when an adventurous new cinema emerged, linking the traditions of classical Hollywood genre filmmaking with the stylistic innovations of European art cinema. This concept of "the new" is predicated on a new audience demographic making its aesthetic preferences felt by opting for a new kind of cinema, alliteratively described by Andrew Sarris as a cinema of "alienation, anomie, anarchy and absurdism".[7]

This account of "the new" is followed quickly by the arrival of the "movie brats," a film-school educated and/or film-critical generation who began making commercial American cinema with an élan that, for some, recalled the emergence of the "French New Wave". The 1960s saw Martin Scorsese graduate from NYU film school (as Jim Jarmusch, Susan Seidelman and Spike Lee would later), Brian De Palma attend Columbia and Sarah Lawrence while on the West Coast Francis Coppola, John Milius, Paul Schrader and George Lucas graduated from UCLA and USC. They were reading the 1960s American film criticism of Pauline Kael, Andrew Sarris and Manny Farber, absorbing the influence of *Cahiers du Cinéma* on Anglo-American film criticism, and admiring the films of Bergman, Fellini, Antonioni, Bertolucci, Truffaut and Godard. Accordingly, some accounts of New Hollywood see this moment as the explicit inscription within American filmmaking of the critical practice of auteurism, resulting in a self-consciously auteur cinema.[8]

Noel Carroll calls this period of American filmmaking a "cinema of allusion" and claims that a shared practice of allusionistic interplay is a distinguishing feature of the work of New Hollywood filmmakers.[9] By "allusion" Carroll means "a mixed lot of practices including quotations, the memorialisation of past genres, homages, and the recreation of 'classic' scenes, shots, plot motifs, lines of dialogue, themes, gestures, and so forth from film history, especially as that history was crystallized and codified in the sixties and early seventies."[10] Steve Neale's description of RAIDERS OF THE LOST ARK (1981) as a film which "uses an idea (the signs) of classical Hollywood in order to promote, integrate and display modern effects, techniques and production values" would support Carroll's view.[11] This notion of a "cinema of allusion" generated by references to other cinematic practices, mainly classical Hollywood cinema and European art cinema, was anticipated by Stuart Byron's claim that John Ford's THE SEARCHERS (1956) was the ur-text of this New Hollywood, a cult movie referred to in Scorsese's TAXI DRIVER (1976), Lucas' STAR WARS (1977), and Schrader's HARDCORE (1978).[12] Similarly, the three films that brought Peter Bogdanovich to prominence, THE LAST PICTURE SHOW (1971), WHAT'S UP DOC? (1972) and PAPER MOON (1973) were loving tributes to the cinema of Howard Hawks and John Ford (about whom he had made the AFI documentary, DIRECTED BY JOHN FORD), and to lapsed classical Hollywood genres such as madcap/screwball comedy. This New Hollywood practice of cinematic citation continued into the 1980s with Schrader's 1982 remake of Tourneur's 1942 horror classic, CAT PEOPLE and AMERICAN GIGOLO (1980) concluding with an homage to Bresson's PICKPOCKET (1959). Schrader also cites Bertolucci's THE CONFORMIST (1969) as a film "I've stolen from ... repeatedly," and says that Nic Roeg/Douglas Cammell's film PERFORMANCE (1970) "is very invigorating visually—if you ever need something to steal, that's a good one to check up".[13]

If we were to add TV as another element in the intertextual-nostalgia-memorialisation process, Carroll could be describing attempts in the 1990s to unify parent and child via a nostalgic cinematic recovery of TV memory: witness such films as THE FUGITIVE, THE FLINTSTONES, THE ADDAMS FAMILY, ADDAMS FAMILY VALUES, MAVERICK, THE BRADY BUNCH, THE BEVERLY HILLBILLIES, MISSION IMPOSSIBLE, THE AVENGERS and THE SAINT. Carroll also claims that this citational cinematic practice assumed a particular reading competence on the part of its cinéliterate audience, resulting in a two-tiered genre film that united a strong action through-line derived from classical Hollywood genres, with some of the more recondite, abstract aspects of European art cinema: "there was the genre film pure and simple, and there was also the art film in the genre film".[14]

Functioning alongside the "movie brat" film school and often overlapping with it was another film school: the Roger Corman exploitation world of AIP and New World Films. Corman's influence on the New Hollywood can scarcely be overestimated. From his time with AIP through to his establishing of New World Films, Corman provided opportunities for such directors as Scorsese, Coppola, Bogdanovich, Monte Hellman, James Cameron, John Sayles, Joe Dante, Jonathan Demme, Jonathan Kaplan, John Milius, Dennis Hopper, Ron Howard, Amy Jones and Stephanie Rothman; and for such actors as Jack Nicholson, Robert DeNiro, Bruce Dern, and Keith Carradine. Carroll credits Corman with having established the "two-tiered" film: "Increasingly Corman's cinema came to be built with the notion of two audiences in mind: special grace notes for insiders, appoggiatura for the cognoscenti, and a soaring, action-charged melody for the rest"[15] and a link with the "Old Hollywood" is apparent in the fact that both Carroll and Jim Hillier note that Corman's workers likened themselves to the "Hollywood professionals" of the studio era, specifically to Raoul Walsh.[16]

Writing a decade earlier than Carroll, Thomas Elsaesser had noted the emergence of a "new liberal cinema" in 1970s America and saw it as breaking away from the classical Hollywood fictional world in which the heroes were "psychologically or morally motivated: they had a case to investigate, a name to clear, a woman (or man) to love, a goal to reach", and moving towards cinematic fictions in which goal-orientation can only figure as nostalgic.[17] According to Elsaesser, 1970s American cinema saw the "affirmative-consequential model" of the classical Hollywood film replaced by a more open-ended, looser-structured narrative. As a result New Hollywood cinema displayed "a kind of malaise already frequently alluded to in relation to the European cinema—the fading confidence in being able to tell a story." But Elsaesser was also quick to say that the New Hollywood cinema achieved its innovations by "shifting and modifying traditional genres and themes, while never quite shedding their support".[18]

After the first two moments of the "New Hollywood"—the brief period of studio uncertainty that allowed experimentation in the early 1970 (under the alibi of the pursuit of the youth audience) and the time of the "movie brats"—the next distinctive moment of "New Hollywood" is one on which ALL critics agree: the period of Hollywood after 1975, after the release of Steven Spielberg's JAWS. David Denby says, "The movie business, perhaps American culture, has never recovered from that electric media weekend in June 1975 when JAWS opened all over the country and Hollywood realized a movie could gross nearly 48 million dollars in three days. Ever since, the only real prestige has come from having a runaway hit."[19] We now know that when JAWS opened at 464 cinemas and went on to become the biggest grossing film of all time (well, for two years, until George Lucas's STAR WARS came along and topped it) we entered the era of high concept and summer hits. As Hoberman puts it, JAWS's "presold property and media-blitz saturation release pattern heralded the rise of marketing men and 'high concept.'"[20] Justin Wyatt would then seem justified in claiming "high concept" as "perhaps *the* central development within post-classical cinema".[21]

Thomas Schatz sees the concentration on the blockbuster as an inglorious distinguishing feature of the New Hollywood period. In the classical Hollywood studio system, he says, "ultimately both blockbuster and B movie were ancillary to first-run feature production, which had always been the studios' strong suit and which the New Hollywood has proved utterly incapable of turning out with any quality or consistency."[22] The post-JAWS world, however, was one in which blockbuster films were conceived as "multi-purpose entertainment machines that breed music videos and soundtrack albums, TV series and videocassettes, video games and theme park rides, novelizations and comic books."[23] The media hype surrounding the theatrical release of films like BATMAN and JURASSIC PARK "creates a cultural commodity that might be regenerated in any number of media forms."[24]

The clarity of this third moment of change is conveyed by the brute commercial fact that post-1975 blockbusters have proved the most profitable films of all time. As Hoberman says, "Hollywood's ten top-grossing films have all been released since 1975. And even if one adjusts the figures to compensate for the dollar's reduced purchasing power, seven of the all-time blockbusters were still made between 1975 and 1985."[25] In *A Cinema Without Walls,* Timothy Corrigan ponders this new situation by looking back on the conglomerate take-overs of the majors in the 1960s and 1970s, the later pressures from video and cable television and the way the status of the blockbuster has come to figure in the corporate thinking of New Hollywood:

> *Far more than traditional epic successes or the occasional predecessor in film history, these contemporary blockbuster movies became the central imperative in an industry that sought the promise of massive profit from large financial investments; the acceptable return on these investments (anywhere from $20 million to $70 million) required, most significantly, that these films would attract not just a large market, but* all *the markets.*[26]

Many critics felt this form of cinema was achieved at the expense of a more meditative, adult cinema that had been present in the first two moments of the New Hollywood. Pauline Kael said that conglomerate control of the studios meant there was less chance for any unusual project to get financed, Andrew Sarris said "the battle was lost when Hollywood realized in 1970 that there was still a huge middle American audience for AIRPORT"[27] and, in a much-quoted phrase, James Monaco said, "Increasingly we are all going to see the same ten movies."[28] Monaco said that in 1979, and we would have to say that the number is now far fewer than ten. The phrase that came to characterize this emphasis in Hollywood's economic-aesthetic strategy was the "film event". As William Paul explains: "At the time of the release of EARTHQUAKE, Jennings Lang, its executive producer, wrote an article for *American Cinematographer* in which he proclaimed that a movie had to be an 'event' in order to succeed in today's market".[29]

But there are other ways in which the exceptional commercial success of films like STAR WARS, ET (1982) and RAIDERS OF THE LOST ARK indicates a change from the first two moments of New Hollywood. If we set aside questions concerning saturation release and merchandising opportunities, the first two moments saw an auteurist cinema explore and stretch genres such as the western (THE WILD BUNCH, MCCABE AND MS MILLER), the gangster film (THE GODFATHER and THE GODFATHER PART 2), and the detective-noir film (CHINATOWN, NIGHT MOVES, THE LONG GOODBYE). This laudable moment of thoughtful metafilmic exploration was then cast aside by the success of the late 1970s and 1980s films of Lucas and Spielberg, which marked a more calculatedly naive relation to classical genres. According to this view Lucas' AMERICAN GRAFFITI (1973) could be regarded as a transitional text. It was adventurous insofar as it took the then-unusual narrative step of basing its forty-five or so scenes around as many pop songs, achieving, through the labors of Walter Murch, an innovative sonic depth of field. But the film's great commercial success (made for less than $1 million and recouping $55 million) foreshadowed the mix of retro-nostalgia and middle-American populism that would be found in most of Lucas's and Spielberg's blockbuster films of the late 1970s and the 1980s. For Hoberman, the success of these films meant that, "as the seventies wore on, it became apparent that the overarching impulse was less an attempt to revise genres than to revive them."[30] Or, as Carroll said, "After the experimentation of the early seventies, genres have once again become Hollywood's bread and butter".[31]

II

Already by the 1990s, the New Hollywood period of 1967 to 1977 and its films had become a benchmark against which developments in contemporary Hollywood cinema could be measured, invoked either to confirm a continuing decline from a time of adventurous commercial cinema or to constitute the most appropriate analogy for any current instances of adventurous American cinema. An example of the latter position is apparent in Quentin Tarantino's 1991 linking of the two periods: "I think right now is the most exciting time in Hollywood since 1971. Because Hollywood is never more exciting than when you don't know,"[32] There are many examples of the former attitude of lament for an aesthetic decline in American cinema. This has been a persistent discourse from the late 1970s to the late 1990s, in articles by William Paul, Jim Hoberman, Pauline Kael, David Denby, Richard Schickel and David Thomson.[33] The choral lament has increased over the past years as industry practitioners and insiders start to endorse the nostalgic narrative first posited by film-cultural critics.

For example, when interviewed in the "Film School Generation" episode of the *American Cinema* TV series, *Variety* editor Peter Bart identified the early 1970s as the moment when "the interior dialogue in Hollywood studios was corrupted irrevocably".[34] Ever since, each film has become "an industry unto itself" as filmmaking becomes a matter of selling the film-as-franchise in "all of its little parts". Judging by two of his recent books, Bart has not changed those opinions. *The Gross: The Hits, The Flops—The Summer that Ate Hollywood* examines the production and reception of the major studio films made for the (northern hemisphere) summer of 1998 by targeting the specific stars, directors, and writers involved in blockbuster films like GODZILLA and ARMAGEDDON and in smaller films like THE TRUMAN SHOW and SOMETHING ABOUT MARY.[35] Bart is encouraged by the unexpected success of these last two films because it helps foster the (necessary) illusion that it is still possible for film-goers to make a hit out of a film that does not bring in big opening weekend dollars. It is always nice when film viewers do not behave as the carefully orchestrated, obedient demographic the Hollywood marketing machine wants them to be.

In *Who Killed Hollywood . . . and Put the Tarnish on Tinseltown?*—a collection of his *Variety* and *GQ* columns—Bart continues his critique of contemporary Hollywood by offering sardonic observations on various filmmaking personnel.[36] Across a series of short chapters on "suits," "stars," "scribes", and "filmmakers", *Who Killed?* laments the influence of globalization on Hollywood filmmaking. Studios no longer are "seedbeds of popular culture" but are "mere appendages of vast multinational corporations grinding out 'content' for their global distribution mills", channeling "new product and ideas into theme-park rides, music, toys, videos, video game emporiums, and all the other ancillary goodies that enhance the revenue streams of their corporate parents."[37]

Bart contrasts the late 1990s context as seen from his position as editor of *Variety* to his moment as a participant in New Hollywood filmmaking in the early 1970s when he worked as a studio executive for Paramount, Lorimar, MGM/UA, and briefly as an independent producer. During this time Bart was involved with the production of such films as Coppola's THE GODFATHER, Hal Ashby's HAROLD AND MAUDE and BEING THERE, Polanski's ROSEMARY'S BABY, Ted Kotcheff's FUN WITH DICK AND JANE, Franklin Schaffner's ISLANDS IN THE STREAM. As an example of how economic-aesthetic decisions were arrived at in the New Hollywood era, Bart recalls his involvement in green-lighting HAROLD AND MAUDE, saying that it was discussed by a handful of executives who admitted they had no idea what it was about but felt they couldn't lose badly on a film that was costing $1.2 million, and so approved it. The film went on to turn "a handsome profit"[38] and to have longevity as a cult object. The cult status of this film would later inspire Douglas Coupland's "Harolding in West Vancouver" chapter in his *Polaroids From the Dead*.[39]

As opposed to this form of decision-making, Bart says the contemporary situation is one in which "scores of executives" debate such things as: "will the movie play well in Europe and Asia? How strong is the video and DVD aftermarket? Will the subject matter attract marketing partners like McDonald's? Will there be tie-ins for toys and other merchandising opportunities? Could the story line inspire a theme-park ride? Could the narrative be captured in a brief TV commercial? Will the star be willing to travel to openings around the world? If the budget is north of $60 million, is co-financing money available? Can the producers fund a completion guarantor who will intercede if overages occur?"[40]

Bart can see no likelihood of a return to a more economically restrained form of Hollywood filmmaking: "Given the monumental resources of the multinational corporations, the demands of stars and star filmmakers will continue to escalate."[41] His lament is supported by one of the most revered screenwriters of the New Hollywood period. In a similarly titled collection, *The Big Picture: Who Killed Hollywood? and Other Essays,* William Goldman says, "Most of the studio guys I've met are really smart, but they don't care much about movies as movies. As slots, yes. As merchandising tie-ins,—oh my—yes. As theme-park rides, you betcha! And that's the problem. They are mostly ex-agents or business school types. They care about slots and profit and product and Burger King cross-promotions."[42] In 1983 Goldman had published *Adventures in the Screen Trade: A Personal View of Hollywood and Screenwriting* to considerable critical acclaim and very healthy sales. In it he offered "nobody knows anything" as the main rule for understanding Hollywood's strange ways of going about its business.[43] In his follow-up volume, *Which Lie Did I Tell?: More Adventures in The Screen Trade,* the anecdote that gives his book its title shows how little his attitudes have changed over the years, and, accordingly, how little some of Hollywood's business practices have altered in the seventeen years between the two *Screen Trade* books. Goldman is in a Las Vegas room with a producer he doesn't like. The producer is showing off, making lots of self-important telephone calls as Goldman reads *Sports Illustrated* to indicate his lack of interest in these conversations. Suddenly the producer asks him, *"which lie did I tell?"*[44] This is presented as one form of Hollywood lying, the mendacity of the money men. On the other hand, of course, there are the beautiful lies fabricated by under-appreciated storytellers-screenwriters (who can tell us this anecdote) and any other Hollywood worker (director, cinematographer) who recognizes the importance of a strong script. Goldman is nearing seventy, and *Which Lie* finds the celebrated New Hollywood screenwriter (who, after all, came to fame with his original screenplay for BUTCH CASSIDY AND THE SUNDANCE KID, a screenplay initially famous for the amount it fetched as much as for the story it told) honouring the classical scriptwriting of a man who worked a generation earlier. Ernest Lehman's eight-minute "cropdusting" sequence for Hitchcock's NORTH BY NORTHWEST is "one of the very best pieces of action adventure" Goldman celebrates—something that wouldn't be possible in the post-MTV world of Hollywood editing, which favours a "blizzard of cuts"—while also analyzing the filmmaking efforts of some of the hipper contemporary types, the brothers Coen (FARGO, THE BIG LEBOWSKI) and Farrelly (THERE'S SOMETHING ABOUT MARY).

III

Any description of the film-cultural world that came *after* the New Hollywood period discussed in this book can easily become a lament for a lapsed mode of being in the world with cinema: a time of movie-going before the predominance of malls and multiplexes, before brands and franchises, synergies, high concept and film as 'event,' a time when the act of going to see a film at a central city "movie palace" or a double-feature at a suburban cinema was the main event. The nostalgia (overt or implied) for this earlier time is implicit in the severity of the critique of a contemporary situation in which Hollywood film industry spokesman Jack Valenti can describe the release of a film as a "platform to other markets", where films are described as being more or less "toyetic" (and where "toyetic'" is regarded as a good thing to be), where watching GODZILLA is as much about "tacos and t-shirts" as it is about an imaginative encounter with a celluloid fiction in a movie theatre. It is a world in which, as Robert C. Allen so succinctly puts it, one's relation to the projecting of celluloid on a big screen jostles for space with a pyjama manufacturer's analysis of the Spielberg-produced animated film AN AMERICAN TALE: FIEVEL GOES WEST: "We think AMERICAN TALE will be strong in sizes 2–7."[45] From this perspective an earlier time in which we could conceive of the Hollywood studio film as a discrete textual object is replaced by an uglier cultural fact: the individual film as simply the first move in a wider game of media market exploitations. The more this cinematic cultural fall is noted, the more some writers worry about a decline in the standards of Hollywood storytelling as kinaesthetic affect overwhelms the earlier tradition of the 'literate script'. One description of this contemporary form of cinema comes in the script rewrite advice Renny Harlin handed to Joan Didion and John Gregory Dunne (on a film that didn't go forward with them as scriptwriters): "First act, better whammies. Second act, whammies mount up. Third act, all whammies."[46]

If many discussions of the mutations effected in Hollywood filmmaking in the 1970s exhibit a strong strain of romanticism and nostalgia, the question remains whether this nostalgia is historically justified. The David Thomson quotation which appears as my second epigraph openly admits to a nostalgic attitude, and Thomson repeats this position in a 1996 piece for *Esquire* by saying of the New Hollywood films: "I look back on the time of first seeing them as one of wonder, excitement, and passion. It was bracing to face such candid, eloquent dismay; enlightenment does not have to be optimistic or uplifting".[47] Citing the ending of Spielberg's THE SUGARLAND EXPRESS (in which the father is shot) he says, "that was the proper ending; in 1974 that's how American films ended. But Spielberg has never risked that tough an ending again. . . ."[48]

For Thomson, Rafelson's FIVE EASY PIECES (1970) and KING OF MARVIN GARDENS (1972), Ashby's THE LAST DETAIL (1973) and Polanski's CHINATOWN (1974)—all with Nicholson—constitute a major cinematic achievement in the history of post-1960s Hollywood cinema, representing a time when "the movies mattered" in a way they haven't since. This early 1970s moment becomes the aesthetic "path not taken". Thomson regrets the passing of that brief half-decade period of productive, innovative uncertainty that enabled a more philosophical, risky, and countercultural cinema. This exciting cultural moment is lost as mainstream genre filmmaking is re-established, often by the very young Turks who supposedly were moving away from traditional forms of cinema towards more "personal" films. In one of the paradoxes of the decade, the already existing practice of "blockbuster cinema" is taken by the movie brats to new levels of profitability.

As we consider changes in modes of distributing and encountering movies from the 1970s to now, it would be hard to better some of Allen's descriptions of this immense cultural shift: "The Happy Meal toy our kids demand *before* the film is released derives its value through its strange metonymic connection (in which the part *precedes* the whole) to a movie that commands our attention as a cinema event because it's already been figured as the inedible part of a Happy Meal."[49] Or, as Jonathan Rosenbaum says in his provocative book, *Movie Wars: How Hollywood and the Media Conspire to Limit What Films We Can See,* "When Disney holds all-day 'seminars' about Native American culture and animation techniques for grade school children in shopping malls as part of its campaign to promote POCAHONTAS, the point at which advertising ends and education begins (or vice-versa) is difficult to pinpoint."[50] Rosenbaum is discussing a cultural context in which it is no longer clear whether in watching a theatrical release of a film one is meant to think of the film as "a viewing experience" or "the central object in a marketing campaign".[51] Of course it is both—as he well knows since he reviews films for the *Chicago Reader*—but Rosenbaum, like many commentators, wants to claim that the latter fact deforms the former experience.

In one sense Rosenbaum's *Movie Wars* pursues a point Jean-Luc Godard made in 1982 when he and Pauline Kael debated "the economics of film criticism" (an encounter organized by and subsequently published in the Californian feminist film journal, *Camera Obscura,*): namely, that there is an obligation on the film critic to practise a form of cultural analysis that distances itself from the many circuits of publicity and advertising masquerading as cultural commentary (e.g. *Details* magazine, *Vanity Fair*'s "Hollywood issue").[52] Godard was referring to "Why are Movies so Bad?, or, the Numbers," an article Kael published in *The New Yorker* (June 23, 1980) which now seems one of the most influential formulations of the position that argues for a continuing decline in American cinema from the late 1970s.[53] Kael took a five-month break from writing her *New Yorker* column on movies to work for Warren Beatty and Paramount as an "executive consultant".[54] She then wrote a piece informed by her insider-knowledge of Hollywood studio film production practices of the late 1970s. Her article reveals its polemical opinion at the outset: "The movies have been so rank the last couple of years that when I see people lining up to buy tickets I sometimes think that the movies aren't drawing an audience—they're inheriting an audience." Kael delivers a familiar lapsarian narrative in which an earlier, foundational era of cinema was presided over by "vulgarian moguls" who were genuinely in touch with a notion of popular entertainment and were ready to face risks that those who replaced them—ex-agents, former TV executives, business school graduates—weren't prepared to take. As a result the quality of the standard studio product goes down. Kael found that the real power in the new, conglomerate Hollywood rested with the advertising and marketing people "who not only determine which movies get financed but which movies they are going to sell".[55] She has a nice description of how a script's status is evaluated in that early 1980s Hollywood: "To put it simply: A good script is a script to which Robert Redford will commit himself. A bad script is a script which Redford has turned down. A script that 'needs work' is a script about which Redford has yet to make up his mind"[56] It's a tribute to Redford's longevity as a star and to the unchanging ways of Hollywood's packaging of films that Kael's comment still stands; we would only have to add a few other names to go along with Redford's.

For Kael the two main enemies of good American cinema are television—the more cinema "televisionises" itself, the more it squanders its aesthetic obligation to perform specifically cinematic work on and with the image—and conglomeratisation: "Part of what has deranged American life in this past decade is the change in book publishing and in magazines and newspapers and in the movies as they have passed out of the control of those whose lives were bound up in them and into the control of conglomerates, financiers, and managers who treat them as ordinary commodities. This isn't a reversible process . . ." Indeed not. The recent memoirs contained in Andre Schiffrin's *The Business of Books: How the Conglomerates took Over Publishing and Changed the Way We Read* and some sections of Jason Epstein's *The Book Business* flesh out the consequences right now of the situation Kael is describing twenty years ago, and Rosenbaum's chapter, "Some Vagaries of Distribution" in *Movie Wars* updates the cinema situation in the US.[57]

For later critics, writing in the 1990s, the decline in quality of American cinema is also the result of the success of the VCR and levels of video rental and purchase. As Janet Wasko says, by 1990 this area of business outgrossed Hollywood theatrical release revenues by 10 billion dollars.[58] By 1996 that figure had risen to almost 12 billion. Writing in 1999, Robert C. Allen encountered an even more intensified version of this situation. Allen notes that in 1992 Disney's Buena Vista Division became the largest and most profitable "film" studio in Hollywood, and points out that Christmas 1998 was the first time the launching of a "video game drew more consumers than the highest grossing feature film. In the last six weeks of 1998 Nintendo's 'The Legend of Zelda: Ocarina of Time' produced $150 million in retail sales, compared with Disney's A Bug's Life, the highest grossing film of the season, which did $114 million."[59]

Hence the crisis for some ways of thinking about the privileged or simply preferred status of Hollywood celluloid and of a lapsed period of moviegoing. Since the 1980s Hollywood films have made far more money from the so-called "ancillary" (syndicated TV, cable, pay per view, etc.) markets than from their social circulation as theatrically released celluloid. Consequently we encounter a slight strangeness of relation between the term "ancillary" and its referent in the world of New Hollywood economics. For of course these ancillary markets are primary and central. Likewise, it seems perverse to refer to the merchandising/franchising elements of a film as an "aftermarket" when they determine much of the structure the film takes in the first place and when they are usually made available to film viewers before the theatrical release of the film.

Allen pushes the issues bound up with different modes of circulation and consumption of films to some kind of philosophical edge when he says, "The, shift that occurs [. . .]— from audience to markets, from film as celluloid experienced in a theatre to film as [film] plus so many other manifestations over so long a period of time—not only alters the logics by which films are made and marketed but alters what the film 'is' in an economic sense, and by extension, in both an ontological and epistemological sense as well." And since it is now the case that theatre owners make more money on "concessions" (the sales at the "candy bar," or "drinks and lollies" as some cultures would say) than on ticket sales, then, as Allen observes, "to theatre owners and managers the most important innovation in recent film exhibition history is not surround-sound or wide-screen but the cup holder."[60]

In the Kael-Godard "economics of film criticism" exchange, Godard said he had prepared for their conversation by reading an article by Kael called "Why is the movie so bad?" Godard then says it should be "the movies"—which in fact it is. He goes on to make many funny, perverse comments, and one of his main points is that, as a film critic, Kael must take responsibility for the state of US cinema. Kael tries to say that critics have little power against advertisers—much as Robert Hughes once responded to the claim that he was a powerful and influential art critic by saying that one might as readily speak of a "powerful beekeeper". If in the short-term Kael's article had the unusual outcome of setting the terms for a debate with one of the greatest of filmmakers, in the longer term it has generated a series of considerations of the health of American cinema. Every five or ten years a prominent film critic takes a sounding and finds that Kael's criticisms still have pertinence. So, when David Denby asked, in 1986, "Can the Movies be Saved?" he was repeating Kael's polemic, and he too attacked conglomerate control by saying, "they want the smash, they're not interested in the modest profit".[61]

IV

In apparent deference to the notion of a "New Hollywood cinema" post 1970s American film sometimes is described as "New New Hollywood." The phrase was used as early as 1978 by David Colker and Jack Virrell in their article on "The *New* New Hollywood," in the Canadian journal, *Take One*.[62] In order to set the ground for their series of interviews with Badham, Kagan, Kleiser, Landis, Weill and Zemeckis/Gale, they said that Coppola "might as well be George Cukor, or Otto Preminger, for that matter." The durability of the category is shown by the fact that an account of contemporary Hollywood filmmaking in October 1995 in *GQ* magazine retains the phrase, "the 'new' Hollywood".[63]

The difficulty in deciding how to remember the period of New Hollywood cinema is indicated by the fact that David Thomson can recall 1970s American cinema as "the decade when movies mattered" while also seeing that decade of film production as one which ushered in "a terrifying spiral . . . whereby fewer films were made, most of them cost more, and a fraction were profitable."[64] Bernardo Bertolucci said of post New Hollywood cinema, "how can an audience desire films if the films themselves do not desire an audience?"[65] In the current context of this collection of writing on New Hollywood cinema we could rephrase Bertolucci's point to say that the film that wants to attract *every* viewer is not the kind of film that is being written about favourably in this book. In a recent piece, Jon Lewis points out that, "as the importance of foreign markets increased, Japanese, French, Australian, Canadian and Italian companies, at one time or another during the decade (the 1990s) took control of a major 'American' film studio. By decade's end the term 'American film' had become relative, perhaps even obsolete."[66] Perhaps this can help (this reader, at least) focus on what to some extent be an exercise in nostalgia. The New Hollywood period might be the last good predominantly *American* time American cinema had. Of course Hollywood has always imported international talent, but the New Hollywood fictions, as Elsaesser's article makes clear, touch on deeply American themes and visions. In the wake of the current crop of internationally financed globalised narratives New Hollywood of the 1970s might represent the last time American cinema was a distinctive, national entity. And as we read the following contributions to our understanding of New Hollywood cinema, we can see that this golden period of filmmaking also challenged film criticism to find a critical language appropriate to New Hollywood's cinematic achievements. This collection of criticism abundantly and inventively meets that challenge. And so the nostalgia is doubled, and also shown to be both real and justified.

Notes

1. David A. Cook, *Lost Illusions: American Cinema in the Shadow of Watergate and Vietnam 1970–1979* (Berkeley: Univ. of California Press, 2002): xvii.
2. David Thomson "The Decade When Movies Mattered," originally *Movieline* (August 1993): 43.
3. William Paul "Hollywood Harakiri," *Film Comment* 13, 2 (1977): 62.
4. Richard Brautigan, *A Confederate General at Big Sur* (New York: Grove/Castle, 1964): 147.
5. Jon Lewis, review of Robert Kolker, *A Cinema of Loneliness: Penn, Stone, Kubrick, Scorsese, Spielberg, Altman (Third Edition)*, in *Scope: An Online Journal of Film Studies* (August 2002) at http://www.nottingham.ac.uk/film/journal/bookrev/booksaugust-02.htm
6. The following argument condenses points made in Noel King, "New Hollywood," in Pam Cook and Mieke Bernink, ed., *The Cinema Book 2nd Edition* (London: BFI, 1999): 98–106.
7. Andrew Sarris, "After THE GRADUATE," *American Film* 3, 9 (1978): 37.
8. James Bernardoni, *The New Hollywood: What the Movies Did with the New Freedom of the Seventies* (Jefferson, N.C.: McFarland and Co, 1991): 8.
9. Noel Carroll, "The Future of Allusion: Hollywood in the Seventies (and Beyond)," *October* 20 (1982): 51–78.
10. Ibid. 56.

11. Steve Neale, "Hollywood Comer," *Framework* 18 (1981): 32.
12. Stuart Byron, *"The Searchers:* Cult Movie of the New Hollywood," *New York Magazine* (March 5,1979): 45–48.
13. Paul Schrader, in Kevin Jackson, ed., *Schrader on Schrader & Other Writings* (London: Faber and Faber, 1990): 210–211.
14. Carroll, 56.
15. Carroll, 74.
16. Jim Hillier, *The New Hollywood* (London: Studio Vista, 1992): 47.
17. Thomas Elsaesser, "The Pathos of Failure," originally published in *Monogram 6* (1975): 13–19.
18. Elsaesser, 14.
19. David Denby, "Can the Movies Be Saved?," *New York Magazine* 19, 28 (1986): 30.
20. J. Hoberman, "Ten Years that Shook the World," *American Film* 10, 8 (1985): 36.
21. Justin Wyatt, *High Concept: Movies and Marketing in Hollywood* (Austin: Univ, of Texas Press, 1994): 8.
22. Thomas Schatz, *The Genius of the System: Hollywood Filmmaking in the Studio Era* (New York: Pantheon, 1988): 492.
23. Schatz, "The New Hollywood," in Jim Collins, et al. (eds.), *Film Theory Goes to the Movies* (London: Routledge, 1993): 9–10. For more recent writing on the blockbuster, see Larry Cross, "Big and Loud," *Sight and Sound* 5, 8 (August, 1995): 6–10; Thomas Elsaesser, "The Blockbuster: Everything Connects, but Not Everything Goes," in Jon Lewis, ed., *The End of Cinema As We Know It: American Cinema in the Nineties* (New York: NYU Press, 2001): 11–22; Sheldon Hall, "Tall Features: The Genealogy of the Modern Blockbuster," in Steve Neale, ed., *Genre and Contemporary Hollywood* (London: BFI, 20(2): 11–26.
24. Schatz, "The New Hollywood", 29.
25. Hoberman, "Ten Years", 58.
26. Timothy Corrigan, *A Cinema Without Walls: Movies and Culture After Vietnam* (London: Routledge, 1991): 12.
27. Sarris, "After The Graduate", 37.
28. James Monaco, *American Film Now: The People, The Power, The Money, The Movies* (New York: OUP, 1979): 393
29. Paul, "Hollywood Harakiri", 59.
30. Hoberman, "Ten Years", 38.
31. Carroll, 56.
32. Quentin Tarantino, in Mim Udovich, "Tarantino and Juliette," *Details* (February, 1996): 117.
33. Apart from the articles already cited in this essay, see Richard Schickel, "The Crisis in Movie Narrative," *Gannett Center Journal* 3 (1989): 1–15; David Denby, "The Moviegoers," *The New Yorker* (April 6,1998): 94–101; David Thomson, "Who Killed the Movies?" *Esquire* (December 1996): 56-63.
34. Bart is interviewed in the "The Film School Generation" episode of the *American Cinema* TV series (Annenberg/CPB Project: 1995: 60 mins).
35. Peter Bart, The Gross: The Hits, The Flops—The Summer that Ate Hollywood (New York: St Martin's Press, 1999).
36. Peter Bart, Who Killed Hollywood?... And Put the Tarnish on Tinseltown? (Los Angeles: Renaissance Books, 1999).
37. Ibid., 17.
38. Ibid., 19.

39. Douglas Coupland, "Harolding in West Vancouver," in his *Polaroids From the Dead* (London: Flamingo, 1996): 101–106.
40. Bart, *Who Killed Hollywood?:* 19–20.
41. Ibid., 22.
42. William Goldman, *The Big Picture: Who Killed Hollywood? and Other Essays* (New York: Applause, 2000): 210–211.
43. Goldman, *Adventures in the Screen Trade: A Personal View of Hollywood and Screenwriting* (New York: Warner Books, 1983).
44. *Which Lie Did I Tell?: More Adventures in The Screen Trade* (New York: Vintage. 2001): x.
45. Robert C. Allen, "The Movie on the Lunch-Box." Abbreviated version available as "Home Alone Together: Hollywood and the 'Family Film'," in Melvyn Stokes and Richard Maltby, ed., *Identifying Hollywood's Audiences: Cultural identity and the Movies* (London: BFI, 1999): 109–131
46. John Gregory Dunne, *Monster Living off the Big Screen* (New York: Vintage, 1997): 37.
47. David Thomson, "Who Killed the Movies"," *Esquire* (December, 1996): 56–63.
48. Ibid., 60.
49. Robert C. Allen, "The Movies on the Lunch-Box" (unpublished manuscript, 21).
50. Jonathan Rosenbaum, *Movie Wars: How Hollywood and the Media Conspire to Limit What Films We Can See* (Chicago: A Cappella, 2001): 10.
51. Ibid., 67.
52. Jean-Luc Godard and Pauline Kael, "The Economics of Film Criticism: A Debate," *Camera Obscura* 8-9-10 (1982): 174–175.
53. Pauline Kael, "Why Are Movies So Bad? or, The Numbers," in Kael, *Taking It All In* (New York: Holt, Rinehart and Winston, 1984): 8–20. The article originally appeared in *The New Yorker* (June 2 1980).
54. See Pat Aufderheide, "Pauline Kael on the New Hollywood," In *These Times* (7–13 May 1980): 12, 23. Reprinted in *Conversations with Pauline Kael*, 41–49.
55. Jean-Luc Godard and Pauline Kael, "The Economics of Film Criticism: A Debate," *Camera Obscura* 8-9-10 (1982): 174–175. Also available in Will Brantley, ed., *Conversations with Pauline Kael* (Jackson: Univ. of Mississippi, 1995): 55–74.
56. Kael, "Why Are Movies So Bad? or, The Numbers": 16.
57. Andre Schiffrin, *The Business of Books: How the Conglomerates took Over Publishing and Changed the Way We Read* (London: Verso, 2001); Jason Epstein, *Book Business: Publishing: Past, Present, and Future* (New York: W. W. Norton & Co, 2001). Jonathan Rosenbaum, "Some Vagaries of Distribution," in his *Movie Wars: How Hollywood and the Media Conspire to Limit What Films We can See* (Chicago: A Cappella, 2001): 39–48.
58. Janet Wasko, *Hollywood in the Information Age* (London: Polity Press, 1994): 114.
59. Robert C. Allen, "The Movies on the Lunch Box": 5, 11.
60. Ibid., 12. See also Thomas Elsaesser, "The Blockbuster: Everything Connects, but not Everything Goes": 14.
61. David Denby, "Can the Movies be Saved?": 34.
62. See Axel Madsen, *The New Hollywood: American Movies in the 70s* (New York: Thomas Y. Crowell Co, 1975); Diane Jacobs, *Hollywood Renaissance: the New Generation of Filmmakers and Their Works* (New York: Delta, 1977/1980); Michael Pye and Lynda Myles, *The Movie Brats: How the Film Generation Took Over Hollywood* (New York: Holt, Rinehart and Winston, 1979); Thomas Schatz, *Old Hollywood/New Hollywood* (UMI Research Press, 1983); *Wide-Angle* 5,4 (1983) is a special issue on "The NEW Hollywood"; Jon Lewis, *Whom God Wishes to Destroy: Francis Coppola and the New Hollywood* (Durham and London: Duke UP,

1995), pp 143–164; David Colker and Jack Virrell, "The *New* New Hollywood," *Take One* 6,10 (August 1978): 19–23.

63. See *GQ* (October 1995), special issue called "The 'New' Hollywood."

64. David Thomson, "The Decade when Movies Mattered," *Movieline* (August 1993) 43–47, 90; David Thomson, *Overexposures: the Crisis in American Filmmaking* (New York: William Morrow & Co, 1981) 27.

65. Bernardo Bertolucci in Enzo Ungari, with Don Ranvaud, BERTOLUCCI ON BERTOLUCCI (London, Plexus, 187) 181.

66. Jon Lewis, "Introduction," to Jon Lewis, ed, *The End of Cinema as We Know It: American Film in the Nineties* (New York: NYU Press, 2001) 2–3.

Taxi Driver

Ian Christie and David Thompson interviewing Martin Scorsese

Brian De Palma introduced me to Paul Schrader. We made a pilgrimage out to see Manny Farber, the critic, in San Diego.[7] I wanted Paul to do a script of *The Gambler* by Dostoevsky for me. But Brian took Paul out for dinner, and they contrived it so that I couldn't find them. By the time I tracked them down, three hours later, they'd cooked up the idea of *Obsession*. But Brian told me that Paul had this script, *Taxi Driver*, that he didn't want to do or couldn't do at that time, and wondered if I'd be interested in reading it. So I read it and my friend read it and she said it was fantastic: we agreed that this was the kind of picture we should be making.

That year, 1974, De Niro was about to win the Academy Award for *The Godfather Part II*, Ellen Burstyn won the Award for *Alice Doesn't Live Here Anymore*, and Paul had sold *The Yakuza* to Warner Brothers, so it was all coming together. Michael and Julia Phillips, who owned the script, had won an Award for *The Sting* and figured there was enough power to get the film made, though in the end we barely raised the very low budget of $1.3 million. In fact, for a while we even thought of doing it on black and white videotape! Certainly we felt it would be a labour of love rather than any kind of commercial success—shoot very quickly in New York, finish it in Los Angeles, release it and then bounce back into *New York, New York*, on which we'd already begun pre-production. De Niro's schedule had to be rearranged anyway, because he was due to film *1900* with Bertolucci.

Much of *Taxi Driver* arose from my feeling that movies are really a kind of dream-state, or like taking dope. And the shock of walking out of the theatre into broad daylight can be terrifying. I watch movies all the time and I am also very bad at waking up. The film was like that for me—that sense of being almost awake. There's a shot in *Taxi Driver* where Travis Bickle is talking on the phone to Betsy and the camera tracks away from him down the long hallway and there's nobody there. That was the first shot I thought of in the film, and it was the last I filmed. I like it because I sensed that it added to the loneliness of the whole thing, but I guess you can see the hand behind the camera there.

The whole film is very much based on the impressions I have as a result of growing up in New York and living in the city. There's a shot where the camera is mounted on the hood of the taxi and it drives past the sign 'Fascination', which is just down from my office. It's that idea of being fascinated, of this avenging angel floating through the streets of the city, that represents all cities for me. Because of the low budget, the whole film was drawn out on storyboards, even down to medium close-ups of people talking, so that everything would connect. I had to create this dream-like quality in those drawings. Sometimes the character himself is on a dolly, so that we look over his shoulder as he moves towards another character, and for a split second the audience would wonder what was happening. The overall idea was to make it like a cross between a Gothic horror and the New York *Daily News*.

There is something about the summertime in New York that is extraordinary. We shot the film during a very hot summer and there's an atmosphere at night that's like a seeping kind of virus. You can smell it in the air and taste it in your mouth. It reminds me of the scene in *The Ten Commandments* portraying the killing of the first-born, where a cloud of green smoke seeps along the palace floor and touches the foot of a firstborn son, who falls dead. That's almost what it's like: a strange disease creeps along the streets of the city and, while we were shooting the film, we would slide along after it. Many times people threatened us and we had to take off quickly. One night, while we were shooting in the garment district, my father came out of work and walked by the set. The press of bodies on the pavement was so thick that, in the moment I turned away from the camera to talk to him, it was impossible to get back. That was typical.

As in my other films, there was some improvisation in *Taxi Driver*. The scene between De Niro and Cybill Shepherd in the coffee-shop is a good example. I didn't want the dialogue as it appeared in the script, so we improvised for about twelve minutes, then wrote it down and shot it. It was about three minutes in the end. Many of the best scenes, like the one in which De Niro says, 'Suck on this,' and blasts Keitel, were designed to be shot in one take. Although every shot in the picture had been drawn beforehand, with the difficulties we encountered, including losing four days of shooting because of rain, a lot of the stuff taken from the car had to be shot as documentary.

We looked at Hitchcock's *The Wrong Man* for the moves when Henry Fonda goes into the insurance office and the shifting points of view of the people behind the counter.[8] That was the kind of paranoia that I wanted to employ. And the way Francesco Rosi used black and white in *Salvatore Giuliano* was the way I wanted *Taxi Driver* to look in colour. We also studied Jack Hazan's *A Bigger Splash* for the head-on framing, such as the shot of the grocery store before Travis Bickle shoots the black guy.[9] Each sequence begins with a shot like that, so before any moves you're presented with an image like a painting.

I don't think there is any difference between fantasy and reality in the way these should be approached in a film. Of course, if you live that way you are clinically insane. But I can ignore the boundary on film. In *Taxi Driver* Travis Bickle lives it out, he goes right to the edge and explodes. When I read Paul's script, I realized that was exactly the way I felt, that we all have those feelings, so this was a way of embracing and admitting them, while saying I wasn't happy about them. When you live in a city, there's a constant sense that the buildings are getting old, things are breaking down, the bridges and the subway need repairing. At the same time society is in a state of decay; the police force are not doing their job in allowing prostitution on the streets, and who knows if they're feeding off it and making money out of it. So that sense of frustration goes in swings of the pendulum, only Travis thinks it's not going to swing back unless he does something about it. It was a way of exorcizing those feelings, and I have the impression that De Niro felt that too.

I never read any of Paul's source materials—I believe one was Arthur Bremer's diary. But I had read Dostoevsky's *Notes from Underground* some years before and I'd wanted to make a film of it; and *Taxi Driver* was the closest thing to it I'd come across. De Niro had tried his hand at scriptwriting on the subject of a political assassin, and he'd told me the story. We weren't very close at this time, I'd just worked with him on *Mean Streets*, but he read the script and said it was very similar to his idea, which he therefore might as well drop. So we all connected with this subject.

Travis really has the best of intentions; he believes he's doing right, just like St Paul. He wants to clean up life, clean up the mind, clean up the soul. He is very spiritual, but in a sense Charles Manson was spiritual, which doesn't mean that it's good. It's the power of the spirit on the wrong road. The key to the picture is the idea of being brave enough to admit having these feelings, and then act them out. I instinctively showed that the acting out was not the way to go, and this created even more ironic twists to what was going on.

It was crucial to Travis Bickle's character that he had experienced life and death around him every second he was in south-east Asia. That way it becomes more heightened when he comes back; the image of the street at night reflected in the dirty gutter becomes more threatening. I think that's something a guy going through a war, any war, would experience when he comes back to what is supposedly 'civilization'. He'd be more paranoid. I'll never forget a story my father told me about one of my uncles coming back from the Second World War and walking in the street. A car backfired and the guy just instinctively ran two blocks! So Travis Bickle was affected by Vietnam: it's held in him and then it explodes. And although at the end of the film he seems to be in control again, we give the impression that any second the time bomb might go off again.

It wasn't easy getting Bernard Herrmann to compose the music for *Taxi Driver*. He was a marvelous, but crotchety old man. I remember the first time I called him to do the picture. He said it was impossible, he was very busy, and then asked what it was called. I told him and he said, 'Oh, no, that's not my kind of picture title. No, no, no.' I said, 'Well, maybe we can meet and talk about it.' He said, 'No, I can't. What's it about?' So I described it and he said, 'No, no, no. I can't. Who's in it?' So I told him and he said, 'No, no, no. Well, I suppose we could have a quick talk.' Working with him was so satisfying that when he died, the night he had finished the score, on Christmas Eve in Los Angeles, I said there was no one who could come near him. You get to know what you like if you see enough films, and I thought his music would create the perfect atmosphere for *Taxi Driver*.

I was shocked by the way audiences took the violence. Previously I'd been surprised by audience reaction to *The Wild Bunch,* which I first saw in a Warner Brothers screening room with a friend and loved. But a week later I took some friends to see it in a theatre and it was as if the violence became an extension of the audience and vice versa. I don't think it was all approval, some of it must have been revulsion. I saw *Taxi Driver* once in a theatre, on the opening night, I think, and everyone was yelling and screaming at the shoot-out. When I made it, I didn't intend to have the audience react with that feeling, 'Yes, do it! Let's go out and kill.' The idea was to create a violent catharsis, so that they'd find themselves saying, 'Yes, kill'; and then afterwards realize, 'My God, no'—like some strange Californian therapy session. That was the instinct I went with, but it's scary to hear what happens with the audience.

All around the world people have told me this, even in China. I was there for a three-week seminar and there was a young Mongolian student who spoke some English following me around Peking; and he would talk about *Taxi Driver* all the time. He said, 'You know, I'm very lonely,' and I'd say, 'Yes, basically we all are.' Then he said, 'You dealt with loneliness very well,' and I thanked him. Then he'd come round again and ask me, 'What do I do with the loneliness?' He wasn't just weird, he was a film student who was really interested. I said, 'Very often I try to put it into the work.' So a few days later he came back and said, 'I tried putting it into the work, but it doesn't go away.' I replied, 'No, it doesn't go away, there's no magic cure.'

People related to the film very strongly in terms of loneliness. I never realized what that image on the poster did for the film—a shot of De Niro walking down the street with the line, 'In every city there's one man.' And we had thought that audiences would reject the film, feeling that it was too unpleasant and no one would want to see it!

I wanted the violence at the end to be as if Travis had to keep killing all these people in order to stop them once and for all. Paul saw it as a kind of Samurai 'death with honour'—that's why De Niro attempts suicide—and he felt that if he'd directed the scene, there would have been tons of blood all over the walls, a more surrealistic effect. What I wanted was a *Daily News* situation, the sort you read about every day: 'Three men killed by one man who saves young girl from them'. Bickle chooses to drive his taxi anywhere in the city, even the worst places, because it feeds his hate.

I was thinking about the John Wayne character in *The Searchers*. He doesn't say much, except 'That'll be the day' (from which Buddy Holly did the song). He doesn't belong anywhere, since he's just fought in a war he believed in and lost, but he has a great love within him that's been stamped out. He gets carried away, so that during the long search for the young girl, he kills more buffalo than necessary because it's less food for the Comanche—but, throughout, he's determined that they'll find her, as he says, 'as sure as the turning of the Earth'.

Paul was also very influenced by Robert Bresson's *Pickpocket*. I admire his films greatly, but I find them difficult to watch. In *Pickpocket* there's a wonderful sequence of the pickpockets removing wallets with their hands, a lot of movement in and out, and it's the same with Travis, alone in the room practicing with his guns. I felt he should talk to himself while doing this, and it was one of the last things we shot, in a disused building in one of the roughest and noisiest areas of New York. I didn't want it to be like other mirror sequences we'd seen, so while Bob kept saying, 'Are you talking to me?' I just kept telling him, 'Say it again.' I was on the floor wearing headphones and I could hear a lot of street noise, so I thought we wouldn't get anything, but the track came out just fine.

I was also very much influenced by a film called *Murder by Contract* (1958), directed by Irving Lerner, who worked on *New York, New York* as an editor and to whom the film was dedicated following his death. I saw *Murder by Contract* on the bottom half of a double bill with *The Journey,* and the neighborhood guys constantly talked about it. It had a piece of music that was like a theme, patterned rather like *The Third Man,* which came round and round again. But above all, it gave us an inside look into the mind of a man who kills for a living, and it was pretty frightening. I had even wanted to put a clip of it into *Mean Streets,* the sequence in a car when the main character describes what different sizes of bullet do to people, but the point had really been made. Of course, you find that scene done by me in *Taxi Driver.*

Notes

1. 'Slate' is normal slang for the clapperboard which is included in every shot for identification and bears at least the working title of the film.
2. Sam Fuller (b. 1911) was a juvenile crime reporter and country-wide traveller before he began writing pulp stories and film scripts in the mid-thirties. After distinguished service in the Second World War, he began to produce and direct his own scripts in 1949, with *I Shot Jesse James*. Other notable films include *The Steel Helmet* (1950), *Park Row* (1952), *Pickup on South Street* (1953), *Run of the Arrow* (1956), *Forty Guns* (1957), *Underworld USA* (1960) and *Shock Corridor* (1963). Described by Sarris as 'an authentic American primitive', Fuller has a graphic—if not tabloid—style, making much use of bizarre point-of-view shots, long identificatory tracks and energetic cross-cutting.
3. *Park Row* (1952) was Fuller's very personal tribute to the spirit of the early American newspaper business, for which he built a lavish studio replica of New York's 'Fleet Street'. This film also features some of his most bravura tracking shots: for one which follows a running fight in and out of many taverns he greased the seat of the operator's trousers so that he could slide smoothly along the bars!
4. A grip is the handyman on the film set, with such duties as laying tracks and moving heavy camera equipment.
5. Russell Metty (1906–78) worked with many major directors in a long career as cinematographer, including Hawks *(Bringing Up Baby)* and Welles *(The Stranger, A Touch of Evil)*. He also photographed Douglas Sirk's three great Technicolor melodramas: *Magnificent Obsession, Written on the Wind* and *Imitation of Life*.
6. William Cameron Menzies (1896–1957) was one of Hollywood's most respected art directors *(The Thief of Bagdad,* 1924) before he took up direction as well in the thirties. His most prestigious projects of the thirties were Korda's spectacular *Things to Come* (1936), which he directed and part-designed, and *Gone with the Wind* (1939) for which he was art director. But his later low-budget science fiction movies have a cult following especially *Invaders from Mars* (1953), in which both the adult world and a flying saucer invasion are seen from a child's point of view.
7. Manny Farber coined the phrase 'termite art' to cover the unselfconscious action cinema that he valued highly, alongside avant-garde work, as a critic working against the grain of respectability. One of the first to celebrate Fuller among other genre- and B-movie specialists, he is also a painter and teacher and has latterly given up writing criticism in favour of allusive 'movie paintings'.
8. Hitchcock's *The Wrong Man* (1956) has a rare documentary-style quality and sense of real New York locations amid his more flamboyantly theatrical works and is also one of his most overtly Catholic. An innocent man (Fonda) falsely accused of homicide is eventually vindicated after a religious experience in prison.
9. Jack Hazan's *A Bigger Splash* (1975) took its title from the painting by its subject, David Hockney. A kind of fantasy documentary on Hockney, his work and his life, the film's lush colour photography and precise, clean framing reflected the artworks which, on occasion, it reproduced exactly.

The Conglomerate Era

LESSON THIRTEEN

The Contemporary Hollywood Blockbuster

The New Hollywood

Thomas Schatz

Among the more curious and confounding terms in media studies is "the New Hollywood." In its broadest historical sense the term applies to the American cinema after World War II, when Hollywood's entrenched "studio system" collapsed and commercial television began to sweep the newly suburbanized national landscape. That marked the end of Hollywood's "classical" era of the 1920s, 1930s, and early 1940s, when movies were mass produced by a cartel of studios for a virtually guaranteed market. All that changed in the postwar decade, as motion pictures came to be produced and sold on a film-by-film basis and as "watching TV" rapidly replaced "going to the movies" as America's preferred ritual of habituated, mass-mediated narrative entertainment.[1]

Ensuing pronouncements of the "death of Hollywood" proved to be greatly exaggerated, however; the industry not only survived but flourished in a changing media marketplace. Among the more remarkable developments in recent media history, in fact, is the staying power of the major studios (Paramount, MGM, Warners, et al.) and of the movie itself—that is, the theatrically released feature film—in an increasingly vast and complex "entertainment industry." This is no small feat, considering the changes Hollywood has faced since the late 1940s. The industry adjusted to those changes, and in the process its ways of doing business and of making movies changed as well—and thus the difficulty in defining the New Hollywood, which has meant something different from one period of adjustment to another.

The key to Hollywood's survival and the one abiding aspect of its postwar transformation has been the steady rise of the movie blockbuster. In terms of budgets, production values, and market strategy, Hollywood has been increasingly hit-driven since the early 1950s. This marks a significant departure from the classical era, when the studios turned out a few "prestige" pictures each year and relished the occasional runaway box-office hit, but relied primarily on routine A-class features to generate revenues. The exceptional became the rule in postwar Hollywood, as the occasional hit gave way to the calculated blockbuster.

The most obvious measure of this blockbuster syndrome is box-office revenues, which have indeed surged over the past forty years.[2] In 1983, *Variety* commissioned a study of the industry's all-time commercial hits in "constant dollars"—that is, in figures adjusted for inflation—which placed only two films made before 1950, *Gone With the Wind* (1939) and *Snow White and the Seven Dwarfs* (1937), in the top 75.[3] In other words, of the 7,000 or so Hollywood features released before 1950, only two enjoyed the kind of success that has become routine since then—and particularly in the past two decades. According to *Variety*'s most recent (January, 1992) update of the all-time "film rental champs," 90 of the top 100 hits have been produced since 1970, and all of the top 20 since *Jaws* in 1975.[4]

The blockbuster syndrome went into high gear in the mid-1970s, despite (and in some ways because of) the concurrent emergence of competing media technologies and new delivery systems, notably pay-cable TV and home video (VCRs). This was the first period of sustained economic vitality and industry stability since the classical era. Thus this post-1975 era best warrants the term "the New Hollywood," and for essentially the same reasons associated the "classical" era. Both terms connote not only specific historical periods, but also characteristic qualities of the movie industry at the time—particularly its economic and institutional structure, its mode of production, and its system of narrative conventions.

This is not to say that the New Hollywood is as stable or well integrated as the classical Hollywood, however. As we will see, the government's postwar dismantling of the "vertically integrated" studio system ensured a more competitive movie marketplace, and a more fundamentally disintegrated industry as well. The marketplace became even more fragmented and uncertain with the emergence of TV and other media industries, and with the massive changes in lifestyle accompanying suburban migration and the related family/housing/baby boom. In one sense the mid-1970s ascent of the New Hollywood marks the studios' eventual coming-to-terms with an increasingly fragmented entertainment industry—with its demographics and target audiences, its diversified "multimedia" conglomerates, its global(ized) markets and new delivery systems. And equally fragmented, perhaps, are the movies themselves, especially the high-cost, high-tech, high-stakes blockbusters, those multi-purpose entertainment machines that breed music videos and soundtrack albums, TV series and videocassettes, video games and theme park rides, novelizations and comic books.

Hollywood's mid-1970s restabilization came after some thirty years of uncertainty and disarray. I would suggest, in fact, that the movie industry underwent three fairly distinct decade-long phases after the War—from 1946 to 1955, from 1956 to 1965, and from 1966 to 1975. These phases were distinguished by various developments both inside and outside the industry, and four in particular: the shift to independent motion picture production, the changing role of the studios, the emergence of commercial TV, and changes in American lifestyle and patterns of media consumption. The key markers in these phases were huge hits like *The Ten Commandments* in 1956, *The Sound of Music* in 1965, and *Jaws* in 1975 which redefined the nature, scope, and profit potential of the blockbuster movie, and which lay the foundation for the films and filmmaking practices of the New Hollywood.

To understand the New Hollywood, we need to chart these postwar phases and the concurrent emergence of the blockbuster syndrome in American filmmaking. Our ultimate focus, though, will be on the post-1975 New Hollywood and its complex interplay of economic, aesthetic, and technological forces. If recent studies of classical Hollywood have taught us anything, it is that we cannot consider either the filmmaking process or films themselves in isolation from their economic, technological, and industrial context. As we will see, this interplay of forces is in many ways even more complex in the New Hollywood, especially when blockbusters are involved. In today's media marketplace, it has become virtually impossible to identify or isolate the "text" itself, or to distinguish a film's aesthetic or narrative quality from its commercial imperatives. As Eileen Meehan suggests in a perceptive study of *Batman,* to analyze contemporary movies "we must be able to understand them as always and simultaneously text and commodity, intertext and product line."[5]

The goal of this essay is to situate that "understanding" historically, tracing the emergence and the complex workings of the New Hollywood. The emphasis throughout will be on the high-cost, high-tech, high-stakes productions that have driven the postwar movie industry—and that now drive the global multimedia marketplace at large. While one crucial dimension of the New Hollywood is the "space" that has been opened for independent and alternative cinema, the fact is that these mainstream hits are where stars, genres, and cinematic innovations invariably are established, where the "grammar" of cinema is most likely to be refined, and where the essential qualities of the medium—its popular and commercial character—are most evident. These blockbuster hits are, for better or worse, what the New Hollywood is about, and thus are the necessary starting point for any analysis of contemporary American cinema.

Hollywood in Transition

The year 1946 marked the culmination of a five-year "war boom" for Hollywood, with record revenues of over $1.5 billion and weekly ticket sales of 90 to 100 million.[6] The two biggest hits in 1946 were "major independent" productions: Sam Goldwyn's *The Best Years of Our Lives* and David O. Selznick's *Duel in the Sun.* Both returned $11.3 million in rentals, a huge sum at the time, and signaled important changes in the industry—though Selznick's *Duel* was the more telling of the two.[7] Like his *Gone With the Wind*, it was a prototype New Hollywood blockbuster: a "pre-sold" spectacle (based on a popular historical novel) with top stars, an excessive budget, a sprawling story, and state-of-the-art production values. Selznick himself termed *Duel* "an exercise in making a big-grossing film," gambling on a nationwide promotion-and-release campaign after weak sneak previews.[8] When the gamble paid off, he proclaimed it a "tremendous milestone in motion picture merchandising and exhibition."

That proved to be prophetic, given Hollywood's wholesale postwar transformation, which was actually well under way in 1946. The Justice Department's pursuit of Hollywood's major powers for antitrust practices began to show results in the courts that year, and culminated in the Supreme Court's May 1948 *Paramount* decree, which forced the major studios to divest their theater chains and to cease various tactics which had enabled them to control the market. Without the cash flow from their theaters and a guaranteed outlet for their product, the established studio system was effectively finished. The studios gradually fired their contract personnel and phased out active production, and began leasing their facilities for independent projects, generally providing co-financing and distribution as well. This shift to "one-film deals" also affected the established relations of power, with top talent (and their agents and attorneys) gaining more authority over production.[10]

The studios' new role as financing-and-distribution entities also jibed with other industry developments. The war boom had ended rather suddenly in 1947 as the economy slumped and, more importantly, as millions of couples married, settled down, and started families—many of them moving to the suburbs and away from urban centers, where movie business thrived. Declining attendance at home was complemented by a decline in international trade in 1947–1948, notably in the newly reopened European markets where "protectionist" policies were initiated to foster domestic production and to restrict the revenues that could be taken out of the country. This encouraged the studios to enter into co-financing and co-production deals overseas, which complemented the changing strategy at home and fueled the general postwar rise in motion picture imports as well as independent production.

Another crucial factor on the domestic front was, of course, television. Early on, the major studios had met the competition head on with efforts to differentiate movies from TV programs. There was a marked increase in historical spectacles, Westerns, and biblical epics, invariably designed for a global market and shot on location with international casts. These were enhanced by the increased use of Technicolor and by innovations in technology, notably widescreen formats and 3-D. These efforts soon began paying off despite TV's continued growth, as *Fortune's* Freeman Lincoln pointed out in a 1955 piece aptly titled, "The Comeback of the Movies." Lincoln noted that, traditionally, "any picture that topped $5 million worldwide was a smash hit," and he estimated that only about 100 Hollywood releases had ever reached that total. "In September, 1953, 20th Century-Fox released *The Robe*, which has since grossed better than $20 million around the world and is expected to surpass $30 million," wrote Lincoln, and pointed out that "in the 17 months since *The Robe* was turned loose nearly 30 pictures have grossed more than the previously magic $5 million."[11]

As Hollywood's blockbuster mentality took hold in 1955, the majors finally ventured into television. MGM, Warners, and Fox, taking a cue from Disney and the lesser Hollywood powers already involved in "telefilm" series production, began producing filmed series of their own in the Fall of 1955.[12] And late that year the majors also began to sell or lease their pre-1948 features to TV syndicators. In 1956 alone, some 3,000 feature films went into syndication; by 1958, all of the majors had unloaded hundreds of pre-1948 films.[13] In 1960, the studios and talent guilds agreed on residual payments for post-1948 films, leading to another wave of movie syndication and to Hollywood movies being scheduled in regular prime-time. Telefilm production was also on the rise in the late 1950s, as the studios relied increasingly on TV series to keep their facilities in constant operation, since more and more feature films were shot on location. The studios also had begun realizing sizable profits from the syndication of hit TV series, both as reruns in the U.S. and as first-run series abroad. As the studios upgraded series production and as the preferred programming format shifted from live video to telefilm—despite the introduction of videotape in 1957—the networks steadily shifted their production operations from New York to Los Angeles. By 1960 virtually all prime-time fictional series were produced on film in Hollywood, with the traditional studio powers dominating this trend.

Meanwhile the blockbuster mentality intensified. Lincoln had suggested in his 1955 *Fortune* piece, "The beauty of the big picture nowadays is, of course, that there seems to be no limit to what the box office return may be."[14] The ensuing decade bore this out with a vengeance, bracketed by two colossal hits: *The Ten Commandments* in 1956, with domestic rentals of $43 million (versus *The Robe's* $17.5 million), and *The Sound of Music* in 1965, with rentals of $79.9 million. Other top hits from the decade included similarly "big" all-star projects, most of them shot on location for an international market:

> *Around the World in 80 Days* (1956; $23 million in rentals)
> *The Bridge on the River Kwai* (1957; $17.2 million)
> *South Pacific* (1958; $17.5 million)
> *Ben-Hur* (1959; $36.5 million)
> *Lawrence of Arabia* (1962; $17.7 million)
> *The Longest Day* (1962; $17.6 million)
> *Cleopatra* (1963; $26 million)
> *Goldfinger* (1964; $23 million)
> *Thunderball* (1965; $28.5 million)
> *Dr. Zhivago* (1965; $46.5 million)

While these mega-hits dominated the high end of Hollywood's output, the studios looked for ways beyond TV series production to diversify their media interests. Besides the need to hedge their bets on high-stakes blockbusters, this impulse to diversify was a response to the postwar boom in entertainment and leisure activities, the increasing segmentation of media audiences in a period of general prosperity and population growth, and the sophisticated new advertising and marketing strategies used to measure and attract those audiences. MCA was the clear industry leader in terms of diversification, having expanded from a music booking and talent agency in the 1930s and 1940s into telefilm production and syndication in the 1950s, eventually buying Decca Records and then Universal Pictures in the early 1960s.

The 1950s and 1960s also saw diversified, segmented moviegoing trends, most of them keyed to the immense, emergent "youth market." With the baby boom generation reaching active consumer status and developing distinctive interests and tastes, there was a marked surge in drive-in moviegoing, itself a phenomenon directed associated with postwar suburbanization and the family boom. With the emergent youth market, drive-in viewing fare turned increasingly to low-budget "teen–pics" and "exploitation" films. The "art cinema" and foreign film movements also took off in the late 1950s and early 1960s, as neighborhood movie houses and campus film societies screened alternatives to mainstream Hollywood and as film courses began springing up on college campuses. These indicated a more "cine-literate" generation—with that literacy actually enhanced by TV, which had become a veritable archive of American film history.

While the exploitation and art cinema movements produced a few commercial hits—Hitchcock's *Psycho* and Fellini's *La Dolce Vita* in 1960, for instance—the box office was dominated well into the 1960s by much the same blockbuster mentality as in previous decades. Indeed, the biopics, historical and biblical epics, literary adaptations, and transplanted stage musicals of the 1950s and 1960s differed from the prestige pictures of the classical era only in their oversized budgets, casts, running times, and screen width. If the emergent youth culture and increasingly diversified media marketplace were danger signs, they were lost on the studios—particularly after the huge commercial success of two very traditional mainstream films in 1965, *The Sound of Music* and *Dr. Zhivago*.

Actually, Hollywood was on the verge of its worst economic slump since the War—fueled to a degree by those two 1965 hits, because they led to a cycle of expensive, heavily promoted commercial flops. Fox, for instance, went on a blockbuster musical binge in an effort to replicate its success with *The Sound of Music,* and the results were disastrous: losses of $11 million on *Dr. Dolittle* in 1967, $15 million on *Star!* in 1968, and $16 million in 1969 on *Hello Dolly,* at the time the most expensive film ever made.[15] Fox then tightened its belt, avoiding bankruptcy thanks to two relatively inexpensive, offbeat films: *Butch Cassidy and the Sundance Kid* (1969; $46 million in rentals), and *MASH* (1970; $36.7 million).

Those two hits were significant for a number of reasons besides the reversal of Fox's fortunes, reasons which signaled changes of aesthetic as well as economic direction in late-1960s Hollywood. With the blockbuster strategy stalled, the industry saw a period of widespread and unprecedented innovation, due largely to a new "generation" of Hollywood filmmakers like Robert Altman, Arthur Penn, Mike Nichols, and Bob Rafelson, who were turning out films that had as much in common with the European art cinema as with classical Hollywood. There was also a growing contingent of international auteurs—Bergman, Fellini, Trauffaut, Bertolucci, Polanski, Kubrick—who, in the wake of the 1966 success of Antonioni's *Blow-Up* and Claude Lelouch's *A Man and a Woman,* developed a quasi-independent rapport with Hollywood, making films for a Euro-American market and bringing art cinema into the mainstream.

Thus an "American film renaissance" of sorts was induced by a succession of big-budget flops and successful imports. Its key constituency was the American youth, by now the most dependable segment of regular moviegoers as attendance continued to fall despite the overall increase in population. Younger viewers contributed heavily to the success of sizable hits like *Bonnie and Clyde* (1967; rentals of $22.8 million), *2001: A Space Odyssey* (1968; $25.5 million), and *The Graduate* (1968; $43 million), and they were almost solely responsible for modest hits like *Easy Rider* (1969; $19 million) and *Woodstock* (1970; $16.4 million). As these films suggest, the older baby boomers were reaching critical mass as a target market and were something of a countercultural force as well, caught up in the antiwar movement, civil rights, the sexual revolution, and so on. And with the 1966 breakdown of Hollywood's Production Code and the emergence in 1968 of the new ratings system—itself a further indication of the segmented movie audiences—filmmakers were experimenting with more politically subversive, sexually explicit, and/or graphically violent material.

As one might suspect, Hollywood's cultivation of the youth market and penchant for innovation in the late 1960s and early 1970s scarcely indicated a favorable market climate. On the contrary, they reflected the studios' uncertainty and growing desperation. Film historian Tino Balio has written about "the Recession of 1969" and its aftermath, when "Hollywood nearly collapsed."[16] *Variety* at the time pegged combined industry losses for 1969–1971 at $600 million, and according to an economic study by Joseph Dominick, studio profits fell from an average of $64 million in the five-year span from 1964 to 1968, to $13 million from 1969 to 1973.[17] Market conditions rendered the studios ripe for takeover, and in fact a number of the studios were absorbed in post-1965 conglomerate wave. Paramount was taken over by Gulf & Western in 1966, United Artists by Transamerica in 1967, and Warner Bros. by Kinney National Services in 1969, the same year MGM was bought out by real-estate tycoon Kirk Kerkorian. This trend proved to be a mixed blessing for the studios. The cash-rich parent company relieved much of the financial pressures and spurred diversification, but the new owners knew little about the movie business and, as the market worsened, tended to view their Hollywood subsidiaries as troublesome tax write-offs.

One bright spot during this period was the surge in network prices paid for hit movies. Back in 1961, NBC had paid Fox an average of $180,000 for each feature shown on *Saturday Night at the Movies;* that year 45 features were broadcast in prime time. By 1970, the average price tag per feature was up to $800,000, with the networks spending $65 million on a total of 166 feature films. That total jumped to 227 for the 1971–1972 season, when movies comprised over one quarter of all prime-time programming. The average price went up as well, due largely to ABC's paying $50 million in the Summer of 1971 for a package of blockbusters, including $5 million for *Lawrence of Arabia,* $3 million for the 1970 hit, *Love Story,* and $2.5 million each for seven James Bond films.[18] Significantly enough, however, these big payoffs were going only to top Hollywood hits as all three networks began producing their own TV—movies. Hollywood features comprised only half of the movies shown on network TV in the 1971–1972 season, and that percentage declined further in subsequent years, as made-for-TV movie production increased.

The network payoff for top movie hits scarcely reversed the late-sixties downturn, as *The Graduate* in 1968 was the only release between 1965 and 1969 to surpass even $30 million in rentals. *Butch Cassidy, Airport,* and *Love Story* in 1969–1970 all earned $45 to $50 million, carrying much of the freight in those otherwise bleak economic years. *Airport* was especially important in that it generated a cycle of successful "disaster pictures" like *The Poseidon Adventure, The Towering Inferno,* and *Earthquake,* all solid performers in the $40 to $50 million range, though they were fairly expensive to produce and not quite the breakaway hits that the industry so desperately needed.

The first real sign of a reversal of the industry's sagging fortunes came with *The Godfather,* a 1972 Paramount release that returned over $86 million. *The Godfather* was that rarest of movies, a critical and commercial smash with widespread appeal, drawing art cinema connoisseurs and disaffected youth as well as mainstream moviegoers. Adapted from Mario Puzo's novel while it was still in galleys, the project was scarcely mounted as a surefire hit. Director Francis Ford Coppola was a debt-ridden film school product with far more success as a writer, and star Marlon Brando hadn't had a hit in over a decade. The huge sales of the novel, published while the film was in production, generated interest, as did well-publicized stories of problems on the set, cost overruns, and protests from Italian-American groups. By the time of its release, *The Godfather* had attained "event" status, and audiences responded to Coppola's stylish and highly stylized hybrid of the gangster genre and family melodrama. Like so many 1970s films, *The Godfather* had a strong nostalgic quality, invoking the male ethos and patriarchal order of a bygone era—and putting its three male co-stars, Al Pacino, James Caan, and Robert Duvall, on the industry map.

The Godfather also did well in the international market, thus spurring an upturn in the overseas as well as the domestic market. Domestic theater admissions in 1972 were up roughly 20 percent over 1971, reversing a 7-year slide, and total box-office revenues surged from the $1 billion range, where they had stagnated for several years, to $1.64 billion. While *The Godfather* alone accounted for nearly 10 percent of those gross proceeds, other films clearly were contributing; revenues for the top ten box-office hits of 1972 were up nearly 70 percent over the previous year. That momentum held through 1973 and then the market surged again in 1974, nearing the $2 billion mark—and thus finally surpassing Hollywood's postwar box-office peak. Key to the upturn were the now-predictable spate of disaster films, though these were far outdistanced by three hits which, in different ways, were sure signs of a changing industry.

One was *American Graffiti,* a surprise Summer 1973 hit written and directed by Coppola protégé George Lucas. A coming-of-age film with strong commercial tie-ins to both TV and rock music, the story's 1962 setting enabled Lucas to circumvent (or rather to predate) the current socio-political climate and broadened its appeal to older viewers. Two even bigger hits were late-1973 releases, *The Sting* and *The Exorcist* ($78 million and $86 million, respectively). *The Sting* was yet another nostalgia piece, a 1930s-era gangster/buddy/caper hybrid, reprising the Newman–Redford pairing of five years earlier—something like "Butch and Sundance meet the Godfather." The nostalgia and studied innocence of both *The Sting* and *American Graffiti* were hardly evident in *The Exorcist,* William Friedkin's kinetic, gut-wrenching, effects-laden exercise in screen violence and horror. While *Psycho* and *Rosemary's Baby* had proved that horror thrillers could attain hit status, *The Exorcist* pushed the logic and limits of the genre (and the viewer's capacity for masochistic pleasure) to new extremes, resulting in a truly monstrous hit and perhaps the clearest indication of the emergent New Hollywood.

Jaws and the New Hollywood

If any single film marked the arrival of the New Hollywood, it was *Jaws,* the Spielberg-directed thriller that recalibrated the profit potential of the Hollywood hit, and redefined its status as a marketable commodity and cultural phenomenon as well. The film brought an emphatic end to Hollywood's five-year recession, while ushering in an era of high-cost, high-tech, high-speed thrillers. *Jaws'* release also happened to coincide with developments both inside and outside the movie industry in the mid-1970s which, while having little or nothing to do with that particular film, were equally important to the emergent New Hollywood.

Jaws, like *Love Story, The Godfather, The Exorcist,* and several other recent hits, was presold via a current best-selling novel. And like *The Godfather,* movie rights to the novel were purchased before it was published, and publicity from the deal and from the subsequent production helped spur the initial book sales—of a reported 7.6 million copies before the film's release in this case—which in turn fueled public interest in the film.[19] The *Jaws* deal was packaged by International Creative Management (ICM), which represented author Peter Benchley and handled the sale of the movie rights. ICM also represented the producing team of Richard Zanuck and David Brown, whose recent hits included *Butch Cassidy* and *The Sting,* and who worked with ICM to put together the movie project with MCA/Universal and *wunderkind* director Steven Spielberg.[20]

Initially budgeted at $3.5 million, *Jaws* was expensive by contemporary standards (average production costs in 1975 were $2.5 million), but it was scarcely a big-ticket project in that age of $10 million musicals and $20 million disaster epics.[21] The budget did steadily escalate due to logistical problems and Spielberg's ever-expanding vision and confidence; in fact problems with the mechanical shark pushed the effects budget alone to over $3 million. The producers managed to parlay those problems into positive publicity, however, and continued to hype the film during postproduction. The movie was planned for a Summer 1975 release due to its subject matter, even though in those years most calculated hits were released during the Christmas holidays. Zanuck and Brown compensated by spending $2.5 million on promotion, much of it invested in a media blitz during the week before the film's 464-screen opening.[22]

The print campaign featured a poster depicting a huge shark rising through the water toward an unsuspecting swimmer, while the radio and TV ads exploited John Williams's now-famous "Jaws theme." The provocative poster art and Williams's pulsating, foreboding theme conveyed the essence of the film experience and worked their way into the national consciousness, setting new standards for motion picture promotion. With the public's appetite sufficiently whetted, *Jaws'* release set off a feeding frenzy as 25 million tickets were sold in the film's first 38 days of release. After this quick start, the shark proved to have "good legs" at the box office, running strong throughout the summer en route to a record $102.5 million in rentals in 1975. In the process, *Jaws* became a veritable subindustry unto itself via commercial tie-ins and merchandising ploys. But hype and promotion aside, *Jaws'* success ultimately centered on the appeal of the film itself; one enduring verity in the movie business is that, whatever the marketing efforts, only positive audience response and favorable word-of-mouth can propel a film to genuine hit status.

Jaws was essentially an action film and a thriller, of course, though it effectively melded various genres and story types. It tapped into the monster movie tradition with a revenge-of-nature subtext (like *King Kong, The Birds,* et al.), and in the film's latter stages the shark begins to take on supernatural, even Satanic, qualities à la *Rosemary's Baby* and *The Exorcist.* And given the fact that the initial victims are women and children, *Jaws* also had ties to the high-gore "slasher" film, which had been given considerable impetus a year earlier by *The Texas Chainsaw Massacre.* The seagoing chase in the latter half is also a buddy film and a male initiation story, with Brodie the cop, Hooper the scientist, and Quint the sea captain providing different strategies for dealing with the shark and different takes on male heroic behavior.

Technically, *Jaws* is an adept "chase film" that takes the viewer on an emotional roller coaster, first in awaiting the subsequent (and increasingly graphic) shark attacks, then in the actual pursuit of the shark. The narrative is precise and effectively paced, with each stage building to a climactic peak, then dissipating, then building again until the explosive finale. The performances, camera work, and editing are all crucial to this effect, as is John Williams's score. This was in fact the breakthrough film for Williams, the first in a run of huge hits that he scored (including *Star Wars, Close Encounters of the Third Kind, Raiders of the Lost Ark,* and *E.T.*) whose music is absolutely essential to the emotional impact of the film.

Many critics disparaged that impact, dismissing *Jaws* as an utterly mechanical (if technically flawless) exercise in viewer manipulation. James Monaco cites *Jaws* itself as the basis for the "Bruce aesthetic" (named after the film crew's pet name for the marauding robotic shark), whose ultimate cinematic effect is "visceral–mechanical rather than human." More exciting than interesting, more style than substance, *Jaws* and its myriad offspring, argues Monaco, are mere "machines of entertainment, precisely calculated to achieve their effect."[23] Others have argued, however, that *Jaws* is redeemed by several factors, notably the political critique in the film's first half, the essential humanity of Brodie, and the growing camaraderie of the three pursuers.

Critical debate aside, *Jaws* was a social, industrial, and economic phenomenon of the first order, a cinematic idea and cultural commodity whose time had come. In many ways, the film simply confirmed or consolidated various existing industry trends and practices. In terms of marketing, *Jaws'* nationwide release and concurrent ad campaign underscored the value of saturation booking and advertising, which placed increased importance on a film's box-office performance in its opening weeks of release. "Front-loading" the audience became a widespread marketing ploy, since it maximized a movie's event status while diminishing the potential damage done to weak pictures by negative reviews and poor word of mouth. *Jaws* also confirmed the viability of the "summer hit," indicating an adjustment in seasonal release tactics and a few other new moviegoing trends as well. One involved the composition and industry conceptualization of the youth market, which was shifting from the politically hip, cineliterate viewers of a few years earlier to even younger viewers with more conservative tastes and sensibilities. Demographically, this trend reflected the aging of the front-end baby boomers and the ascendance not only of their younger siblings but of their children as well—a new generation with time and spending money and a penchant for wandering suburban shopping malls and for repeated viewings of their favorite films.

This signaled a crucial shift in moviegoing and exhibition that accompanied the rise of the modern "shopping center." Until the mid-1970s, despite suburbanization and the rise of the drive-in, movie exhibition still was dominated by a select group of so-called "key run" bookings in major markets. According to Axel Madsen's 1975 study of the industry, over 60 percent of box-office revenues were generated by 1,000 key-run indoor theaters—out of a total of roughly 11,500 indoor and 3,500 outdoor theaters in the U.S.[24] Though Madsen scarcely saw it at the time, this was about to change dramatically. Between 1965 and 1970, the number of shopping malls in the U. S. increased from about 1,500 to 12,500; by 1980 the number would reach 22,500.[25] The number of indoor theaters, which had held remarkably steady from 1965 to 1974 at just over 10,000, began to increase sharply in 1975 and reached a total of 22,750 by 1990, due largely to the surge of mall-based "multi-plex" theaters.[26]

With the shifting market patterns and changing conception of youth culture, the mid-1970s also saw the rapid decline of the art cinema movement as a significant industry force. A number of films in 1974–1975 marked both the peak and, as it turned out, the waning of the Hollywood renaissance—Altman's *Nashville*, Penn's *Night Moves*, Polanski's *Chinatown*, and most notably perhaps, Coppola's *The Conversation*. The consummate American auteur and "godfather" to a generation of filmmakers, Coppola's own artistic bent and maverick filmmaking left him oddly out of step with the times. While Coppola was in the Philippines filming *Apocalypse Now*, a brilliant though self-indulgent, self-destructive venture of Wellesian proportions, his protégés Lucas and Spielberg were busy refining the New Hollywood's Bruce aesthetic (via *Star Wars* and *Close Encounters*), while replacing the director-as-author with a director-as-superstar ethos.

The emergence of star directors like Lucas and Spielberg evinced not only the growing salaries and leverage of top talent, but also the increasing influence of Hollywood's top agents and talent agencies. The kind of packaging done by ICM on *Jaws* was fast becoming the rule on high stakes projects, with ICM and another powerful agency, Creative Artists Associates (CAA), relying on aggressive packaging to compete with the venerable William Morris Agency. Interestingly enough, both ICM and CAA were created in 1974—ICM via merger and CAA by five young agents who bolted William Morris and, led by Michael Ovitz, set out to revamp the industry and upgrade the power and status of the agent-packager. For the most part they succeeded, and consequently top agents, most often from CAA or ICM, became even more important than studio executives in putting together movie projects. And not surprisingly, given this shift in the power structure, an increasing number of top studio executives after the mid-1970s came from the agency ranks.

Yet another significant mid-1970s industry trend was the elimination of tax loopholes and write-offs which had provided incentives for investors, especially those financing independent films. This cut down the number of innovative and offbeat films, although by now the critical mass of cinephiles and art cinema theaters was sufficient to sustain a vigorous alternative cinema. This conservative turn coincided with an upswing in defensive market tactics, notably an increase in sequels, series, reissues, and remakes. From 1964 to 1968, sequels and reissues combined accounted for just under five percent of all Hollywood releases. From 1974 to 1978, they comprised 17.5 percent. *Jaws,* for instance, was reissued in 1976 (as was *The Exorcist*), generating another $16 million in rentals, and in 1978 the first of several sequels, *Jaws 2,* was released, returning $49.3 million in rentals and clearly securing the Jaws "franchise."[27]

Another-crucial dimension of the New Hollywood's mid-1970s emergence was the relationship between cinema and television, which was redefined altogether by three distinct developments. The first involved TV advertising which, incredibly enough, had not been an important factor in movie marketing up to that time. A breakthrough of sorts occurred in 1974 with the reissue of a low-budget independent 1971 feature, *Billy Jack,* whose director and star, Tom Laughlin, successfully sued Warner Bros. for not sufficiently promoting the film on its initial release. For the 1974 reissue, according to *Variety,* "Laughlin compelled Warners to try what was then a revolutionary marketing tactic: 'Billy Jack' received massive amounts of tv advertising support, an unheard of practice at the time."[28] The film went on to earn $32.5 million in rentals, after generating only $4 million in its initial release. This tactic gained further credibility with the *Jaws* campaign and others, soon becoming standard practice and taking motion picture marketing into a new era.

A second crucial development grew out of the FCC's 1972 Report and Order on Cable Television and the 1975 launch of SATCOM I, which effectively ended the three-network stranglehold over commercial television.[29] Pay-cable services started slowly after the 1972 ruling, but the launching of America's first commercially available geo-stationary orbit satellite—and the August 1975 decision by Home Box Office (HBO) to go onto SATCOM—changed all that. HBO immediately became a truly nationwide "movie channel" and a key player in the ancillary movie market. Cable TV proved to be a boon to Hollywood in another way as well, thanks to the FCC's "Must Carry" and "Prime Time Access" rules which increased the demand for syndicated series and movies. That in turn sent syndication prices soaring, providing another windfall for those studios producing TV series.

An even more radical change in Hollywood's relationship with television came with the introduction in 1975 of Sony's Betamax videotape recorder, thus initiating the "home-video revolution." In 1977 Matsushita, the Japanese parent company of Pioneer, JVC, and other consumer electronics companies, introduced its "video home system" (VHS), setting off a battle for the home-video market. Matsushita's VHS format prevailed for several reasons: VHS was less expensive (though technically inferior), more flexible and efficient in off-the-air recording, and Matsushita was more savvy and aggressive in acquiring "software" (i.e., the rights to movie titles) as a means of pushing its hardware.[30]

While Hollywood's initial response to the "Japanese threat" was predictably (and characteristically) negative, it became increasingly evident that the key home-video commodity was the Hollywood film—and particularly the blockbuster hit with its vast multi-media potential. And there was plenty to drive these new media industries, as Hollywood's blockbuster mentality reestablished itself with a vengeance in 1977–1978. Total domestic grosses, which had reached $2 billion for the first time in 1975, surged to $2.65 billion in 1977 and $2.8 billion in 1978, a 40 percent climb in only three years, with hits like *Star Wars, Grease, Close Encounters, Superman,* and *Saturday Night Fever* doing record business. From *The Sound of Music* in 1965 through 1976, only seven pictures (including *Jaws*) had returned $50 million in rentals; in 1977–1978 nine films surpassed that mark.

While *Star Wars* was the top hit of the period, doing $127 million in rentals in 1977 and then another $38 million as a reissue in 1978, *Saturday Night Fever* was, in its own way, an equally significant and symptomatic New Hollywood blockbuster. The film did well at the box office ($74 million in rentals) and signaled both the erosion of various industry barriers and also the multimedia potential of movie hits. The film starred TV sitcom star John Travolta, the first of many "cross-over" stars of the late seventies and eighties. The Bee Gees soundtrack dominated the pop charts and album sales, and along with the film helped spur the "disco craze" in the club scene and recording industry. *Saturday Night Fever* also keyed the shift from the traditional Hollywood musical to the "music movie," a dominant eighties form, and was an obvious precursor to MTV.

In terms of story, *Saturday Night Fever* was yet another male coming-of-age film, centering on the Travolta character's quest for freedom, self expression, and the Big Time as a dancer on Broadway. The age-old male initiation rite had found new life in Hollywood with the success of *The Graduate* and the emergent youth market, and proved exceptionally well suited to changes in the industry and the marketplace during the 1970s. One measure of its adaptability and appeal was *Star Wars*, which charts Luke Skywalker's initiation into manhood in altogether different terms—though here too the coming-of-age story, while providing the spine of the film, is developed in remarkably superficial terms. Indeed, *Star Wars* is so fast-paced ("breathtaking," in movie ad-speak) and resolutely plot driven that character depth and development are scarcely on the narrative agenda.

This emphasis on plot over character marks a significant departure from classical Hollywood films, including *The Godfather* and even *Jaws*, wherein plot tended to emerge more organically as a function of the drives, desires, motivations, and goals of the central characters. In *Star Wars* and its myriad successors, however, particularly male action-adventure films, characters (even "the hero") are essentially plot functions. *The Godfather* and *Star Wars*, for example, are in many ways quite similar but ultimately very different kinds of stories. Like *Star Wars*, *The Godfather* is itself a male action film, a drama of succession, and a coming-of-age story centering on Michael's ascension to warrior status by fighting the "gang wars." Both films have a mythic dimension, and are in fact variations on the Arthurian legend. But where *Star Wars* is so obviously and inexorably plot-driven, *The Godfather* develops its story in terms of character—initially Don Corleone, then sons Sonny and Michael, and finally Michael alone—whose decisions and actions define the narrative trajectory of the film.

This is not to say that *Star Wars* does not "work" as a narrative, but that the way it works may indicate a shift in the nature of film narrative. From *The Godfather* to *Jaws* to *Star Wars*, we see films that are increasingly plot-driven, increasingly visceral, kinetic, and fast-paced, increasingly reliant on special effects, increasingly "fantastic" (and thus apolitical), and increasingly targeted at younger audiences. And significantly enough, the lack of complex characters or plot in *Star Wars* opens the film to other possibilities, notably its radical amalgamation of genre conventions and its elaborate play of cinematic references. The film, as J. Hoberman has said, "pioneered the genre pastiche—synthesizing a methology so soulless that its most human characters were a pair of robots."[31] The hell-bent narrative careens from one genre-coded episode to another—from Western to war film to vine-swinging adventure—and also effectively melds different styles and genres in individual sequences. The bar scene early on which introduces Han Solo's character, for instance, is an inspired amalgam of Western, film noir, hardboiled detective, and sci fi. Thus the seemingly one-dimensional characters and ruthlessly linear chase-film plotting are offset by a purposeful incoherence which actually "opens" the film to different readings (and readers), allowing for multiple interpretive strategies and thus broadening the potential audience appeal. This is reinforced by the film's oddly nostalgic quality, due mainly to its evocations of old movie serials and TV series (*Flash Gordon, Captain Video,* and so on), references that undoubtedly are lost on younger viewers but relished by their cineliterate parents and senior siblings.

Like *Jaws*, Lucas's space epic is a masterwork of narrative technique and film technology. It too features an excessive John Williams score and signature musical theme, and Lucas's general attention to sound and audio effects was as widely praised as the visuals. Indeed, while the film was shut out in its major Oscar nominations (best picture, director, and screenplay), it won Academy Awards for editing, art direction, costume design, visual effects, and musical score, along with a special achievement award for sound effects editing. And although *Star Wars* was the twenty-first feature to be released with a Dolby soundtrack, it was the first to induce theater owners to install Dolby sound systems.[32] There were countless commercial tie-ins, as well as a multi-billion dollar licensing and merchandising bonanza. And strictly as a movie franchise it had tremendous legs, as this inventory of its first decade well indicates:

May 1977 *Star Wars* released
July 1978 *Star Wars* reissue #1
May 1979 *Star Wars* reissue #2
May 1980 *Star Wars* sequel #1: *The Empire Strikes Back*
Apr 1981 *Star Wars* reissue #3
May 1982 *Star Wars* available on videocassette
Aug 1982 *Star Wars* reissue #4
Feb 1983 *Star Wars* appears on pay-cable TV
May 1983 *Star Wars* sequel #2: *Return of the Jedi*
Feb 1984 *Star Wars* on network TV
Mar 1985 *Star Wars* trilogy screened in 8 cities
Jan 1987 "Star Tours" opens at Disneyland[33]

The promise of *Jaws* was confirmed by *Star Wars,* the only other film at the time to surpass $100 million in rentals. *Star Wars* also secured Lucas's place with Spielberg as charter member of "Hollywood's delayed New Wave," as J. Hoberman put it, a group of brash young filmmakers (Brian DePalma, John Landis, Lawrence Kasdan, John Carpenter, et al.) steeped in movie lore whose "cult blockbusters" and genre hybrids elevated "the most vital and disreputable genres of their youth . . . to cosmic heights."[34] Perhaps inevitably, Lucas and Spielberg decide to join forces—a decision they made, as legend has it, while vacationing in Hawaii in May 1977, a week before the release of *Star Wars,* and during a break between the shooting and editing of *Close Encounters.* Lucas was mulling over an idea for a movie serial about the exploits of an adventurer-anthropologist; Spielberg loved the idea, and he convinced Lucas to write and produce the first installment, and to let him direct.[35]

The result, of course, was *Raiders of the Lost Ark,* the huge 1981 hit that established the billion-dollar Indiana Jones franchise and further solidified the two filmmakers in the New Hollywood pantheon. Indeed, whether working together or on their own projects—notably Spielberg on *E.T.* and Lucas on the *Star Wars* sequels—the two virtually rewrote the box-office record books in the late 1970s and 1980s. With the release of their third Indiana Jones collaboration in 1989, Lucas and Spielberg could claim eight of the ten biggest hits in movie history, all of them surpassing $100 million in rentals.[36] Seven of those hits came out in the decade following the release of *Jaws,* a period that Hoberman has aptly termed "ten years that shook the world" of cinema, and that A.D. Murphy calls "the modern era of super-blockbuster films."[37]

Into the 1980s

The importance of the Lucas and Spielberg super-blockbusters can hardly be overstated, considering their impact on theatrical and video markets in the U.S., which along with the rapidly expanding global entertainment market went into overdrive in the 1980s. After surpassing $2 billion in 1975, Hollywood's domestic theatrical revenues climbed steadily from $2.75 billion in 1980 to $5 billion in both 1989 and 1990. And remarkably enough, this steady theatrical growth throughout the 1980s was outpaced rather dramatically by various "secondary markets," particularly pay-cable and home video. During the 1980s, the number of U.S. households with VCRs climbed from 1.85 million (one home in 40) to 62 million (two-thirds of all homes). Pre-recorded videocassette sales rose from only three million in 1980 to 220 million in 1990—an increase of 6,500 percent—while the number of cable households rose from 19.6 million in 1980 to 55 million in 1990, with pay subscriptions increasing from 9 million to 42 million during the decade.[38]

This growth has been a tremendous windfall for Hollywood, since both the pay-cable and home-video industries have been driven primarily by feature films, and in fact have been as hit-driven as the theatrical market. Through all the changes during the 1980s, domestic theatrical release remained the launching pad for blockbuster hits, and it established a movie's value in virtually all other secondary or ancillary markets. Yet even with the record-setting box-office revenues throughout the 1980s, the portion of the Hollywood majors' income from theater rentals actually declined, while total revenues have soared. According to Robert Levin, president of international motion picture marketing for Disney, the domestic box office in 1978 comprised just over half (54 percent) of the majors' overall income, with a mere 4 percent coming from pay-cable and home video combined. By 1986, box-office revenues comprised barely one quarter (28 percent) of the majors' total, with pay-cable and home video combining for over half (12 percent and 40 percent respectively).[39] Home-video revenues actually exceeded worldwide theatrical revenues that year, 1986, and by decade's end cassette revenues alone actually doubled domestic box-office revenues.[40]

Another crucial secondary market for Hollywood has been the box office overseas, particularly in Europe. While the overseas pay-TV and home-video markets are still taking shape, European theatrical began surging in 1985 and reached record levels in 1990, when a number of top hits—including *Pretty Woman, Total Recall, The Little Mermaid,* and *Dances With Wolves*—actually did better box office in Europe than in the U.S.[41] And *Forbes* magazine has estimated that the European theatrical market will double by 1995, as multiplexing picks up in Western Europe and as new markets open in Eastern Europe.[42]

With the astounding growth of both theatrical and video markets and the continued stature of the Hollywood-produced feature, the American movie industry has become increasingly stable in the late 1980s. What's more, the blockbuster mentality seems to have leveled off somewhat. In the early 1980s, one or two huge hits tended to dominate the marketplace, doing well over $100 million and far outdistancing other top hits. From 1986–1990, however, the number of super-blockbuster hits dropped while the number of mid-range hits earning $10 million or more in rentals increased significantly, as did the number returning $50 million or more—still the measure of blockbuster-hit status. From 1975 to 1985 ten films earned $100 million or more in rentals; there have been only four since. Meanwhile, the number of films earning $50 million or more has climbed considerably. From 1965 to 1975, only six reached this mark; from 1976 to 1980 there were 13; from 1981 to 1985 there were 17. From 1986 to 1990, 30 films surpassed $50 million in rentals.

As the economic stakes have risen so have production and marketing costs. The average "negative cost" (i.e., money spent to complete the actual film) on all major studio releases climbed from $9.4 million in 1980 to $26.8 million in 1990. Over the same period, average costs for prints and advertising rose from $4.3 million per film in 1980 to $11.6 million in 1990.[43] The rise in production costs is due largely to two dominant factors: an increased reliance on special effects and the soaring salaries paid to top talent, especially stars. The rise in marketing costs reflects Hollywood's deepening commitment to saturation booking and advertising, which has grown more expensive with the continued multiplex phenomenon and the increased ad opportunities due to cable and VCRs. The number of indoor theaters in the U.S. increased from about 14,000 in 1980 to over 22,000 in 1990, which meant that widespread nationwide release required anywhere from 1,000 to 2,700 prints, at roughly $2,500 per print. But the primary reason for rising marketing costs is TV advertising, particularly for high-stakes blockbusters. In 1990, for example, well over $20 million was spent on TV ads alone for *Dick Tracy, Total Recall,* and *Die Hard 2*.[44]

While this may seem like fiscal madness, there is method in it. Consider the performance of the three top hits of the "blockbuster Summer" in 1989, Hollywood's single biggest season ever. In a four-week span beginning Memorial Day weekend, *Indiana Jones and the Last Crusade, Ghostbusters II,* and *Batman* enjoyed successive weekend releases in at least 2,300 theaters in the U.S. and Canada after heavy TV advertising. Each of these pre-sold entertainment machines set a new box-office record for its opening weekend, culminating in *Batman's* three-day ticket sales of $40.5 million. In an era when $100 million in gross revenues is one measure of a blockbuster hit, it took *Indiana Jones* just 19 days to reach that total; it took *Batman* 11. And like so many recent hits, all three underwent a "fast burn" at the box office. Compare these week-to-week box-office revenues on Hollywood's two all-time summer hits, *E.T.* (1982) and *Batman,* which well indicate certain crucial 1980s market trends.[45]

	wk 1	2	3	4	5	6	7	8	9	10
E.T.	$22m	22	26	24	23	23	19	19	16	15
Batman	70	52	30	24	18	13	11	8	5	4

E.T. earned another $100 million at the box office, which in 1982 was its only serious source of domestic income, while *Batman* was pulled from domestic theatrical for the home-video market—where it generated another $179 million in revenues." Few recent films match *Batman's* home-video performance, and for that matter, few match its box-office legs, either. In 1990, no saturation summer releases except *Ghost* and *Pretty Woman* had any real pull beyond five weeks, although a number of films (*Total Recall, Die Hard 2, Dick Tracy*) grossed over $100 million at the box office.

The three top hits of 1990, *Home Alone, Ghost,* and *Pretty Woman,* bucked the calculated blockbuster trend and demonstrated why Hollywood relies on a steady output of "smaller" (i.e., less expensive) films which, mainly via word of mouth rather than massive pre-selling and promotion, might emerge as surprise hits. Such "sleepers" are most welcome, of course, even in this age of high-cost, high-tech, high-volume behemoths, and they invariably are well exploited once they begin to take off—as were those three surprise hits of 1990. And each undoubtedly will spawn a sequel of calculated blockbuster proportions, with the studio hoping not only for a profitable follow-up but for the kind of success that MGM/UA had with *Rocky,* a modest, offbeat sleeper in 1976 that became a billion-dollar entertainment franchise.

Many have touted the three 1990 hits as a return to reason in Hollywood filmmaking, including Disney production chief Jeffrey Katzenberg in a now legendary interoffice memo of January 1991. Katzenberg warned of "the 'blockbuster mentality' that has gripped our industry," and encouraged a return to "the kind of modest, story-driven movie we tended to make in our salad days."[47] The memo was leaked to the press and caused quite a stir, but scarcely signaled any real change at Disney or anywhere else. *Variety* subtly underscored this point by running excerpts from the memo directly below an even more prominent story with the banner headline, "Megabudgets Boom Despite Talk of Doom." That story inventoried the numerous high-cost Hollywood films "still being greenlighted," including several at Disney.[48]

In one sense, Katzenberg's memo was a rationale for *Dick Tracy,* the 1990 Disney blockbuster that cost $46 million to produce and another $55 million to market and release, with $44 million spent on advertising and promotion alone. Those figures were disclosed some two months before Katzenberg's memo and startled many industry observers, since by then the film had run its theatrical course and returned only about $60 million to Disney in rentals. But Hollywood insiders (including Katzenberg, no doubt) well understood the logic, given today's entertainment marketplace. As one competing executive told the *New York Times,* Disney had to "build awareness" of the Tracy story and character not simply to sell the film, but to establish "the value of a new character in the Disney family . . . so that it could be brought back in a sequel and used in Disney's theme parks."[49]

The future of the Tracy franchise remains to be seen, but one can hardly fault Disney for making the investment. Lip service to scaled-down moviemaking aside, Hollywood's blockbuster mentality is more entrenched now than ever, the industry is more secure, and certain rules of the movie marketplace are virtually set in stone. The first is William Goldman's 1983 axiom, "nobody knows anything," which is quoted with increasing frequency these years as it grows ever more evident that, despite all the market studies and promotional strategies, the kind of public response that generates a bona fide hit simply cannot be manufactured, calculated, or predicted.[50] The studios have learned to hedge their bets and increase the odds, however, and thus these other rules—all designed not only to complement but to counter the Goldman Rule.

The most basic of these rules is that only star vehicles with solid production values have any real chance at the box office (and thus in secondary markets as well). Such films nowadays cost $20 to $30 million, and will push $50 million if top stars, special effects, and/or logistical difficulties are involved. The next rule concerns what is termed the "reward risk" factor, and holds that reaping the potential benefits of a hit requires heavy up-front spending on marketing as well as production. A corollary to this is that risk can be minimized via pre-sold pictures, and today the most effective pre-selling involves previous movie hits or other familiar media products (TV series, pop songs, comic books). An aesthetic corollary holds that films with minimal character complexity or development and by-the-numbers plotting (especially male action pictures) are the most readily reformulated and thus the most likely to be parlayed into a full-blown franchise.

Another cardinal rule is that a film's theatrical release, with its attendant media exposure, creates a cultural commodity that might be regenerated in any number of media forms: Perhaps in pop music, and not only as a hit single or musical score; note that *Batman* had two soundtrack albums and *Dick Tracy* had three. Perhaps as an arcade game, a $7 billion industry in 1990; note that *Hook* and *Terminator 2* both were released simultaneously as movies and video games. Perhaps as a theme park ride; note that Disney earns far more on its theme parks than on motion pictures and television, and that the hottest new Disney World attraction is "Toon Town," adapted from *Who Framed Roger Rabbit?*[51] Perhaps as a comic book or related item; note that the Advance Comics Special Batlist offered 214 separate pieces of *Batman*-related paraphernalia.[52] Perhaps in "novelized" form, with print (and audiocassette) versions of movie hits regularly becoming worldwide best-sellers; note that Simon and Schuster, a Paramount subdivision and the nation's largest bookseller, has devoted an entire division to its Star Trek publications.

These rules are evident not only in today's multimedia worldwide blockbusters, but also in the structure and operations of international corporate giants that produce and market them. Competing successfully in today's high-stakes entertainment marketplace requires an operation that is not only well financed and productive, both also diversified and well coordinated. John Mickelthwait of the *Economist* has written that an entertainment company "needs financial muscle to produce enough software to give itself a decent chance for bringing in a hit, and marketing muscle to make the most of that hit when it happens."[53] Thus there has been a trend toward "tight diversification" and "synergy" in the recent merger-and-acquisitions wave, bringing movie studios into direct play with television production companies, network and cable TV, music and recording companies, and book, magazine, and newspaper publishers, and possibly even with games, toys, theme parks, and electronics hardware manufacturers as well.

So obviously enough, diversification and conglomeration remain key factors in the entertainment industry, though today's media empires are much different than those of the 1960s and 1970s like Gulf & Western, Kinney, and Transamerica. Those top-heavy, widely diversified conglomerates sold out, "downsized," or otherwise regrouped to achieve tighter diversification. Gulf & Western, for instance, sold all but its media holdings by the late 1980s and changed its corporate name to Paramount Communications. Kinney created a media subsidiary in Warner Communications, which also downsized in the early 1980s—only to expand via a $13 billion marriage with Time in 1989 (to avoid a hostile $12 billion takeover by Paramount), thereby creating Time Warner, the world's largest multimedia company and a model of synergy, with holdings in movies, TV production, cable, records, and book and magazine publishing. Because movies drive the global multimedia marketplace, a key holding for any media conglomerate is a motion picture studio; but there is no typical media conglomerate these days due to the widening range of entertainment markets and rapid changes in media technology.

Conglomeration has taken on another new dimension in that several studios have been purchased by foreign media companies: Fox by Rupert Murdoch's News Corporation in 1985, Columbia by Sony in 1989, and MCA/Universal by Matsushita in 1990. The Fox purchase may have greater implications for TV than cinema, given the creation of a "fourth network" in American and its expansion into Europe. The Sony and Matsushita buyouts take the cinema-television synergy in yet another direction, since this time the two consumer electronics giants are battling over domination of the multi-billion-dollar high definition television (HDTV) market. Columbia and MCA gave the two firms sizable media libraries and active production companies, which may well give them an edge in the race not only to develop but to sell HDTV.

The Sony-Columbia and Matsushita-MCA deals are significant in terms of "talent" as well. Beyond the $3.5 billion Sony paid for Columbia, the company also spent roughly $750 million for the services of Peter Guber and Jon Peters, two successful producers (*Batman, Rain Man,* et al.) then under contact to Warners. This underscored the importance of corporate and studio management in the diversified, globalized, synergized marketplace. Indeed, the most successful companies in the mid-to-late 1980s—Paramount, Disney, Warners, and Universal—all enjoyed consistent, capable executive leadership. Successful studio management involves not only positioning movies in a global multimedia market, but also dealing effectively with top talent and their agents, which introduces other human factors into the New Hollywood equation. These factors were best indicated by the role of Michael Ovitz in both the Sony and Matsushita deals. Co-founder and chief executive of CAA, Ovitz is the most powerful agent in Hollywood's premiere agency. He was a key advisor in the Sony-Columbia deal, and in fact he packaged *Rain Man* during the negotiations and later helped arrange the Guber-Peters transaction. And Ovitz quite literally brokered the Matsushita-MCA deal, acting as the sole go-between during the year-long negotiations.[54]

Ovtiz's rise to power in the New Hollywood has been due to various factors: CAA's steadily expanding client list, its packaging of top talent in highly desirable movie packages, and its capacity to secure favorable terms for its clients when cutting movie deals. In perhaps no other industry is the "art of the deal" so important, and in that regard Ovitz is Hollywood's consummate artist. He also is a master at managing relationships—whether interpersonal, institutional, or corporate, as the Columbia and MCA deals both demonstrate. And more than any other single factor, Ovitz's and CAA's success has hinged on the increasingly hit-driven nature of the entertainment industry, and in turn on the star-driven nature of top industry products.

The "star system" is as old as the movie industry itself, of course. "Marquee value," "bankable" talent, and "star vehicles" have always been vital to Hollywood's market strategy, just as the "star persona" has keyed both the narrative and production economies of moviemaking. In the classical era, in fact, studios built their entire production and marketing operations around a few prime star-genre formulas. In the New Hollywood, however, where fewer films carry much wider commercial and cultural impact, and where personas are prone to multimedia reincarnation, the star's commercial value, cultural cache, and creative clout have increased enormously. The most obvious indication of this is the rampant escalation of star salaries during the 1980s—a phenomenon often traced to Sylvester Stallone's $15 million paycheck in 1983 for *Rocky IV*.[55] Interestingly enough, many (if not most) of the seminal New Hollywood blockbusters were not star-driven; in fact many secured stardom for their lead actors. But as the blockbuster sequels and multimedia markets coalesced in the early 1980s, both the salary scale and narrative agency of top stars rose dramatically—to a point where Stallone, Arnold Schwarzenegger, Bruce Willis, Michael Douglas, Eddie Murphy, Sean Connery, and Kevin Costner earn seven or even eight figures per film, having become not only genres but franchises unto themselves, and where "star vehicles" are often simply that: stylish, careening machines designed for their star-drivers which, in terms of plot and character development, tend to go nowhere fast.

Not surprisingly, the studios bemoan their dwindling profit margins due to increased talent costs while top talent demand—and often get—"participation" deals on potential blockbusters. CAA's package for *Hook* gave Dustin Hoffman, Robin Williams, and Steven Spielberg a reported 40 percent of the box-office take, and Jack Nicholson's escalating 15 to 20 percent of the gross on *Batman* paid him upwards of $50 million.[56]

While studio laments about narrowing margins are understandable, so too are agency efforts to secure a piece of the box-office take for their clients, particularly in light of the limited payoff for stars and other talent in ancillary markets and in licensing and merchandising deals. And given the potential long-term payoff of a franchise-scale blockbuster, the stars' demands are as inevitable as the studios' grudging willingness to accommodate them. As Geraldine Fabrikant suggests in a *New York Times* piece on soaring production costs: "Some studios can more easily justify paying higher prices for talent these days because, with the consolidation of the media industry and the rise of integrated entertainment conglomerates that distribute movies, books, recordings, television programming and magazines, they have more outlets through which to recoup their investments."[57]

The Economics and Aesthetics of the New Hollywood

This brings us back, yet again, to the New Hollywood blockbuster's peculiar status as what Eileen Meehan has aptly termed a "commercial intertext." As Meehan suggests, today's conglomerates "view every project as a multimedia production line," and thus *Batman* "is best understood as a multimedia, multimarket sales campaign."[58] Others have noted the increased interplay of moviemaking and advertising, notably Mark Crispin Miller in a cover story for the *Atlantic*, "Hollywood: The Ad." Miller opens with an indictment of the "product placement" trend in movies (a means of offsetting production costs which, as he suggests, often brings the narrative to a dead halt), and he goes on to discuss other areas where movies and advertising—especially TV advertising—have begun to merge. Like TV ads, says Miller, movies today aspire to a total "look" and seem more designed than directed, often by filmmakers segueing from studio to ad agency. And now that movies are more likely to be seen on a VCR than a theater screen, cinematic technique is adjusted accordingly, conforming with the small screen's "most hypnotic images," its ads. Visual and spatial scale are downsized, action is repetitiously foregrounded and centered, pace and transitions are quicker, music and montage are more prevalent, and slick production values and special effects abound.[59]

While Miller's view of the cinema as the last bastion of high culture under siege by the twin evils of TV and advertising displays a rather limited understanding of the contemporary culture industries, there is no question but that movie and ad techniques are intermingling. In fact, one might argue that the New Hollywood's calculated blockbusters are themselves massive advertisements for their product lines—a notion that places a very different value on their one-dimensional characters, mechanical plots, and high-gloss style. This evokes that New Hollywood buzzword, "high concept," a term best defined perhaps by its chief progenitor, Steven Spielberg, in an interview back in 1978: "What interests me more than anything else is the idea. If a person can tell me the idea in twenty-five words or less, it's going to be a good movie."[60] And a pretty good ad campaign as well—whether condensed into a 30-second movie trailer or as a feature-length plug for any number of multimedia reiterations.

This paradoxical reduction and reiteration of blockbuster movie narratives points up the central, governing contradiction in contemporary cinema. On the one hand, the seemingly infinite capacity for multimedia reiteration of a movie hit redefines textual boundaries, creates a dynamic commercial intertext that is more process than product, and involves the audience(s) in the creative process—not only as multimarket consumers but also as mediators in the play of narrative signification. On the other hand, the actual movie "itself," if indeed it can be isolated and understood as such (which is questionable at best), often has been reduced and stylized to a point where, for some observers, it scarcely even qualifies as a narrative.

Critic Richard Schickel, for instance, has stated: "In the best of all possible marketing worlds the movie will inspire some simple summarizing graphic treatment, adaptable to all media, by which it can be instantly recognized the world over, even by subliterates."[61] The assembly-line process in the studio era demanded that story ideas be progressively refined into a classical three-act structure of exposition, complication, and resolution. But nowadays, says Schickel, "Hollywood seems to have lost or abandoned the art of narrative.... [Filmmakers] are generally not refining stories at all, they are spicing up 'concepts' (as they like to call them), refining gimmicks, making sure there are no complexities to fur our tongues when it comes time to spread the word of mouth." Schickel argues that all genres have merged into two meta-categories, comedies and action-adventure films, both of which offer "a succession of undifferentiated sensations, lucky or unlucky accidents, that have little or nothing to do with whatever went before or is about to come next," with a mere "illusion of forward motion" created via music and editing.[62]

Schickel excuses his "geriatric grumble" while demeaning "youthful" moviegoers for their lack of "very sophisticated tastes or expectations when it comes to narrative," and his nod to audience fragmentation along generational lines raises a few important issues.[63] To begin with, younger viewers—despite "grownup" biases about limited attention spans, depth of feeling, and intellectual development—are far more likely to be active multimedia players, consumers, and semioticians, and thus to gauge a movie in intertextual terms and to appreciate in it a richness and complexity that may well be lost on middle-aged movie critics. In fact, given the penchant these years to pre-sell movies via other popular culture products (rock songs, comic books, TV series, etc.), chances are that younger, media-literate viewers encounter a movie in an already-activated narrative process. The size, scope, and emotional charge of the movie and its concurrent ad campaign certainly privilege the big screen "version" of the story, but the movie itself scarcely begins or ends the textual cycle.

This in turn raises the issue of narrative "integrity," which in classical Hollywood was a textual feature directly related to the integrity of both the "art form" and the system of production. While movies during the studio era certainly had their intertextual qualities, these were incidental and rarely undermined the internal coherence of the narrative itself. While many (perhaps most) New Hollywood films still aspire to this kind of narrative integrity, the blockbuster tends to be intertextual and purposefully incoherent—virtually of necessity, given the current conditions of cultural production and consumption. Put another way, the vertical integration of classical Hollywood, which ensured a closed industrial system and coherent narrative, has given way to "horizontal integration" of the New Hollywood's tightly diversified media conglomerates, which favors texts strategically "open" to multiple readings and multimedia reiteration.

These calculated blockbusters utterly dominate the movie industry, but they also promote alternative films and filmmaking practices in a number of ways. Because the majors' high-cost, high-stakes projects require a concentration of resources and limit overall output, they tend to foster product demand. This demand is satisfied, for the most part, by moderately priced star vehicles financed and distributed by the majors, which may emerge as surprise hits but essentially serve to keep the industry machinery running, to develop new talent, and to maintain a steady supply of dependable mainstream product. Complementing these routine features, and far more interesting from a critical and cultural perspective, are the low-cost films from independent outfits like Miramax and New Line Cinema. In fact, the very market fragmentation which the studios' franchise projects are designed to exploit and overcome, these independents are exploiting in a very different way via their small-is-beautiful, market-niche approach.

Miramax, for instance, has carved out a niche by financing or buying and then distributing low-budget art films and imports like *sex, lies and videotape, My Left Foot, Cinema Paradiso,* and *Tie Me Up, Tie Me Down* to a fairly consistent art film crowd. New Line's strategy is more wide-ranging, targeting an array of demographic groups and taste cultures from art film aficionados and environmentalists to born-again Christians and wrestling fans. If any one of New Line's products takes off at the box office, it's liable to be a teen pic like *Teenage Mutant Ninja Turtles,* which returned $67 million in rentals in 1990. While fully exploiting that hit was a real challenge for a company like New Line, an even bigger challenge, no doubt, was resisting the urge to expand their operations, upgrade their product, and compete with the majors—an impulse that proved disastrous for many independent companies during the 1980s.[64]

Thus we might see the New Hollywood as producing three different classes of movie: the calculated blockbuster designed with the multimedia marketplace and franchise status in mind, the mainstream A-class star vehicle with sleeper-hit potential, and the low-cost independent feature targeted for a specific market and with little chance of anything more than "cult film" status. These three classes of movie have corresponding ranks of auteurs, from the superstar directors at the "high end" like Spielberg and Lucas, whose knack for engineering hits has transformed their names into virtual trademarks, to those filmmakers on the margins like Gus Van Sant, John Sayles, and the Coen brothers, whose creative control and personal style are considerably less constrained by commercial imperatives. And then there are the established genre auteurs like Jonathan Demme, Martin Scorsese, David Lynch, and Woody Allen who, like Ford and Hitchcock and the other top studio directors of old, are the most perplexing and intriguing cases—each of them part visionary cineaste and part commercial hack, whose best films flirt with hit status and critique the very genres (and audiences) they exploit.

Despite its stratification, the New Hollywood is scarcely a balkanized or rigidly class-bound system. On the contrary, these classes of films and filmmakers are in a state of dynamic tension with one another and continually intermingle. Consider, for instance, the two recent forays into that most contemptible of genres, the psycho-killer/stalk-and-slash film, by Jonathan Demme in *The Silence of the Lambs* and Martin Scorsese in *Cape Fear.* Each film took the genre into uncharted narrative and thematic territory; each was a cinematic tour-de-force, enhancing both the aesthetic and commercial value of the form; and each thoroughly terrified audiences, thereby reinforcing the genre's capacity to explore the dark recesses of the collective American psyche and underscoring the cinema's vital contact with its public.

Besides winning the Oscar for "Best Picture of 1991," *Silence of the Lambs* emerged as a solid international hit, indicating the potential global currency of the genre while raising some interesting questions about the New Hollywood's high-end products vis-à-vis the American cultural experience. With the rapid development of multiplex theaters and home video in Europe and the Far East, and the concurrent advances in advertising and marketing, one can readily foresee the "global release" of calculated blockbusters far beyond the scale of a *Batman* or *Terminator 2*, let alone a surprise hit like *The Silence of the Lambs*. This may require a very different kind of product, effectively segregating the calculated blockbuster from the studios' other feature output and redefining the Hollywood cinema as an American culture industry. But it's much more likely that the New Hollywood and its characteristic blockbuster product will endure, given the social and economic development in the major overseas markets, the survival instincts and overall economic stability of the Hollywood studios, and the established global appeal of its products.

Notes

1. Recent studies of "classical" Hollywood and the "studio system" include *The Classical Hollywood Cinema: Film Style and Mode of Production to 1960,* David Bordwell, Janet Staiger, and Kristin Thompson (New York: Columbia University Press, 1985); *The Hollywood Studio System,* Douglas Gomery (New York: St. Martin, 1986); and *The Genius of the System: Hollywood Filmmaking in the Studio Era.* Thomas Schatz (New York: Pantheon, 1988).

2. Here and throughout this essay, I will be referring to *"rentals"* (or "rental receipts") and also to *"gross revenues"* (or "box-office revenues"). This is a crucial distinction, since the gross revenues indicate the amount of money actually spent at the box office, whereas rental receipts refer, as *Variety* puts it, to "actual amounts received by the distributor"—i.e., to the moneys returned by theaters to the company (usually a "studio") that released the movie. Unless otherwise indicated, both the rentals and gross revenues involve only the "domestic box office"—i.e., theatrical release in the U.S. and Canada.

    All of the references to box-office performance and rental receipts in this article are taken from *Variety,* most of them from its most recent (January 11–17, 1989; pp. 28–74) survey of "All-Time Film Rental Champs," which includes all motion pictures returning at least $4 million in rentals. Because this survey is continually updated, the totals include reissues and thus may be considerably higher than the rentals from initial release. In these cases I try to use figures from earlier *Variety* surveys for purposes of accuracy.

3. "'Gone With the Wind' Again Tops All-Time List," *Variety* (May 4, 1983), p. 15.

4. "Top 100 All-Time Film Rental Champs," *Variety* (January 6, 1992), p. 86.

5. Eileen R. Meehan, "'Holy Commodity Fetish, Batman!': The Political Economy of a Commercial Intertext," in *The Many Lives of the Batman,* Roberta E. Pearson and William Uricchio, eds. (New York: BFI-Routledge, 1991), p. 62.

6. Christopher H. Sterling and Timothy R. Haight, *The Mass Media: Aspen Institute Guide to Communications Industry Trends* (New York: Praeger, 1978), pp. 187 and 352. Unless otherwise noted, the statistics on attendance, ticket sales, etc., are from this reliable compendium of statistical data on the movie industry.

7. "All-Time Film Rental Champs," *Variety* (January 11–17, 1989), pp. 28–74.

8. Personal correspondence from Selznick to Louis B. Mayer, September 16, 1953; David O. Selznick Collection, Humanities Research Center, University of Texas at Austin.

9. Rudy Behlmer, ed., *Memo from David O. Selznick* (New York: Viking, 1972), p. 373.

10. See Janet Staiger, "Individualism Versus Collectivism," *Screen* 24 (July–October, 1983), pp. 68–79.

11. Freeman Lincoln, "The Comeback of the Movies," *Fortune* (February, 1955), p. 127.

12. See Robert Vianello, "The Rise of the Telefilm and the Networks' Hegemony Over the Motion Picture Industry," *Quarterly Review of Film Studies* (Summer, 1984) pp. 204–18.

13. See William Lafferty, "Feature Films on Prime-Time Television," in *Hollywood in the Age of Television*, Tino Balio, ed. (Boston: Unwin Hyman, 1990), pp. 235–256.
14. Lincoln, "Comeback," p. 131.
15. Stephen M. Silverman, *The Fox That Got Away* (Secaucus, N.J.: Lyle Stuart Inc., 1988), pp. 323–329.
16. Tino Balio, "Introduction to Part II" of *Hollywood in the Age of Television*, pp. 259–260.
17. Joseph R. Dominick, "Film Economics and Film Content: 1964–1983," in *Current Research in Film* (Norwood, N.J.: Ablex, 1987), p. 144.
18. Lafferty, "Feature Films," pp. 245–248.
19. Michael Pye and Lynda Myles, *The Movie Brats* (New York: Holt, Rinehart and Winston, 1979), p. 236.
20. Carl Gottlieb, *The Jaws Log* (New York: Dell, 1975), pp. 15–19. Note that Dell is a subdivision of MCA.
21. Gottlieb, *Jaws Log,* p. 62.
22. Pye and Myles, *Movie Brats,* p. 232.
23. James Monaco, *American Film Now* (New York: New American Library, 1979), p. 50.
24. Axel Madsen, *The New Hollywood* (New York: Thomas Y. Crowell, 1975), p. 94.
25. Balio, "Introduction to Part I," *Hollywood in the Age of Television,* p. 29.
26. "Theatrical Data" section in "1990 U.S. Economic Review" (New York: Motion Picture Association of America, 1991), p. 3.
27. Dominick, "Film Economics," p. 146.
28. Jennifer Pendleton, "Fast Forward, Reverse," *Daily Variety* (58th Anniversary Issue, "Focus on Entertainment Marketing," October, 1991), p. 14.
29. Michelle Hilmes, "Breaking the Broadcast Bottleneck," in Balio, *Hollywood,* pp. 299–300.
30. See Hilmes, "Breaking," and also Bruce A. Austin, "Home Video: The Second-Run 'Theater' of the 1990s," in Balio, *Hollywood,* pp. 319–349.
31. J. Hoberman, "Ten Years That Shook the World," *American Film* 10 (June, 1985); p. 42.
32. Jim McCullaugh, "*Star Wars* Hikes Demand for Dolby," *Billboard* (July 9, 1977), p. 4.
33. "*Star Wars:* A Cultural Phenomenon," *Box Office* (July, 1987), pp. 36–38.
34. Hoberman, "Ten Years," pp. 36–37.
35. "Behind the Scenes on *Raiders of the Lost Ark.*" *American Cinematographer* (November, 1981), p. 1096. See also Tony Crawley, *The Steven Spielberg Story* (New York: Quill, 1983), p. 90.
36. "Top 100 All-Time Film Rental Champs," *Variety* (January 11–17, 1989), p. 26.
37. Hoberman; "Ten Years," and A. D. Murphy, "Twenty Years of Weekly Film Ticket Sales in U.S. Theaters," *Variety* (March 15–21, 1989), p. 26.
38. Figures from "Theatrical Data" and "VCR and Cable" sections in MPAA's "1990 U.S. Economic Review."
39. Robert B. Levin and John H. Murphy, unpublished case study of Walt Disney Pictures' 1986 marketing strategies, for use in an advertising course taught by Professor Murphy.
40. Richard Natale, "Hollywood's 'new math': Does it still add up?," *Variety* (September 23, 1991), pp. 1, 95.
41. Terry Ilott, "Yank pix flex pecs in new Euro arena," *Variety* (August 19, 1991), pp. 1, 60.
42. John Marcon, Jr., "Dream Factory to the World," *Forbes* (April 29, 1991), p. 100.
43. Figures from "Prints and Advertising Costs of New Features" in MPAA's "1990 U.S. Economic Review."

44. Charles Fleming, "Pitching costs out of ballpark: Record pic-spending spells windfall for tv," *Variety* (June 27, 1990), p. 1.
45. "Week-by-week domestic b.o. gross," *Variety* (January 7, 1991), p. 10.
46. "Video and Theatrical Revenues," *Variety* (September 24, 1990), p. 108.
47. "The Teachings of Chairman Jeff," *Variety* (February 4, 1991), p. 24. Article contains excerpts of the January 11 memo.
48. Charles Fleming, "Megabudgets Boom Despite Talk of Doom," *Variety* (February 4, 1991), pp. 5ff.
49. Geraldine Fabrikant, "In Land of Big Bucks, Even Bigger Bucks," *New York Times* (October 18, 1990), p. C5.
50. William Goldman, *Adventures in the Screen Trade* (New York: Warner Books, 1983), p. 39.
51. "Disney's profits in park: Off 23%," *The Hollywood Reporter* (November 15, 1991), pp. 1, 6.
52. Meehan, "Holy Commodity," p. 47.
53. John Mickelthwait, "A Survey of the Entertainment Industry," *The Economist* (December 23, 1989), p. 5.
54. For an excellent overview of both the Sony and Matsushita deals, and Ovitz's role in each, see Connie Bruck, "Leap of Faith," *New Yorker* (September 9, 1991), pp. 38–74.
55. Lawrence Cohn, "Stars' Rocketing Salaries Keep Pushing Envelope," *Variety* (September 24, 1990), p. 3.
56. Spielberg/Hoffman/Williams deal reported in Geraldine Fabrikant, "The Hole in Hollywood's Pocket," *New York Times* (December 10, 1990), p. C7. Nicholson deal in Ben Stein, "Holy Bat-Debt!," *Entertainment Weekly* (April 26, 1991), p. 12.
57. Fabrikant, "The Hole in Hollywood's Pocket," p. C7.
58. Meehan, "'Holy Commodity," p. 52.
59. Mark Crispin Miller, "Hollywood: The Ad," *Atlantic Monthly* (April, 1990), pp. 49–52.
60. Quoted in Hoberman, "Ten Years," p. 36.
61. Richard Schickel, "The Crisis in Movie Narrative," *Gannett Center Journal* 3 (Summer, 1989), p. 2.
62. Schickel, "Crisis," pp. 3–4.
63. Schickel, "Crisis," p. 3.
64. See Joshua Hammer, "Small Is Beautiful," *Newsweek* (November 26, 1990), pp. 52–53, and William Grimes, "Film Maker's Secret Is Knowing What's Not for Everyone," *New York Times* (December 2, 1991), pp. B1+.

Batman

Mark Salisbury Interviewing Tim Burton

The movie rights to Bob Kane's comic strip character had been secured from DC Comics in 1979 by producers Benjamin Melniker and Michael Uslan, who had hired Superman *screenwriter Tom Mankiewicz to write a script which focused on the Dark Knight's origins. Eventually, Melniker and Uslan relinquished production duties to Peter Guber and Jon Peters, and throughout the early eighties a number of film-makers, including Joe Dante and Ivan Reitman, were linked to the property, though it remained in development until a satisfactory script was found. Following the success of* Pee-Wee's Big Adventure, *the project, which was in development at Warner Bros, was offered to Burton. His* Frankenweenie *producer, Julie Hickson, wrote a thirty-page treatment, before Burton brought in Sam Hamm, a comic book fan and screenwriter with only one produced credit,* Never Cry Wolf.

They had had the project for ten years and had had several directors attached to it. After *Pee-Wee,* they asked me if I was interested in directing *Batman,* and I was. But they didn't give the okay officially until after the first weekend's grosses from *Beetlejuice* came in. It was kind of charming in a way, because Sam and I would meet on weekends to discuss the early writing stages, and we had a great script, but they kept saying there were other things involved. They were just waiting to see how *Beetlejuice* did. They didn't want to give me that movie unless *Beetlejuice* was going to be okay. They wouldn't say that, but that was really the way it was. So, after that first weekend, it got the magical green-light.

Hamm and Burton fashioned a dark, brooding, deeply psychological story for the Caped Crusader which, like Mankiewicz's script, pitted him against The Joker but was set in a dark, hellish vision of Gotham City that eschewed the campness of the Batman *TV series of the sixties and instead went back to Kane's original comic strips of the forties. Helping sell Warners on the script's noirish approach was the comic book/graphic novel explosion of the mid-eighties, and the resurgence of interest in Batman that had been initiated by comic book artist/writer Frank Miller's* The Dark Knight Returns, *a graphic novel which delved into the darker side of Batman's psyche, and Alan Moore's* The Killing Joke, *which featured Batman battling against The Joker.*

I was never a giant comic book fan but I've always loved the image of Batman and The Joker. The reason I've never been a comic book fan—and I think it started when I was a child—is because I could never tell which box I was supposed to read. That's why I loved *The Killing Joke*, because for the first time I could tell which one to read. It's my favourite. It's the first comic I've ever loved. And the success of those graphic novels made our ideas more acceptable.

So, while I was never a big comic book fan, I loved Batman, the split personality, the hidden person. It's a character I could relate to. Having those two sides, a light side and a dark one, and not being able to resolve them—that's a feeling that's not uncommon. So while I can see it's got a lot of Michael Keaton in it because he's actually doing it, I also see certain aspects of myself in the character.

Otherwise, I wouldn't have been able to do it. I mean, this whole split personality thing is so much a part of every person that it's just amazing to me that more people don't consciously understand it. Everybody has several sides to their personality, no one is one thing. Especially in America, people often present themselves as one thing, but are really something else. Which is symbolic of the Batman character.

While the casting of Jack Nicholson as The Joker received almost unanimous acceptance, that of Michael Keaton in the dual role of Bruce Wayne and Batman sparked off an unprecedented amount of controversy. It was producer Jon Peters who first suggested Keaton for the role, and when the news was announced Bat-fans the world over were horrified, with 50,000 letters flooding into Warner Bros' offices to protest at the decision. In fact, the negative reaction reached such proportions that Warners' share price slumped, outraged fans tore up offending publicity material at comic conventions and the Wall Street Journal *covered the crisis on page one. One appalled aficionado wrote in the* Los Angeles Times *that, 'By casting a clown, Warner Bros and Burton have defecated on the history of Batman.' Even Adam West, who had camped up the Caped Crusader in the TV series of the sixties, thought himself a better choice than Keaton.*

In my mind I kept reading reviews that said, 'Jack's terrific, but the unknown as Batman is nothing special.' So I saw a zillion people and the thing that kept going through my mind when I saw these action-adventure hero types come into the office was, 'I just can't see them putting on a bat-suit. I can't see it.' I was seeing these big macho guys, and then thinking of them with pointy eyes, and it was, 'Why would this big, macho, Arnold Schwarzenegger-type person dress up as a bat for God's sake?' A bat is this wild thing. I'd worked with Michael before and so I thought he would be perfect, because he's got that look in his eye. It's there in *Beetlejuice*. It's like *that* guy you could see putting on a bat-suit; he does it because he *needs* to, because he's not this gigantic, strapping macho man. It's all about transformation. Then it started to make sense to me: All of a sudden the whole thing clicked, I could see the pointy ears; the image and the psychology all made sense. Taking Michael and making him Batman underrscored the whole split personality thing which is really what I think the movie's all about.

With all this controversy, the studio was a little apprehensive. It was like, 'That wasn't what we were thinking.' But they quickly understood. Obviously, there was a lot of negative response from comic book people. I think they thought we were going to make it like the TV series, and make it campy, because they all thought of Michael from *Mr Mom* and *Night Shift* and stuff like that. But that never bothered me because I knew we weren't doing that. Whatever the movie would be, I knew we weren't making a joke of the material.

When I was at school I went to a comic book convention in San Diego a few months before *Superman* was due to be released, and someone from Warner Bros came down and gave a presentation, and the fans tore him to shreds. That was the first time I really saw the intensity and passion that comic book fans have. They didn't like the fact that Superman changed into his costume on the edge of a building. This one guy stood up and said, 'I'm going to boycott this movie and tell everyone you are destroying the legend', and there was this huge round of applause. I never forgot that.

I remember when I first met Bob Kane, he was very pleased with what Sam Hamm and I had done with the script, but he was as freaked out as the rest of them about certain choices in it. Michael Keaton is not the image of Bruce Wayne, but in the comic books the image of The Joker is this really thin so-and-so, so it's a bit elitist to say Jack Nicholson's perfect. Well, he *is* perfect, but he's certainly not the comic book image. So people's bibles seemed to change. If you look at the *Batman* encyclopedia, the fucking thing changes every fucking week. Because, if you think about the reality of it, comic book writers say, 'God, what are we going to do this week? Let's change the history of how Robin was created.' There's no such thing as a bible. I always react against the single-mindedness that you find in Hollywood a lot. You can't think about it. I thought about being true to what I loved about the original idea, and I think in the spirit of it, it's close to Bob Kane. If you look at Michael, he's got all those wheels and that wild energy in his eyes which would compel him to put on a bat-suit. It's like, if he had gotten therapy he wouldn't be putting on a bat-suit. He didn't, so this is his therapy.

But there was no way to satisfy everybody. What you just had to hope for was that you were true to the spirit. And luckily comic books had gone through a phase where they had become much more acceptable. They had made things darker. They had taken Batman into the psychological domain. To me it was very clear: the TV series was campy; the regeneration, the new comics, were totally rebelling against that. I just had to be true to the spirit of it and what I got out of it: the absurdity of it.

Part of what interested me was that it's a human character who dresses up in the most extremely vulgar costumes. The first treatment of *Batman*, the Mankiewicz script, was basically *Superman*, only the names had been changed. It had the same jokey tone, as the story followed Bruce Wayne from childhood through to his beginnings as a crime fighter. They didn't acknowledge any of the freakish nature of it, and I found it the most frightening thing I'd ever read. They didn't acknowledge that he was a man who puts on a costume. They just treated it as if he's doing it for good and that was it. You can't do that. I never felt there had been a totally successful comic book movie ever made. At least not one that I had seen. I thought *Superman* was well done, but in terms of capturing the very specific feel of a comic book, it really didn't do it.

The Mankiewicz script made it more obvious to me that you couldn't treat *Batman* like *Superman* or treat it like the TV series, because it's a guy dressing up as a bat and no matter what anyone says that's weird. And you've got to go along with that, to some degree. If you want it to be bright and light you either do *Superman* or Cotton Candy Man, you don't do *Batman*.

The TV series was something else, and I grew up on that. I remember running home to be there on opening night on TV. I was prepared. But they'd *done* that, so there was no point in doing that again. And then, as the movie got closer, the comic book explosion clicked in, which I thought was very healthy for everybody because comics, even though I still didn't really read them, are part of American mythology.

Batman *was filmed at Pinewood Studios in England during the winter of 1988/9 where the entire backlot was turned, at a cost of $5.5 million, into a vision of Gotham City that was described in Sam Hamm's script as 'if Hell had sprung up through the pavements and kept on going'. The man responsible was British production designer Anton Furst, who had previously worked on* The Company of Wolves *and* Full Metal Jacket, *and who Burton had tried to employ for* Beetlejuice.

To do a big movie you either do it in LA or you do it in London, due basically to the facilities. I mean, the dollar wasn't even great at the time, but at Pinewood there was nothing going on and it had a big outdoor area which we could build on. So it made sense. The characters were so extreme that I felt we had to set them somewhere that was designed for them. Because *Superman* had been filmed on New York locations, I don't think it captured the right comic book feel. I was very happy we did it at Pinewood, just to get away from all that stuff with the casting and the hype and the pressure. The British press were intense too, but that didn't bother me as much. I liked being there, I liked working there, I liked a lot of the people, a lot of great artists; I made some friends and it was nice.

Design is very important to me and there are very few designers that I get excited about. Anton was a great designer. I had liked *The Company of Wolves,* and I thought he was one of the most individual ones around. I had met him before *Beetlejuice* and tried to get him to work on that, but he was working on something else. Because of my background, design is the one area I'm very critical about. Working with someone like Anton, who had a real talent, is a luxury. It excites me and it has always been important for me to like designers as friends.

For Gotham City we looked at pictures of New York. *Blade Runner* had come out, and any time there's a movie like that, that's such a trend setter, you're in danger. We had said early on that any city we were going to do was going to get the inevitable *Blade Runner* comparison. So we decided there was nothing we could do about it. We just said, 'This is what's happening to New York at the moment. Things are being added and built on and design is getting all over the place.' We decided to darken everything and build vertically and cram things together and then just go further with it in a more cartoon way. It has an operatic feel, and an almost timeless quality, which I think is similar to *Beetlejuice*.

Every time I do anything I start with the character. Batman's character likes the dark and wants to remain in the shadows, so it's a city at night without many day scenes. Everything is meant to support these characters, so every decision we make is based on that, running it by the character almost, and making sure it's okay with what that character's about.

In addition to the casting of Keaton, comic book fans were also outraged by the redesign of the batsuit by costume designer Bob Ringwood, who changed its colour from blue to black and incorporated fake musculature into the design.

We just took off from the psychology of saying 'Here's a guy who doesn't look like Arnold Schwarzenegger, so why is he doing this?' He's trying to create an image for himself, he's trying to become something that he's not. Therefore, every decision that we made was based upon that. What's he trying to achieve? Why do you dress up as a bat? You're trying to scare criminals, you're putting on a show, you are trying to scare and intimidate people. The idea was to humanize the character.

Despite Warners' initial faith in Hamm's screenplay, the script went through another two writers— Beetlejuice's *Warren Skaaren and Charles McKeown, co-writer of Terry Gilliam's* The Adventures of Baron Münchausen—*and also required rewrites on set.*

I don't understand why that became such a problem. We started out with a script that everyone liked, although we recognized it needed a little work. Everyone thought the script was great, but they *still* thought it needed a total rewrite. Obviously it was a big movie, and it represented an enormous investment by Warners, so I understood why we had to make it right. But what made the situation worse was that there was all this fuss about making the script better and suddenly we were shooting.

There were so many changes and fixes that it was like unravelling a ball of yarn. It gets to a point where you're *not* helping it any more. We were shooting a scene leading up to the bell-tower and Jack's walking up the steps, but we didn't know why. He said to me that day, 'Why am I going up the steps?' And I said, 'I don't know, we'll talk about it when you get up the top.' You're always working on something, you're always trying to make it better, that happens all the way through, but in this case I felt I wasn't making it better. That pressure is really lousy because you don't have your own strong foundation to stand on like you usually do. I like improvising, but not that way. *Beetlejuice* was amorphous, but it didn't matter because it wasn't as expensive, and it wasn't as big a dinosaur.

The first time you direct a movie on that scale it's kind of surreal. You're not fearful because you don't know. You only have to fight things off after you've been through it once or twice. It's a weird kind of conditioning. If you give somebody a little electrical jolt, the first time they won't know what's coming. After that, they'll be thinking about that little jolt. It's a similar kind of thing.

I was very lucky because I didn't go into it with a fear of 'Oh my God, Jack Nicholson!' And he was great to me. He was very supportive. With Jack a lot of the work was done early on in terms of how he felt about me. He was very cool. He helped me a lot when there was trouble on the movie and the studio freaked out. He was very calming and helpful and would just say, 'Get what you need, get what you want, and just keep going.' He's so great. He'll do like six takes and each take he'll give it something else. He was fascinating that way, and you'd almost wish you could play all six takes in the movie. He was very exciting to watch.

Charles McKeown came in and we did some work on The Joker character. He was The Joker and he needed more jokes, not for the sake of more jokes, but because that was his character. He needed more of that identification. He's the best character and besides Catwoman he's the clearest villain. I just love the idea of a person who's turned into a clown and is insane. The film is like the duel of the freaks. It's a fight between two disfigured people. That's what I love about it. I was always aware of how weird it was, but I was never worried about it in any way. The Joker is such a great character because there's a complete freedom to him. Any character who operates on the outside of society and is deemed a freak and an outcast then has the freedom to do what they want. The Joker and Beetlejuice can do that in a much more liberating way than, say, Edward Scissorhands, or even Pee-Wee, because they're deemed disgusting. They are the darker sides of freedom. Insanity is in some scary way the most freedom you can have, because you're not bound by the laws of society.

We tried to put Robin in, to make that relationship work in a real way. In the TV series he's just *there*. We tried a slightly more psychological approach, but I felt unless you're going to focus on that and give it its due, it's like 'Who is this guy?' Sam and I spent a lot of time going over that, anguishing over it. It's a good thing we didn't do it, because it would have cost a lot, and when we were getting ready to shoot the movie it was the easiest lift. Again, I just went back to the psychology of a man who dresses up as a bat; he's a very singular, lonely character, and putting him with somebody just didn't make sense. It didn't make sense in the next one either; we tried it there too. But it's just too much. There's too much material with these characters.

As with Pee-Wee's Big Adventure *and* Beetlejuice, *Burton called upon Danny Elfman to provide* Batman's *dark, orchestral score. This time, however, Elfman's soundtrack album was complemented by one from Prince, who had initially been commissioned to provide two songs for the movie.*

We needed two numbers—one for when The Joker goes into the museum, and the other for the parade sequence, and I actually used music by Prince for those scenes when we shot them. But what happened was it snowballed. It got bigger. He really got into the movie and wrote a bunch of songs. Guber and Peters had this idea of getting Michael Jackson to do the love theme, Prince to do The Joker theme, and Danny would just tie it all together. They can make that work for *Top Gun,* but my stuff isn't like that. It needs to be finessed a bit more. And I don't think those songs work. It doesn't have anything to do with Prince's music, it has more to do with their integration into the film. I liked them on their own, but I'm not proficient enough to make something like that work if it's not right.

I love Prince. I saw him twice at Wembley when I was shooting the movie. I think he's incredible. Here was a guy who was looking at a movie and doing his thing to it. It's like what comic book people do, it's their impression. I love that. I wish there was more of that kind of thing. It's cool to have crossover things like that. But I couldn't make the songs work, and I think I did a disservice to the movie and to him. But the record company wanted those things to be in there. Obviously, they made a lot of money from it, so I guess in that respect they achieved something. But I don't feel I made it work very well. The songs bring it too much into a specific time frame.

Batman *opened in the USA on 21 June 1989 and became the first film to break $100 million in its first ten days of release. It eventually became not only the top money-maker of 1989, with a worldwide gross in excess of $500 million, and the biggest film in Warner Bros's history, but also a multimedia merchandising and cultural phenomenon, the hype of which had never been seen before; until the release of* Jurassic Park *in 1993, it was the blockbuster against which all subsequent blockbusters had to be measured.*

The interesting thing about hype is that everyone thought the studio was creating it, when in fact you can't create hype; it's a phenomenon that's beyond a studio, it has a life of its own. The most negative thing to me was working on something that gained so much hype, because I'm the type of person—and there is a percentage of the population out there like myself—who if I hear too much about something gets turned off by it. And it was odd to be working on something that, if I was a normal person, I'd have gone, 'Shut the fuck up. I'm sick of hearing about this thing. I won't go see it, 'cos I've heard too much about it.' That was the most disturbing thing. But there was no way to control it. And then you get the inevitable backlash to that. My main concern was that the movie be judged on its own merits and not become this *thing*. But there's nothing you can do about it. It helped being in England, even with the press attention there, because it wasn't my country, and so I just focused on making the movie and didn't think too much about anything else.

Batman *won Anton Furst an Oscar for his design work, but was criticized in some quarters for being 'too dark'. Many critics also felt that Burton was more interested in The Joker than in the title character.*

That's not true, but there is an inherent problem with these characters. It was similar to the criticism that Adam and Barbara Maitland were boring. That's not true either. But there is an inherent difference in the characters of Batman and The Joker: The Joker is an extrovert and Batman an introvert. So no matter what you do, you can't match the energy, the balance. You have this character who always wants to remain in the shadows, to remain hidden. If these two were standing on the street, Batman would always be wanting to hide, whereas The Joker would be, 'Look at me. Look at me.' So that's part of what the energy of it was. I certainly wasn't less interested in Batman, it's just that he is who he is, and The Joker is who he is. Right or wrong, I sort of let these things play themselves out. Some people got it, some people understood that. Obviously, a lot of people thought The Joker was the thing, but a lot of people found Michael to be more compelling because of that. He captured a certain subtle sadness in his character. It was as if he was thinking, 'Look at this guy. He gets to go out there and jump around and be a clown, and I have to remain in the shadows.' And there was a pent-up, bottled-up feeling to him which I think works with the Batman character.

It's funny, that whole dark and light thing. In fact, I've gotten more confused by it in a way. It was so weird on the second *Batman* because I would do those big press junkets where you're seeing a zillion people—every six minutes somebody new—and it became like a joke. I felt I was on *Candid Camera*, because one person would come in and go, 'The film is much lighter than the last one', and then the next person would come up and say, 'It's much darker than the first movie.' I felt like a psycho because I never think of things as dark or light. I've always felt that you couldn't even pull apart light and dark, they're so intertwined. I felt that way growing up, and I feel that way now. Sometimes I'll watch something that people don't see anything weird about and I'll find it deeply subversive and scary and dark. And then people will look at something that I've done and go, 'That's really dark', and I don't see it. It's like the end of *Vincent* when they said they wanted him to live and walk off with his dad. That felt darker to me, because the other ending felt more beautiful and more like what was in his mind, which is what the thing was about. It was about somebody's spirit, and to make it literal was, I felt, making it darker, ultimately. So what is perceived as light and dark is completely open to interpretation.

During the shooting of Batman, *Burton met Lena Gieseke, a German painter, and they were married in February 1989 while he was completing post-production in England.*

LESSON FOURTEEN

Independents: Miramax and Black Film

sex, lies and marketing: Miramax and the Development of the Quality Indie Blockbuster

Alisa Perren

The origins of an American Beauty *are in 1989 with Steven Soderbergh doing that kind of movie.* —Harvey Weinstein, 2000[1]

In 1989, the world of independent distribution was in disarray. While the appearance of the video market in the 1980s had helped spur the emergence and expansion of a number of independent distributors, by the end of the decade several of these same companies—including Vestron, Island, and Cinecom—had overextended themselves by investing heavily in larger budget, in-house productions. Consequently, by 1989, many within the industry were predicting the death of the independent distributor. However, what seemed to be the decline of independent distribution was actually an "independent shakedown," a label presciently attached to the period by *Los Angeles Times* writer Daniel Cerone in June 1989.[2] Cerone saw that it was a transitional time within the independent world. While the vast majority of independent distributors who had thrived in the 80s were forced to declare bankruptcy by the end of the decade, a few companies were positioned to make a significant mark on the industrial structure and aesthetics of low-budget filmmaking in the 90s. At the head of the pack was Miramax.

The August 1989 release of *sex, lies and videotape* by Miramax marked a turning point in American independent cinema. In fact, the film should be perceived as central to the development of New Hollywood aesthetics, economics, and structure.[3] *sex, lies and videotape* ushered in the era of the "indie blockbusters"—films that, on a smaller scale, replicate the exploitation marketing and box-office performance of the major studio high-concept event pictures.[4] On a cost-to-earning ratio, Steven Soderbergh's creation—with its $1.1 million dollar budget and $24 million plus in North American box office—was a better investment than *Batman,* which—at an investment of $50 million—returned $250 million in domestic box office.[5]

These figures begin to suggest how *sex, lies and videotape* helped to set the standard for low-budget, niche-based distribution in the 90s and to lay the groundwork for a bifurcation within the entertainment industry.[6] In the ten years following the release of *sex, lies and videotape,* each major studio or media conglomerate created or purchased at least one specialty division. These divisions generally operated relatively autonomously from the studio in terms of production and distribution. In the wake of Disney's April 1993 purchase of Miramax, a number of studio-based niche operations emerged, including Universal Focus, Paramount Classics, and Fox Searchlight. The studios focused predominantly on the distribution of big-budget spectacles, while studio-based subsidiaries (which Miramax became in 1993, when Disney purchased the company) focused predominantly on smaller-scale quality pictures that centered on the foibles of well developed characters.[9] While the majors favored projects such as *The Rock* (1996), *Con Air* (1997), and *Enemy of the State* (1998), studio subsidiaries developed such films as *Shine* (1996), *Good Will Hunting* (1997), and *The Cider House Rules* (1999). But it was *sex, lies and videotape,* in the skillful hands of Miramax, that redefined the label of "independence" as it was used by the press and the entertainment industry. During the years that followed its release, a number of films would replicate its financial success and media attention. And the vast majority of these would be theatrically distributed in the U.S. by Miramax.

Miramax in the 1980s

Founded in downtown Buffalo, New York, in 1979 by brothers Harvey and Robert (Bob) Weinstein, Miramax began, like many low-budget distributors of the late 70s and early 80s, by booking live rock-and-roll acts as well as exhibiting classic films and concert movies. But the Weinsteins soon branched out, first with film festivals that screened cult favorites and foreign-language films, and then by moving into production and distribution. They made the kinds of movies that the studios weren't interested in but that had developed into profitable ventures by virtue of the emergence of the home video market. As they slowly expanded during the course of the 80s, the Weinsteins and their staff grew increasingly adept at selling positive images of themselves and their company along with their films. They became known for employing exploitation marketing tactics to promote their movies, with publicity stunts ranging from encouraging *Erendira* (1983) actress Claudia Ohana to pose for *Playboy* to setting up actor Daniel Day-Lewis, who portrayed cerebral palsy sufferer Christy Brown in *My Left Foot* (1989), to testify before Congress on behalf of the Americans With Disabilities Act.

Because the company's executives were so skilled at selling positive images of themselves and their films (including *sex, lies and videotape),* reconstructing a history of Miramax becomes a complicated task. It is often hard to distinguish legitimate claims from exaggeration. Yet in spite of Miramax's effective integration of myth and fact, a number of details about the contours of the company's development can be untangled from the mix.

During the 80s, Miramax consistently released three to four films per year. Except for a few failed efforts in production, including the 1986 co-directorial effort *Playing for Keeps* (released through Universal), the company focused mainly on acquiring and distributing films produced by outside companies. Miramax was interested in a range of documentary, foreign-language, and art house-oriented films, basing their choices on three criteria. First, they selected movies that could be promoted as quality pictures—films that aspired to the status of "art" in terms of style and narrative construction. These movies were often promoted at least in part on the merits of their director's unique vision. Such films—examples are Lizzie Borden's *Working Girls* (1987), Bille August's *Pelle the Conquerer* (1987), and Errol Morris's *The Thin Blue Line* (1988)—had the potential for garnering critical support from the outset, a crucial component for distributors working with limited advertising budgets. Second, Miramax selected nonclassical films that focused on unconventional subjects and styles: *Working Girls* was a hard-edged critique of prostitution, while *The Thin Blue Line* was a documentary about a man on death row whom Morris proved to be wrongly accused. Both films' documentary aesthetic also set them apart from most slick, glossy Hollywood product. Third, Miramax found marketing hooks that could help the films transition from the art house to the multiplex. With *Working Girls,* for example, the Weinsteins "determined how to sell the sex in a film that was utterly, demonstrably unsexy," while with *The Thin Blue Line* Harvey Weinstein pledged, "Never has Miramax had a movie where a man's life hangs in the balance."[8]

Thus, by appealing to multiple niches and using sex, violence, and controversy as sales strategies, the Weinsteins gained a foothold in an increasingly competitive marketplace and attracted the attention of producers and financiers looking for a distributor. As much as Miramax's success can be interpreted as an accident or side effect of a more broadly shifting industrial structure, such an interpretation must be balanced by attention to the business savvy and acute judgment of Miramax executives, led by the Weinstein brothers. Other strategies developed by the Weinsteins throughout the late 80s further aided the company's growth even as most other independent distributors failed. The Weinsteins limited their spending, opted for continuing in acquisitions rather than producing their own films, and restricted their release schedule. The factor that finally motivated the brothers to go into production was an infusion of money in 1988 from Midland Montague Ventures, an arm of the London-based Midland Bank. With a $25 million debt/equity package, the brothers moved from acquiring and distributing films to producing them. Their first in-house production through this arrangement was the aptly titled *Scandal* (1989), a film about British defense minister John Profumo's affair with teenager Christine Keeler. The controversy, with its rumors of the betrayal of state secrets, may have contributed to the fall of the Conservative government in 1963, but it helped Miramax produce a hit. Costing $7 million in a co-venture with Britain's Palace Pictures, the film grossed $30 million worldwide, in part due to a poster that featured a nude Joanne Whalley-Kilmer as Keeler provocatively straddling a chair, and in part due to a promotional/talk-show tour by Keeler herself.

With the success of *Scandal* and the help of good reviews, shrewd marketing, strong festival screenings, and extensive promotions, Miramax began a string of hits that peaked with *Cinema Paradiso, My Left Foot,* and, of course, *sex, lies and videotape,* which played a particularly important role in redefining low-budget filmmaking and marketing. The company rapidly rose from being a mid-level independent distributor to become one of the few surviving independent distributors of the 80s. Even as companies such as Orion, MCEG, and Vestron disappeared from the film scene, Miramax thrived, turning the very label of independent into a sign of distinction. In this process of differentiation, independent films earned more money—and gained more interest from the studios.

sex, lies and videotape: The Beginning of the Indie Boom

It is notable that Miramax played no role in the initial development of *sex, lies and videotape*. In fact, the company did not have any involvement with the movie until it premiered at the U.S. Film Festival (later renamed the Sundance Film Festival) in 1989. The film was co-financed by RCA/Columbia Home Video and Virgin; RCA/Columbia obtained domestic video rights while Virgin retained foreign video. The producers were free to seek a theatrical distributor if RCA/Columbia rejected it upon "first look." This expectation of earning the investment back by video sales and rentals was a holdover from the early 80s, before the consolidation of the video rental industry.

Although the financiers expected to make back their money through rentals, this did not imply that they approved of the presence of the word "videotape" in the film's title. Even before they saw it, according to Soderbergh, the marketing people at RCA/Columbia had asked for a change, believing that "the vendors would *say* that the buying public would *think* that the film was shot on videotape."[9] The film's marketers—even before Miramax—obviously believed that an independent movie carried connotations bearing specific "qualities," but although these qualities may have included the more controversial (and hence salable) elements of sex and lies, they did not include the suggested "low-quality" appearance of videotape. The use of the word in the title was, however, probably more of a boon than a bane. As producer John Pierson explains, the word resonated symbolically: "By using videotape in the title . . . and in the film itself, Soderbergh almost literally ushered in the new era of the video-educated filmmaker."[10] Thus a film in which women confess their sexual histories and anxieties on videotape to help a central male character satisfy himself sexually was marked as timely and distinct for both technological and social reasons. The themes of impotence and sexual paranoia rang true in the late 80s, when AIDS panics were leading the news.

The film gained in popularity throughout the festival (which at this time had 30,000 visitors and was a much more low-profile event than would be the case in later years), screening in front of sold-out audiences and receiving rave reviews. Soderbergh more modestly observed that the "praise is getting out of hand,"[11] but *sex, lies and videotape* left the festival with the Dramatic Competition Audience Award and theatrical distribution offers from several independent distributors as well as one major studio. Yet in spite of extensive praise lavished on the film by the press and festival-goers alike, North American theatrical rights for *sex, lies and videotape* were not sold until a few weeks later, when Miramax purchased them at the American Film Market in Los Angeles. According to Soderbergh, Harvey Weinstein said that he would not go back to New York until he had the movie.[12] By 1989, Miramax had already established a reputation for outbidding the rest of the independent distributors. Yet when Miramax later reflected on how they "won" the rights to *sex, lies and videotape,* "the Weinsteins maintain[ed] that their marketing plan was as crucial as their cash advance."[13]

It is because marketing is as significant as content in the building of the quality independent blockbuster that Miramax's role can be seen as crucial in determining the film's box-office success. Ultimately, the interest created in the film as a result of Miramax's skillful distribution cannot be distinguished from the interest created in it by virtue of its subject matter and storyline. The company played up *sex, lies and videotape* to the press in ways that helped the film move out of the so-called art-house ghetto. In the process of marketing *sex, lies and videotape* as a quality independent as opposed to an art-house entity, Miramax also played itself up to the press in ways that helped to construct the company as the primary force in the film's development and financial success.

The marketing of the film began months before its August opening. According to Bob Weinstein, Miramax started to develop the pre-release buzz for *sex, lies and videotape* at the Cannes Film Festival in May 1989.[14] The film was initially screened for the main competition, but it was rejected and subsequently placed in the Director's Fortnight, the venue for new films from up-and-coming directors. However, a last-minute cancellation from another American film placed *sex, lies and videotape* back in the main competition. Soderbergh worried about the movie being lost in the shuffle, particularly as it was competing against Spike Lee's high-profile *Do the Right Thing*. Yet his film ended up playing to standing ovations and shutting out Lee's film for awards. By the conclusion of the Cannes festival, *sex, lies and videotape* had won the prestigious Palme d'Or, given Soderbergh and his film enormous free publicity, and added to the cachet of festivals as valuable sites for building word of mouth.

Cannes marked just the beginning of the summer marketing blitz initiated by Miramax. The original 1989 press kit for *sex, lies and videotape* hints at the image the company tried to craft to the press and public: "The Weinstein brothers built their company with an aggressive marketing and distribution strategy, individually tailoring each film's release to suit its particular strengths." The very notion of "tailoring" a film on the basis of its strengths reveals the company's dependence on niche marketing. "Marketing is not a dirty word," Harvey Weinstein told the *Los Angeles Times* in May 1989. He continued, in what may be seen as a shorthand manifesto for Miramax as well as a more emphatic articulation of previous conceptions of quality independents:

> *Although we market artistic films, we don't use the starving-artist mentality in our releases. Other distributors slap out a movie, put an ad in the newspaper—usually not a very good one—and hope that the audience will find it by a miracle. And most often they don't. It's the distributors' responsibility to find the audience.*[15]

For *sex, lies and videotape,* this amounted to an attempt to give the film the specialized attention that Soderbergh so desired, packaged as if it was a major studio release. Just one of the means by which Miramax accomplished this was by tapping into the high concept in even the lowest-budgeted film.[16] Thus when Soderbergh developed his own trailer, Miramax quickly rejected it, telling him it was "arthouse death." Although Soderbergh saw his trailer containing "a mood perfectly emulat[ing] the mood of the film . . . [and] not like any other trailer [he'd] ever seen," Miramax demurred. Soderbergh finally reached a compromise with Miramax in which the company used its own trailer, but also filled in some additional footage shot by Soderbergh as a transitional device.

All this suggests that although Miramax may have sold each film on its merits, the company nonetheless had certain ideas about what worked in promoting niche films. Clearly avant-garde trailers were not part of the company's conception of good marketing. An analysis of one of the print advertisements for *sex, lies and videotape* reveals several characteristics of Miramax marketing. In the one-sheet for the film's domestic theatrical distribution, Miramax tried to appeal to several markets simultaneously. First they pursued the art-house audience—a group consisting of cine-literate baby boomers who had grown up on a blend of international art cinema and New American Cinema. This niche, which was presumed to be knowledgeable of the status of festivals as sites for the celebration of global cinema, was sought through the text of the advertisement. At the top of the one-sheet, the most significant festival honors bestowed on the film were listed. Below the list of awards, a number of positive press responses were listed, including opinions from some of the best-known reviewers from the *New York Times,* the *Chicago Sun-Times,* and *Time* magazine.

The second niche targeted by Miramax was the youth audience—college students and twenty somethings. The largest print in the ad, aside from the film's title, came from two critics' statements that constructed two different visions of the film. The first comment, "One of the Best of 1989," associated the movie with the kinds of films that usually receive kudos, such as dramas. Meanwhile, the second comment, "An Edgy, Intense Comedy," suggested a lighter movie well suited for the August release date. The movie was thus differentiated as being more serious than its summer blockbuster counterparts even as it was drawn closer to studio product by its association with comedy. Meanwhile, the images depicted in the advertisement—of multiple couples embracing and kissing—contributed to the film's edgy mystique. Along with the film's title, these images conveyed raciness, excitement, something more adult—and not coincidentally, something more commercial. These images also conformed to the "exploitation" marketing tactics so characteristic of the company at this point in its development. As one reporter observed of Miramax's effective print ads, the company eagerly hinted at sexual desires that were not necessarily apparent in the films themselves. [17]

To many within the industry, Miramax's attempts to find the high concept in low-budget films— while still targeting specific niches in the market—was a welcome approach to a then-struggling independent film scene. As one public relations spokesman stated, in a manner that summed up the sentiments of many, "The marketers of quality independent films aren't doing as effective a job as they might be doing."[18] Hence the logic of Bob Weinstein declaring that "Some guys run from controversy, we run toward it."[19] By establishing this renegade image, Miramax differentiated itself within the marketplace.

The Weinsteins may have penetrated multiplexes in 1989, but they nonetheless remained aware of their position relative to the studios. Specifically, they recognized that their films had to complement rather than compete with the studios' product. They had no illusions that they could match the studios in terms of either financial investment or marketing scale. Thus they relied heavily on free publicity, word of mouth, and counter-programming strategies.[20] While they eventually released *sex, lies and videotape* on about 350 screens, they opened it slowly and let it build on positive reviews and reactions over more than six months. They scheduled a platform release for the film, opening it first only in Los Angeles and New York, and then later moving it into nationwide release by the end of the month. Thus *sex, lies and videotape* had its broadest opening in the time period when the studio blockbusters were fading and quality product was in short supply.

Press and Industry Discourse on *sex, lies and videotape*

To Steven Soderbergh, the overall impact of his film was jarring. In 1990, he returned to Sundance to find a far different scene, one to which he responded negatively. "I'm a little concerned by what *sex, lies* might have wrought here," Soderbergh told the Associated Press, adding, "this can become more of a film market than a film festival." Soderbergh's opinion seemed to be in the minority, however. Many more of those working for independents, as well as those writing about them, looked favorably at the mutually beneficial relationship developing between independents and festivals. Few could have anticipated that this relationship would evolve to the point where the pervasive attitude at Sundance 2000 would be described as "Buy low, *but buy, dammit.* Fail to snap up a certain movie and you might miss out on the next $140 million dollar cash cow. Turn up your nose at a trend and the future might pass you by."[21]

What is apparent in retrospect is that the "small is beautiful" mentality that was beginning to become omnipresent at festivals as well as for promotional purposes was, in fact, the beginning of a larger industrial shift. Rather than *Batman* and *sex, lies and videotape* representing anomalies at both the mass-market and niche levels respectively, they were signals of broader structural and aesthetic changes afoot in New Hollywood. Even as the studios were reviving the same high-concept formulas with such 1990 releases as *Rocky V, Predator 2, Back to the Future III,* and *Days of Thunder,* the independents seemed comparatively fresh and cutting-edge with such films as *Longtime Companion, Pump Up the Volume, Henry V,* and *The Grifters.* The dichotomy between these two types of films indicates the widening split in the kinds of films being produced. The movies that were starting to return the most profits with the smallest risks were either the high-budget, high-concept franchises that had broad international appeal, or low-budget independents that could be targeted to a number of audiences and promoted relatively inexpensively through festivals, word of mouth, and positive critical response.

Thus, although independent releases were down 15 percent in 1989 from the previous year, and box-office receipts were down 7 percent, the slump was short-lived. The continuing global expansion of the industry, rather than contributing to what many predicted would be the demise of independent and/or low-budget filmmaking, actually contributed to their growth. The conditions of social diversity, along with a post-Fordist market structure, similarly led to the development of niche markets as byproducts of the film industry's ever-expanding global orientation. At the same time that many industry analysts predicted the inevitable demise of all but the high-concept blockbuster, then-Cinecom president Amir Malin explained more precisely why niche films would remain attractive culturally and economically:

> *Just because someone sees* Indiana Jones *doesn't mean they won't want to see a sophisticated film like* sex, lies and videotape *or* Scenes from the Class Struggle [of Beverly Hills]. *The fallout will occur with the standard studio fare that cannot compete with the* Raiders, Ghostbusters *and* Batmans.[22]

Malin's comments were prescient for two reasons. First, on the level of industrial structure, he suggests why standard studio fare (or the so-called middle-class films) would be the least cost-effective. Such movies, which at the time of *sex, lies and videotape* included thrillers such as *Pacific Heights* (1990) and romances such as *Joe Versus the Volcano* (1990), based their appeal primarily on their stories or their stars. The studios' event films, conversely, based their appeal on action, special effects, superstars, and simple marketing hooks.[23] Event pictures drove up the marketing, production, and distribution costs of all studio films. However, from the mid-70s onward, the studios increasingly viewed them as worthwhile because of their broader international appeal and synergistic potential.

To a growing number of industry executives, middle-level films did not offer the same global opportunities as event films. If event films failed at home, they could still make money abroad; a Stallone film—typically an event due to his superstar presence—could easily be translated across the globe, guaranteeing international box-office success even if its fate was uncertain in the U.S. If middle-level films failed at home, they were not likely to perform any better abroad, since they had neither the effects and action nor the simple marketing hooks that were the high-concept foundations of the globally oriented Hollywood product. With Disney estimating that by 1996, 60 percent of studio revenues were coming from abroad, and with many executives predicting that the international box office could increase to 80 percent of total entertainment revenues by the first decade of the millennium, event films continued to become more desirable. Meanwhile, middle-level star-genre vehicles—the types of films that were the staple of the Hollywood studio era—continued to lose value.

The second reason for the foresight in Malin's comments comes from his exploitation of the rhetoric of quality. In using the label "sophisticated" to describe *sex, lies and videotape,* Malin employed language in a manner similar to the Weinsteins. In other words, he depicted these movies as special films rather than as industry products. More important than the actual industrial circumstances within which a movie such as *sex, lies and videotape* was produced is the manner in which it was constructed by its marketing team and the press. Companies such as Miramax could take terms such as "independent," "quality," "specialty," and "sophisticated" and use them as points of distinction, helped by the fact that in the late 80s the studios were frequently portrayed in the media as ever-expanding monoliths cranking out cookie-cutter sequels with excessive action and minimal plots.

Miramax's rapid growth stemmed largely from making itself and its films favorites of the press with its emphasis on how films such as *sex, lies and videotape* were different from Hollywood product. Yet at the same time, the company broadened the audience of these same movies by portraying them as what Hollywood had to offer *and more:* full of sex, violence, and risky content.[24] This marketing sleight of hand, in which the films were at once similar and different from Hollywood, helped Miramax and other low-budget distributors carve out an often financially lucrative and aesthetically viable space for independent cinema from the late 80s and into the 90s.

The $24 million earned by *sex, lies and videotape* in its U.S. theatrical release was, however, a small sum compared to the $80 million-plus earned by the quality indie blockbuster hits released later in the decade—movies that included *Pulp Fiction* (1994), *Good Will Hunting,* and *The Talented Mr. Ripley* (1999). Artisan's *The Blair Witch Project,* released almost exactly ten years after *sex, lies and videotape,* represented the culmination of the 1990s independent blockbuster trend. In its cost-to-profit ratio, its application of exploitation marketing tactics, its cinéma-vérité aesthetic, and its use of the discourse of independence to differentiate itself, *The Blair Witch Project* could be considered the cinematic descendant of Soderbergh's 1989 film.

If a strict structural definition of quality indie blockbusters were to apply, then very few independent films would qualify for it. Clearly, from an industrial standpoint, *Pulp Fiction, Good Will Hunting,* and *The Talented Mr. Ripley* are not independent; aesthetically, their independence is also questionable. In the New Hollywood as it evolved in the age of Miramax, indie films increasingly employed established stars and featured classical filmmaking and scripts from established talent. In other words, 1990s indies—if such Miramax movies as *Citizen Ruth* (1996), *Copland* (1997), and *Rounders* (1998) are included—could be considered a hybrid of the studio system's A picture and the post studio-era exploitation film. This suggests the extent to which "independence" (or its hip offspring, "indie") served as a discursive tool employed by the press and the industry. In addition, such indie examples provide further proof that, by the late 90s, the industry's focus was divided between two types of films: niche-targeted and high-concept. Within this context, the niche arena functioned as the key site in which new styles and modes of storytelling were blended to varying degrees; all the while, established talent merged with newer, up-and-coming actors, writers, and directors.

Thus a term that was introduced by the press during the late 80s as a descriptive label to explain structural and aesthetic changes afoot in the New Hollywood morphed in the next decade into a publicity tool for Miramax and its many imitators. The surprising fact was that even though by the mid-90s the label no longer held any definitional value, the press continued to celebrate the companies and the films as if they were guerrillas and renegades fighting Evil Hollywood. The most blatant example of this came from the consistent declaration by the mainstream press that "Independents Day" was afoot during the 1995 Oscar nominations. In this oft-titled "Year of the Independents," four low-budget indies—The *English Patient* (Miramax/Disney), *Breaking the Waves* (October/Universal), *Fargo* (Gramercy/Polygram), and *Shine* (Fine Line/Time Warner)—allegedly trounced the studios, which could only muster up one nominee, *Jerry Maguire* (Columbia). The irony was that all of these independents were released by subsidiaries owned by major media corporations. Yet attention to this shift came much more slowly. During most of the 90s, the mainstream press continued to depict the relationship between independents and majors in terms of conflict and opposition. It was not until Miramax tried to promote *Shakespeare in Love* (1998) as an independent that the tide truly started to turn. It was at this point that a significant portion of the press began to question the use of the label of independence by specialty divisions—and by themselves.

sex, lies and videotape: The Template for the Distribution of the 90s Niche Film

The critical and financial success of *sex, lies and videotape* not only served as an initial step in Miramax's ascendance to the status of top specialty distributor of the 90s, it was also an indication of a changing industry. The bifurcation of the industry came with some repercussions. First, the two Hollywoods each developed interrelated but fundamentally distinct aesthetics. While superstars and super explosions defined the high-concept films, quality independents became defined by well-known actors working for scale because of their belief in the script's explosive subject matter. If high-concept films became known primarily for their glossy look and high production values, quality independents were distinguished by virtue of their gritty look or edgy content. Following in the tradition established by *sex, lies and videotape,* independents of the 90s often stood out either because of an excessiveness in style, sex, and violence, or because of a minimalist aesthetic that emphasizes dialogue over camerawork.

Second, as these films developed in the hands of studio-based specialty divisions, they needed to have a clearly defined niche—whether it was teens, African-Americans, Latinos, women, or the art-house audience. In the process, there was a decline not only in the types of low-budget films that attained distribution, but also in the production of the so-called middle-range product—the standard star-genre formulations that were the bread and butter of the studio system. By the late 90s, such films were typically only placed into production based on the influence wielded by such powerful stars as Jim Carrey, Tom Hanks, and Julia Roberts.

At the beginning of the new millennium, Miramax—as well as the independent scene that it fostered—has changed dramatically. After years of financial support from Disney, the company has grown from an independent to an industry powerhouse in its own right. Miramax regularly releases more than 25 films a year. Films like *Scary Movie, Scream,* and *Chocolat* help the company bring in over $500,000,000 at the box office annually. Occasionally Miramax acquires smaller, independently produced pictures like *Human Traffic* and *Committed*; however, such films are no longer a priority for the company's executives, nor are they the focus of its marketing muscle. Miramax now focuses on developing its own stable of talent—writers, producers, and filmmakers with whom the company had nurtured relationships during the 1990s. Many of these people, including Quentin Tarantino, Kevin Williamson, Robert Rodriguez, Wes Craven, Anthony Minghella, and John Madden, have seen their careers blossom in large part due to Miramax's support.

The company, as well as much of the talent it has supported, has long since moved beyond the boundaries of the independent film world. The styles, subjects, and talent that defined the quality indie scene of the early 90s have now been incorporated into the Hollywood system. Films that earlier might have been labeled quality indies are now regularly produced by studio subsidiaries such as Fox Searchlight, Fine Line Pictures, and of course, Miramax. The content and distribution of *Boys Don't Cry, Dancer in the Dark,* and Soderbergh's own *Traffic* replicate that of *sex, lies and videotape*. And, as Harvey Weinstein observes, *American Beauty* is a direct cinematic descendant of *sex, lies and videotape*. These films continue the tradition established by Miramax in the late 80s and early 90s: aesthetically and topically challenging films can be commercially successful with skillful marketing.

The future, however, does not seem quite so bright for many newer filmmakers and independent distributors struggling to find a space in today's marketplace. With the industry now dominated by a combination of studios releasing big-budget films and specialty distributors handling niche films, independent distributors such as Cowboy Booking International, Winstar, and New Yorker Films are fighting to acquire films and secure available screens. Meanwhile, several of the most influential independent distributors, including Trimark and The Shooting Gallery, have succumbed to today's market pressures and ceased to exist. All of this translates into a much more competitive and uncertain terrain for filmmakers working outside of the studio environment. While Miramax led the way in transforming Hollywood aesthetics, economics, and structure during the 90s, the company has now become a crucial part of the system. It remains to be seen what the next *sex, lies and videotape* will be—and what as yet unidentified company will help drive its success.

Notes

1. Jeff Gordinier, "Defy and Conquer," *Entertainment Weekly Special Edition: Our 10th Anniversary,* Spring 2000, p. 31.
2. Daniel Cerone, "Independent Film Makers, Marketers, Confront Box-Office Crisis," *Los Angeles Times,* 15 September, 1989, sec. 6, p. 4.

3. I employ the New Hollywood label as it is used by Thomas Schatz, "The New Hollywood," in *Film Theory Goes to the Movies,* ed. Jim Collins, Hillary Radner, and Ava Preacher Collins (New York: Routledge, 1998), pp. 25–32. For an extensive discussion of the intersection of aesthetics and marketing of big-budget Hollywood films, see Justin Wyatt, *High Concept: Movies and Marketing in Hollywood* (Austin, TX: University of Texas Press, 1994).

4. The term "indie" has been widely used by trade journalists to include films from studio specialty and niche subsidiaries such as Miramax, Fine Line, and Paramount Classics.

5. Paul D. Colford, "Movies Are Their Game; Miramax Steers Small Films into the Public Consciousness," *Newsday,* 20 February, 1990, part II, p. 8.

6. Scholars and journalists have acknowledged that there has been a split within the industry in recent years between low-budget niche films and high-concept event films, but in general, scholarly work on the emergence of independents and specialty houses has been limited. The majority of attention has been on the evolution of the high-concept blockbuster and big-budget product of the major studios. For examples, see Tino Balio, " 'A Major Presence in All the World's Important Markets,': The Globalization of Hollywood in the 1990s," in *Contemporary Hollywood Cinema,* ed. Steve Neale and Murray Smith (London: Routledge, 1993), pp. 8–36, and Schatz, "The Return of the Hollywood Studio System," in *Conglomerates and the Media,* ed. Erik Barnouw (New York: The New York Press, 1997), pp. 73–106. While Balio, Schatz, and others have addressed the growth of specialty houses to an extent, Justin Wyatt has done the majority of work on low-budget product. For examples, see his discussions of Miramax and New Line in "Economic Constraints/Economic Opportunities: Robert Altman as Auteur," *The Velvet Light Trap* 38 (Fall 1996): pp. 51–67; "The Formation of the 'Major Independent' " Miramax, New Line and the New Hollywood," in *Contemporary Hollywood Cinema,* pp. 74–90; and "From Roadshowing to Saturation Release: Majors, Independents and Marketing/Distribution Innovations," in *The New American Cinema,* ed. Jon Lewis (Durham, N.C.: Duke University Press, 1998), pp. 64–86.

7. I use the word "quality" throughout in much the same way it is used by Jane Feuer, Paul Kerr, and Tise Vahimagi in *MTM 'Quality Television'* (London: BFI, 1984). In "The MTM Style," Feuer, for example, writes that "The very concept of 'quality' is itself ideological. In interpreting an MTM programme as a quality programme, the quality audience is permitted to enjoy a form of television which is seen as more literate, more stylistically complex and more psychologically 'deep' than ordinary fare. The quality audience gets to separate itself from the mass audience and can watch TV without guilt, and without realising that the double-edged discourse that they are getting is also ordinary TV" (56). Quality independent films functioned in a similar sense for theatrical features released in the hands of Miramax.

8. John Pierson, *Spike, Mike, Slackers and Dykes: A Guided Tour Across a Decade of Independent American Cinema* (New York: Hyperion/Miramax Books, 1995), pp. 84, 87.

9. Steven Soderbergh, *sex, lies and videotape* (New York: Harper & Row, 1990), p. 21. In the decade between the release of *sex, lies and videotape* and *The Blair Witch Project* (1999), this attitude shifted to a certain extent. By the end of the 1990s, it often became a means of product differentiation that a movie was shot on digital video.

10. Pierson, p.131.

11. Aljean Harmetz, "Independent Films Get Bigger but Go Begging," *New York Times,* 1 February, 1989, p. C17.

12. Soderbergh, p. 225.

13. Colford, p. 8.

14. Ibid.

15. Cerone, "Taking an Independent Path," *Los Angeles Times,* 3 May, 1989, part 6, p. 1.

16. I apply the label "high concept" in much the same manner as it is applied by Wyatt in *High Concept.* He writes: "High concept can be conceived . . . as a product differentiated through

the emphasis on style in production and through the integration of the film with their marketing" (23).

17. Colford, p. 8.
18. Cerone, "Independent Film Makers, Marketers Confront Box-Office Crisis," p. 4.
19. Cerone, "Taking an Independent Path," p. 1.
20. These tactics would change significantly by the late 90s as Miramax became the prominent studio subsidiary with a solid stable of prominent talent such as Quentin Tarantino, Wes Craven, and Kevin Williamson. At this point, both their product as well as their financial output altered somewhat, as vast sums of money were directed at marketing more commercially viable genre films such as *Scream* (1996), *Jackie Brown* (1997), and *The Faculty* (1998). Yet in terms of quality independents, Miramax's strategies remained remarkably stable during the 90s, altering only to the extent that the company had more capital to invest in production and marketing.
21. Jeff Gordinier and Chris Nashawaty, "Film's Next Frontier," *Entertainment Weekly,* 11 February, 2000, p. 20.
22. Cerone, "Smaller Films Seek a Summer Place," p. 1.
23. See Wyatt, *High Concept,* chapter 1.
24. The tension between presenting something "different" from the majors—and yet also more of the same—was a crucial element in Miramax's rise and its attractiveness to Disney. Yet paradoxically, it has also been the source of much consternation between Disney and Miramax as well as between Miramax and the press. The subsidiary and its parent have been repeatedly forced to test the threshold of what the public could handle in terms of risky and controversial subject matter on numerous occasions, including most dramatically *Kids* (1994), *Dogma* (1999), and *0* (2001). With both *Kids* and *Dogma,* the public outcry over Disney's relationship to these films compelled Miramax to sell the rights to both projects. With *0,* which portrayed racial conflict and violence in an American high school, Miramax kept the project shelved in the wake of the Columbine incident. There was scarcely any media outcry about Miramax handling this film; rather, the company pre-empted any such public conversation by continually pushing the film's release back until finally independent distributor Lion's Gate took over the film's theatrical distribution. This is just one further example of the way that a corporate parent has played a role in shifting the content and marketing strategies of Miramax in recent years. The same story could easily be told with other studio subsidiaries as well.

Blockbusters and Independents: 1975 to the Present

Jesse Algeron Rhines

In the 1970s, the major studios had yet to recover completely from the debilitating effects of the Paramount Consent Decree, the advent of competition from the recently invented television technology, and the doubling of film production costs between 1962 and 1972. In the 1960s, the first two difficulties caused a crisis in the industry.[1] Between 1959 and 1970, the majors' combined distribution of four hundred dropped to an average of only 250 films per year. This low supply of films hurt exhibitors.[2] The majors' incomes were declining. To combat this decline they changed their strategies. Mass communications scholars Garth Jowett and James Linton observe that there are two strategic options to making money in the feature film industry: (1) minimizing production costs, that is, making a smaller, more specialized movie, or conversely (2) maximizing potential appeal, that is, making a blockbuster.[3] Blaxploitation films are extreme examples of the first strategy. *Shaft* and *Superfly* were very low-budget features targeted at a very narrow market, the African American audience. Between 1970 and 1974, many white filmmakers made handsome profits from the blaxploitation genre film.

However, says film scholar Ed Guerrero, "when Hollywood no longer needed its cheap, black product line for its economic survival, it reverted to traditional and openly stereotypical modes of representation, as the industry eagerly set about unplugging this brief but creatively insurgent black movie boom."[4] From the mid-1970s through the 1980s, blockbuster after blockbuster was released by the majors. The *Star Wars* trilogy, the *Indiana Jones* quartet, *Jaws I, II,* and *III,* and *The Deep* were but a few features with elaborate special effects, shot in exotic locations, and paying stars enormous sums of money. However, the films themselves are not the real story of the majors' phoenix-like recovery in the 1980s. Rather, their success is the product of applied research used to promote these films. Film industry insider James Monaco observes, for example:

> *The real secret to Columbia's success in 1977 was not* Close Encounters *at all, it was* The Deep, *a more conventional package, presold by Peter Benchley's novel followup to* Jaws. *It had a couple of stars, some acceptable adolescent sex (Jackie Bisset in a wet teeshirt), and an outrageously racist plot, where not only are the villains all black but they do strange voodoo sex things to our Jackie.*[5]

At $31 million from its June opening to the end of the year, it was the sixth-highest-grossing film of 1977. Success was based on the way producer Peter Guber sold it.

Guber spent nearly two years devising *The Deep*'s marketing strategy. First hardcover, then paperback books were published. Magazine excerpts and condensations followed. Publicity on the set was constant, and journalists were enticed with a junket to Bermuda. Guber wrote the gossipy *Inside "The Deep,"* which was full of behind-the-scenes "news." The first printing of this book was 124,000 copies released the final two days before the film's premiere. Since most workers get paid on the fifteenth, *The Deep* opened June 17, 1977. Research told Guber that by now each potential moviegoer would have been hit by at least fifteen print, television, or other media exposures of the film.

Saturation booking of eight hundred theaters, or about 6 percent of total American theaters at the time, opened *The Deep* on the same day. Guber reasoned that getting theaters filled quickly would protect the film from bad word of mouth or bad reviews. Monaco says the theory is to "get in quick, get the money, and get out before the bad news trickles down . . . . A see-through blue-vinyl soundtrack album, a treasure-chest contest at supermarkets and shopping malls, department store mannequins dressed in *The Deep* tee shirts," and products from boat, watch, and cosmetics manufacturers tied the public imagination to the upcoming film.[6] In June, while a merchandising campaign was building steam, for advertising as well as to make money from tie-ins, Guber, the film's director, Peter Yates, the book's author, Peter Benchley, and the stars were on all the talk shows.

Columbia allotted $1.5 million for print and $1.3 million for television advertising. Their objective was for the nation's fifty top markets to receive two and a half billion visual advertising impressions during the month of June. The publicity, marketing, and distribution campaign for *The Deep* set the mold for the modern blockbuster film. Another Columbia blockbuster, *Close Encounters,* used a similar strategy with an advertising budget of half the film's $9 million production costs. "Saturation marketing" and "saturation release" were the keys to blockbuster success. As a result, "distribution's share of the domestic market increased from $500 million in 1972 to $1,215 million in 1978 or 143%, while the gross U.S. box-office figures grew only 67%."[7]

The Mass Audience

The Peter Guber marketing approach is a wonderful example of the operation of the mass audience model. Clint Wilson and Felix Gutierrez, the authors of *Minorities and Media,* describe this model as one in which racial minorities are seen at the margins of a coveted American mass audience where they are ignored not only by those in the movie industry but by other media that seek a mass audience as well. In 1978, Otis Chandler, then publisher of the *Los Angeles Times,* was quoted as saying, "We cut out unprofitable circulation, and we arbitrarily cut back some of our low-income circulation." In 1976, a *Detroit News* editor ordered his staff to "aim the newspaper at people who made more than $18,000 a year and were between the ages of 28 and 40." Such stories, the editor wrote, "should be obvious: they won't have a damn thing to do with Detroit and its internal problems." Wilson and Gutierrez argue that newspapers seek a mass audience at the demand of their advertisers, who want to reach more affluent, now suburban readers. They say that some newspaper circulation strategies were designed to make it "difficult, if not impossible for residents of ghettos and barrios to subscribe to newspapers . . . at the same time they were starting or expanding new editions in outlying areas. The strategies were defended as being based on economics, because the low-income characteristics of blacks and Latinos made them undesirable newspaper readers."[8]

This approach also states that media seeking a mass audience will look for "commonalities" or "themes" to which large majorities will respond. Again, racial minority groups and their peculiar "cultures and traditions" will be ignored or, where used, will be presented so as not to offend the mass audience. Minorities will be pictured as "seen through Anglo eyes," or stereotyped in order to present a "common content denominator" to potential viewers.[9] However, the most effective way to avoid confronting nonwhite peoples is to avoid employing members of nonwhite races as much as possible.

In line with the least-common-denominator approach to reaching a mass, mostly Anglo audience, the majors either avoided depiction of nonwhite domestic cultures or stereotyped individual minority group members throughout the blockbuster period. Use of a fairly uniform, generic cultural environment aids in appealing to the largest audience possible, which since the 1950s has been about 75 percent under thirty with the greater portion between fourteen and twenty-five years old.[10]

American Film magazine reported that in the 240 films released in 1981 there were only a dozen major roles for Blacks. Of all "on camera parts in the 4th quarter, ten and two-tenths percent went to blacks and Hispanics." Brock Peters, who starred with Gregory Peck in *To Kill a Mockingbird* (1962), stated, "The only leading roles offered to blacks [were] those that support a white lead. There is a false theory that audiences will not go to see a black star unless that star is accompanied by a white counterpart." Yaphet Kotto, who has played significant roles in such films as *The Thomas Crown Affair*, with Steve McQueen, and *Alien*, with Sigourney Weaver, says it's not racism, it's economics: "People want to be involved in fifteen- to twenty-million-dollar movies, and they want their returns guaranteed. So they go for the Redfords, the Connerys, the Brandos. . . . If they ever scale their expectations down and return to modest, low-budget films, they might just turn to me."[11]

Janet Wasko, author of *Movies and Money*, appears to support Kotto's view that race is not the real issue. She says that the movie industry does not produce pure art or pure communication but, rather, commodities that are produced, distributed, and exhibited under market conditions. Market scrutiny "inevitably" influences who makes films, the type of films made, and the manner of public distribution. James Monaco says investors are more likely to "throw in for a share or two" if, by appealing to a minority audience, a film promises to "make back its investment plus a small profit in a relatively short space of time." So casual a strategy is impossible for the blockbuster, however, because the risks are too high: production and marketing costs of up to $30 million, $50 million, even $100 million demand that research virtually guarantee a market before a film is made.[12]

Jowett and Linton observe that the producer knows that his or her films will be viewed by individuals. But as marketeer, the producer must group these individuals into "diverse 'publics . . .' for *each specific movie.*" Producers try to routinize actions required to make a profit on new movies by using actors and ideas already proved to attract an audience.

> *Faced with [high] uncertainty, moviemakers have generated an implicit philosophy or ideology about movie-making which provides them with an image of their audience and their viewing interests. This "audience image" has tended to narrow the range of subject matter and forms that movies employ, and has caused moviemakers to invoke formulaic approaches and engage in imitations of "breakthrough" successes, in what are known as movie "cycles." As innovations are introduced and the environment changes, the "landscape" of the industry adapts, with the "chameleonlike" majors managing to maintain dominance in the marketplace.*
>
> *. . . [A]dvertising campaigns [sometimes] cost as much as the actual production of the movie itself, and "some recent marketing campaigns have cost as much as twice the negative cost."*[13]

In her book *American Film Distribution*, Suzanne Mary Donahue says that large-scale publicity can so whet public anticipation that "people feel that it is a social necessity to see a film."[14] In recent years even box office grosses are published and touted in advertising to draw further attention to a film. The popular belief, generated by high grosses, that everyone else has seen a movie may make more people feel that seeing it is a social necessity.[15]

The early distribution experience of the 1973 independent film *Hester Street* demonstrates how the majors' preconceptions and risk aversion can miss the opportunities presented by a small film. Director Joan Micklin Silver made this film for only $356,000, but it was very well received at the Cannes Film Festival. From Cannes *Hester Street* sold well in several foreign countries. But in the United States, the film made the rounds of the major Hollywood distribution studios three times and was rejected. When Silver and her husband were informed that the film's black-and-white cinematography, low budget, and ethnic orientation caused the majors to predict a box office failure, they decided to distribute it themselves. Because of the film's success at festivals, some exhibitors were willing to book the picture in a few theaters. When *Hester Street* actress Carol Kane received a Best Actress Academy Award nomination, however, hundreds of smaller exhibitors opened up to it. The picture finally grossed more than $4 million.[16]

Despite such rare stories of success and the general profitability of the blockbuster technique, industry professionals still point out that meeting the public's tastes at a particular time remains a crap shoot. Even big-budget films—*Ishtar* and *Hudson Hawk,* for example—can fail, because the public taste is fickle and what seems a sure bet when shooting starts can be the last thing the public wants to see one year later when the film is released.[17]

The mass audience approach dictates that cultural out-groups will be stereotyped or depicted in ways that will not offend the majority of viewers. John Sayles, producer of such low-budget independent features as *The Return of the Secaucus Seven, Brother from Another Planet,* and *Eight Men Out,* who left a prosperous and productive career as a Hollywood writer to become an independent producer, says, "I co-wrote one movie called *The Challenge,* and the director said, 'Well, I know they're all Chinese in the script, but let's make them all Japanese because I can get Toshiro Mifune and who knows the difference anyway?'"[18]

The primary mission of studio heads and those white males responsible for hiring, and against whom many equal opportunity suits are filed, is to design a homogenized film image that will draw greatest number of viewers. Ironically, as Monona Wali points out in *Black Film Review,* Hollywood may be missing an opportunity to reap even larger profits. "Commercial cinema also ignores one of the fundamental realities of America today—it is increasingly multi-racial, multi-cultural society, and the various races and cultures seek to have their images represented in their full and true dimensions."[19]

Since the mid-1970s, as major distributors have reduced the number of films they finance and/or release per year in an effort to release larger-budget films with greater Anglo, mass appeal and a correspondingly greater short-term box office potential, the use of both nonwhite actors and themes derived from nonwhite people has been deemed potentially alienating to this mass audience and therefore avoided or homogenized, that is, depicted in a way distributors project will be nonthreatening to the greatest pool of potential ticket purchasers. From the mid-1970s through the early 1980s, major studio concentration on blockbuster production and mass marketing techniques ended the industry's financial crisis. This focus on so-called high-concept, almost monoracial movies also limited nonwhite people's access to lead roles, to film production financing, and to channels designed to get film products shown in American theaters. Hollywood executives did not realize, however, that by reducing the number of films released they had provided rare opportunity to a new breed of independent producers and distributors.

Niche Marketing

Independent distributors do not start out competing with the majors. Mass marketing is the furthest thing from their minds and abilities. Independents operate in niche or specialized markets normally ignored or serviced by the majors with "B" or genre films. The market at which a film is aimed is very important, especially for the first-time producer and the small distributor. Astute assessment of the types of productions a particular audience will find entertaining and, therefore, will pay to see is the primary task of the specialized marketeer. In fact, what is entertaining to a specialized market is rarely entertaining to a mass audience.

Genre marketing is the independent distributor's equivalent of the majors' mass marketing technique. Success in this area comes from developing a sustained following for films because of specific attributes, whether or not the film is a critical success. Martial arts and horror are genre categories that have developed such followings. A few of these, *Night of the Living Dead* and *Rocky Horror Picture Show,* for example, have also developed a cult following, which ensures a long-term revenue stream. Certain types of comedies do as well, the *Airplane* and *Police Academy* series, for example. The majors secure a devoted following from mass audiences by featuring big-name actors, stars whom large audiences are inclined to see regardless of the film's quality.

Genre films are not "art" films, however. Art films pose a greater risk for distributors since they present a filmmaker's very personal vision for which no audience has been developed. Early John Waters films fit this category, as do *The Producers, El Norte,* Julie Dash's *Daughters of the Dust,* Hector Babenco's *Kiss of the Spider Woman,* and, some say, Spike Lee's *She's Gotta Have It.* Art films have a more narrow, less predictable market than genre films and are frequently shorter lived and less profitable. They rarely contain elements intended for, or conducive to, sequel development: for example, *Night of the Living Dead,* an early 1970s release, led to sequels into the 1990s; yet none of the films Spike Lee has produced sequels his first, *She's Gotta Have It,* because they do not use elements developed in his original success.

Barbara Kopple's documentary *Harlan County, USA* is said to be the avatar and the beginning of a wave of late-1970s independent American feature films.

> *There are several reasons for this sudden surge of activity. The proliferation of film schools in the late sixties flooded the market with ambitious, often socially conscious, young talents. At the same time, the conglomeration of Hollywood reduced the number of low-budget, "experimental" studio films. Unable (or unwilling) to crack the industry, aspiring filmmakers were forced to create their own opportunities. Movies had achieved a certain prestige as tax write-offs—and, for a time, tax shelters—and, even more important, there was an increasing amount of foundation funding available.*[20]

Independent productions of the 1980s differed from films released by the majors both in terms of the amount of money spent on their production and in the way they "imaged" colored people and/or women. Films like *Who Killed Vincent Chin?, El Norte, Do the Right Thing,* and *Desperately Seeking Susan* all challenged the dominant feature film industry's portrayal of nonwhites and/or women and were deemed "socially conscious" for this reason. Independent filmmakers like Peter Wang or Wayne Wang (they are not related) and the Hudlin brothers do not want to make the same kinds of films Hollywood is making. Hollywood's preference for already proven audience-getters is, generally, not in accord with a social consciousness that seeks to overturn the views on race, class, and gender most white American audiences have traditionally supported at the box office. Examples of the views these new filmmakers wish to express are: female independence in thought and action is good; cross-class unity among Blacks aimed at improving conditions for all Blacks should be encouraged; African America continues to be oppressed by white America, and this oppression has always been the reason for most Black poverty and vice; Black Americans retain and celebrate an African heritage; white supremacy is bad; corporate and financial profiteering continues to divide and impoverish the working class; cultural and racial differentiation is acknowledged and accepted. Therefore, non-Europeans need not assimilate European racial or cultural norms to be co-equal within American pluralism.

Reginald Hudlin, a graduate of Harvard University's film program who is sometimes called the "intellectual gremlin of black independent cinema," makes the point: "For a whole year [after its release] I was asked, 'You're a black filmmaker: What do you think about *The Color Purple?*' And I'd say, 'I think you ought to go see a black independent film: That's what's happening.'"[21] The Hudlin brothers are among a growing number of young Black and non-Black filmmakers who refuse the Hollywood approach to film production.

The Black Filmmaker Foundation

By the late 1970s, Black film distributors TAM and Cinemethics International were dead. Over the next decade, Third World Cinema, Women Make Movies, and other nonprofit organizations began to distribute noncommercial and art films by people of color, but their focus was significantly more independent than Hollywood oriented.

In 1978, Warrington Hudlin, a 1974 graduate of Yale University, co-founded and became president of the Black Filmmaker Foundation (BFF), an incorporated, nonprofit arts organization headquartered in New York City. Warrington Hudlin's film career began with his documentary *Black at Yale* (1974) and his undergraduate thesis project, *Street Corner Stories* (1977), a cinema verité piece on the Black community in New Haven, Connecticut. BFF's original mission was to distribute films made by African Americans to libraries, museums, and colleges and to create a dialogue between Black filmmakers and their audience by showing films at community centers and on community access cable channels. By the mid-1980s, it also served as fiscal agent and was commissioned to administer funds awarded to Black filmmakers by other nonprofit organizations. Author and filmmaker Trey Ellis says that BFF is "one of the first black-arts organizations that couples the creativity of the new black artists themselves with the insider's knowledge of high finance from the current flood of young black investment bankers and lawyers."[22] In fact, Black graduates of both Harvard and Yale law schools and Blacks employed on the business side of corporations such as Home Box Office have been BFF board members since the group's inception. Ellis says that BFF's relationship with these professionals is probably what has made it last so long.

Warrington Hudlin became an outspoken critic of Hollywood's continued reluctance to hire African Americans either as actors or behind the camera. He championed the independent spirit exemplified by Melvin Van Peebles's release of *Sweetback*. BFF became a major influence for aspiring filmmakers, such as Spike Lee, whose grants the organization administered. Warrington and other BFF officers became well-known spokespersons before the media and funding sources, as well as at conferences and film festivals where African American or third world filmmaking was concerned.

Spike Lee's NYU student films were also distributed by BFF. Lee gave talks, showed his films, and participated in panel discussions set up by Warrington and the BFF staff. In fact, BFF members, including Reginald Hudlin, appear in Lee's first feature, *She's Gotta Have It* (1986), and helped him mount the production. Proceeds from the New York premiere were donated, at least in part, to BFF. This film's box office success made it the model for other African American filmmakers and for white film financiers and distributors.

Island Pictures and *She's Gotta Have It*

Lee used "creative financing" to produce *She's Gotta Have It* on a low budget of $175,000, and the independent distributor Island Pictures opened the film in a few theaters nationwide. This film tells the story of Nola Darling, who is romantically involved with three very different men who openly resent one another. Jamie is matter-of-fact and appears steadfast. Greer drives a fancy car, knows he's good looking, and cannot understand why Nola doesn't settle down with him alone. Mars is a wise-cracking, bicycle-riding, gold-necklace-wearing, unemployed homeboy who keeps Nola laughing. Russell Schwartz, then president of Island Pictures, released *She's Gotta Have It* as a comedy/art feature in 1986, and this affected the American film scene like few art releases before or since.

Though written, produced, and directed by African Americans, *She's Gotta Have It* had its initial critical success at the San Francisco Film Festival, where it played before an audience that was more than 90 percent white. Success in this venue was a primary determining factor in Island's picking up the film and in the structure of its release pattern. Although impressed by Lee's vigorous promotion of a Black middle-class audience hungry for a feature depicting their own race/class image, even before meeting with Lee, Island executives had "a hunch that there was a segment of America that was not being catered to in terms of movies, and we identified that as a Black middle class that we felt was out there . . . And after speaking with [Spike] about it we said that this makes a lot of sense."[23] Releasing this film downtown demonstrated a successful attempt to bring distribution of Black films in line with a new and untested American attitude toward race relations:

> *The whole idea was to find and test the limits of a black audience—and to expose them, for the first time in many years at that point—to a film that spoke about relationships, and not one that was standard blaxploitation. . . . Further the reason the film was opened in the Lincoln Center area was to avoid the film being "ghettoized." This was done in full consultation with Spike Lee. The surprise was not that Blacks came, but that WHITES came. Based on this successful opening, we were able to give the film a more commercial playoff throughout Manhattan (including Harlem) and the rest of the country. In effect,* She's Gotta Have It *was a break-through film because it not only attracted a black middle class audience, but a white one as well. If we had opened the film in Harlem initially, we would never have gotten it to cross over.*[24]

Although Island was a young company in the mid-1980s, it was a profitable corporation and had built a reputation distributing a number of well-received art films. Statistics and demographics, however, are not the tools relied on by successful distributors. Dennis Greene, former vice president for production at Columbia Pictures, says that "motion pictures are not made on the basis of audience. They're made on the basis of who you want to be in business with."[25] What stars or directors seem to be up-and-coming is more important to a financing company than what statistics say an audience is likely to pay for. This recalls the statement that numbers had nothing to do with Island's decision to distribute *She's Gotta Have It*. In fact, the decision was based on Island's people having seen the film, Lee's conviction that the film would make it, and a "hunch" that the movie would exhibit "legs," or be able to stand on its own.

New Line Cinema and *House Party*

Starting with a budget of $3,000, Robert Shay, son of a grocer, created New Line Cinema and distributed foreign films to college audiences in the mid-1970s. In the early 1980s, he bought the expired copyright for a 1940s-era government production aimed at young people and designed to discourage their use of marijuana. For late-1980s youth this film, *Reefer Madness,* was a tremendous, unintentionally comedic success, and its distribution was so profitable that Shay expanded beyond the campus into movie houses.

Real success began for Shay with the production and distribution of the horror-film-genre *Nightmare on Elm Street,* then the *Friday the 13th* series. The audience for these films included college-age youth but extended New Line's reach to younger audiences who were even more dedicated moviegoers. These films developed a cult following sufficient to sustain many profitable sequels. Emerging film companies like New Line stick to producing films in a limited number of genres, that is, films with particular, predetermined or formulaic attributes and elements demonstrated to have appeal for a certain audience segment. New Line both financed and released the Hudlin brothers' first feature film, *House Party,* in 1990 as one in a series of rap music comedies.

The Hudlin brothers' financial success with *House Party* was, in large part, the product of close attention paid to the economic structural developments in the U.S. feature film industry. As they worked for ten years distributing Black independent films through the Black Filmmaker Foundation, they studied the distribution and marketing aspects of the business. Warrington Hudlin, intimately aware of difficulties Lee encountered in producing the "no-budget" *She's Gotta Have It,* used this knowledge to advantage in negotiations with potential financiers.

Recommended by Lee to film financiers and distributors after his film's success, the Hudlin brothers got their *House Party* produced by independent distributor New Line Cinema for $2.5 million. In March 1990, the film opened in five hundred theaters nationwide with a television, print, and newspaper advertising budget of about $4 million. *House Party,* a feature-length version of a short film Reginald had made as an undergraduate at Harvard, grossed over $30 million in its first six months. It was perhaps the first Black independent feature to attempt to make use of the saturation release and advertising techniques developed by Peter Guber as part of the blockbuster marketing approach. As a result, Warrington Hudlin says, the film grossed more than any other film by a first time Black feature director and more than any other Black independent film except Spike Lee's *Do the Right Thing* through 1991. The result of this success was quick action on the part of the entertainment industry. The June 27, 1990, issue of *Variety* reported Hudlin brothers contracts with both Tri-Star Pictures and NBC television for multiple productions over the next two or three years.[26]

KJM3: A Black Film Distributor

African Americans, as an audience for feature films, are variously defined and delimited. Jacqueline Bobo reported at the 1992 "Available Visions" film and video conference that in 1988 Blacks spent $1.1 billion on theatrical films. This constituted about one-fourth of $4.5 billion spent nationally.²⁷ Spike Lee saw *She's Gotta Have It* as marketable to a Black middle-class audience. Island Pictures opened it near Lincoln Center to boost its crossover potential. In order to avoid competition with the majors in the current period, many small companies avoid the inner-city or underclass audience to whom, they say, the majors are addressing their Black films. For example, KJM3, which was the marketing company for Julie Dash's *Daughters of the Dust* and has now become a film distributor, believes that trying to market to the Black urban underclass would put them in direct competition with the majors.²⁸ KJM3 does not expect to cater to the Black middle class either, because they choose to market films which they call "authentically Black."²⁹ Professor of African American studies Talmadge Anderson says, "Black arts and literary works are truly authentic when they reflect the condition and experience of African Americans in relation to the broader society and world."³⁰ KJM3 defines a Black film as one in which all three positions of authority (screenwriter, director, and producer) are held by Blacks and the story content presents a "representation of how Black people interact" that is believable to the general African American audience.³¹ Michelle Materre, vice president of KJM3, says that "African American media is that which is produced by African American film and videomakers, rather than that which is produced by others about African Americans."³² Thus, for KJM3, the cultural circumstances within which characters interact are important and must ring true for Black viewers." Such films are not expected to cross over to a white, general audience.

> *KJM3's commitment to the Black audience is a cultural imperative. Our specialized focus on the needs and tastes of the Black audience as a whole puts us in a position to satisfy its entertainment needs. The general market competitors, and the specialized "art house" distributors, are very skilled at targeting the general and specialty markets. However, their traditional approach to reaching out to the Black audience results in those films which reflect the African and African-American experience never achieving their potential performance levels, and an audience hunger that remains unsatisfied. . . . Our releases will be marketed on a market-by-market basis, utilizing a strategy which cross-references the tastes, habits and opinions of the African and African-American viewing audience in order to reach the broadest potential market.³⁴*

Julie Dash provided the chance to demonstrate the validity of this view by bringing KJM3 and Kino International, distributors of *Daughters of the Dust,* together. Dash's lyric storytelling shows how an extended family of Geechees, Blacks descended from Africans who largely remained on the sea islands off the coast of South Carolina after slavery, decided to migrate north. In their local Gullah dialect of mixed English and African languages, generations of Black women powerfully narrate, debate, and act out their forceful, emotional, and secret responses to years of rape and other oppressions by local whites. Two hallmarks of *Daughters* are a clear, celebrated memory link between enslaved Africans and post-slavery Blacks and presentation of both familial and romantic love between young and old, male and female.

KJM3 marketed *Daughters* to a core audience via their "surgical marketing model," a method of cross-referencing tastes, habits, and entertainment consumption patterns of that core audience. A major component of this model is a profile of an identifiable, targetable market segment called the cultural grassroots.³⁵ Persons who fit this category may be in the economic underclass, the middle class, or even the small Black upper class. They may be well educated or have little formal training. They may learn African dance or wear traditional African attire and have a strong image of themselves as African. This target group comprises a comparatively small audience and for this reason may have not been respected by general product and media distributors. Yet, in New York and other major American cities, this audience numbers in the millions, and while many of the cultural grassroots will not attend a film for years at a time, they will stand on line for hours to see a film they have heard delivers a representation of African American culture likely to make them feel comfortable. KJM3 used both traditional and nontraditional marketing techniques not only in New York but in New Jersey and Connecticut to promote the film to the cultural grassroots. It arranged interviews on Black radio and television programs, placed stories in major Black mainstream and arts newspapers and magazines, and enlisted the support of many Black social and political organizations. Materre noted that "KJM3 was able to promote *Daughters of the Dust* to Black churches because they contacted the ministers one on one and had them talk it up to their congregations."[36]

Several advance word-of-mouth screenings were held for influential Black people from diverse backgrounds. In addition, KJM3 distributed leaflets describing the film at a variety of venues—at New York–area Black professional organization events normally held during the Kwanzaa-Christmas holiday season, such as the annual Black Expo and the Malcolm X Cultural Conference, both held in New York City, and other events likely to attract Blacks interested in the cultural and political history of Africa and African America. The opening of *Daughters* was scheduled for January 15 to coincide with the nationwide celebration of the Rev. Dr. Martin Luther King Jr.'s legacy and to precede February's annual nationwide celebration of Black history.

KJM3 executives say that they employed this marketing strategy because *Daughters of the Dust* was conceived and funded as a non-commercial, independent work. Materre defines an independent work as one that is "produced primarily as a result of the vision of director or producer [and] is usually funded 'catch as catch.'"[37] Hollywood has released so few films that carry cultural and Sociopolitical content derived from the lived experiences of diasporic Blacks in Africa, Europe, and the Americas that it has no method for reaching the core audience for *Daughters*. *Daughters of Dust* presents such experiences, and white-American-controlled major and "mini-major" distribution companies have not proved competent to reach an audience for them. One might say that a diasporic African work of this type eschews negative stereotyping of Blacks and is opposed to both implicit and explicit inferences of non-Black and Eurocentric domination in any guise. Such works, even as comedies, are likely to support community, communal defense and development among Black people in any part of the world.

Although KJM3 handled marketing for *Daughters of the Dust,* its premiere distribution effort was with the film *Neria* (1992) by Zimbabwe-born director Godwin Mawuru, which opened at the Biograph Theater in Washington, D.C., in early April. The film follows Neria's fight to hold her family together in the face of traditional cultural customs and rituals of inheritance. It is a modern Zimbabwean story, which the distributor's literature quotes *Variety* as saying "looms as an unusual attraction for African American audience tired of Hollywood exploitation . . . heartwarming." In April and May *Neria* played to sellout crowds at the Lincoln Center's "Modern Days, Ancient Nights: Thirty Years of African Filmmaking" festival in New York City. Another culturally authentic film, *Neria* was promoted using the same marketing strategy that KJM3 used to promote *Daughters:* events attended by the core audience were initially targeted, and word-of-mouth advertising spread interest in the film.

Crossover: Content and Marketing Structure Conflict

Eddie Murphy, one of America's most successful screen personalities, enlisted the Hudlin brothers directing/production team for his film *Boomerang*, to be distributed by Paramount, a major studio. Given the tremendous success of Murphy releases such as *48 Hours* and *Beverly Hills Cop I* and *II*, *Boomerang* received perhaps the largest budget, just under $50 million, of any Black production in history. Although the initial *Boomerang* screenplay was written by whites to attract Murphy's normal audience, Reginald Hudlin altered the film to such an extent that the story became more accessible to Blacks than to whites. The result was that Blacks turned out for the film in large numbers while whites were significantly less inclined to see it. *Los Angeles Times* film reviewer Kenneth Turan, for example, said:

> *You can tell a performer is in trouble when his legal entanglements are more entertaining than his movies. . . . Watching Murphy in "Boomerang" it is almost impossible to remember the sharp, high-spirited exhilaration he brought to comedy in films like "48 HRS" and "Trading Places." . . . [T]he character he plays . . . is no hustler, no scrambler after respectability, he is a polished and successful director of marketing for a successful cosmetics corporation. . . . Watching the best*

> *wisenheimer in the business determinedly turning himself into a sensitive, New Age guy is an exercise in sheer frustration.*[38]

In *Hollywood and the Box Office,* John Izod says that a film must make two and a half times its production costs before it breaks even.[39] Grossing $70 million on a production budget of about $50 million, *Boomerang* is considered a domestic financial failure despite excellent reception in the African American community. *Boomerang* turned out not to be a crossover film. However, the final word on this is yet unspoken.[40]

This case provides evidence that culture has box office significance. It also demonstrates that there may be an upper limit on the size of the return that can be expected from a particular market segment. This has implications for how big a film production budget a market segment can support. In contrast to Dennis Greene and Island executives, KJM3 feels that if it is targeting the Black audience with an "authentically Black" product, it may be unwise to finance a higher budget than that audience can profitably reimburse.

Although on a creative plane screenwriters abhor the thought that audience and financial considerations determine their scripts, distributors and investors are naturally very concerned with who is likely to pay to see their releases. It is therefore the business side of filmmaking that tries to match a script with a profitable viewing audience. A major consideration in this regard is how accessible the film will be to a large white audience approaching two hundred million persons, with potential single-film revenues (at an average four dollars per ticket in 1992) of $800 million, as opposed to a smaller Black audience that may number well under ten million with corresponding single-film potential revenues of $40 million. Thus, even before a production budget can be validly considered, the issue of crossover potential must be addressed.

In today's film industry, *crossover* refers to the potential of a film addressing nonwhite Americans' concerns to secure a significant financial return from white American viewers. While one might argue that a film addressing white concerns can conceptually cross over to a nonwhite audience as well, since the real issue is the film's "legs" or moneymaking ability, the size of the white market can *alone* provide very strong legs, so crossover to nonwhites need not be considered seriously. Culture and finance are intimately interwoven within the crossover concept, and because whites control film financing, nonwhite filmmakers must consider their films' crossover potential to attract white private financing.

Yet, Spike Lee says to nonwhite filmmakers, "No, you don't have to cross over. Not at all. That depends on what the film is. There's no law. Like *School Daze,* I knew going in it was gonna be very hard for a white audience to relate to what happens on a Black college campus. Whereas *She's Gotta Have It* was more accessible to them. Same thing with *Do the Right Thing.*" But when asked why *She's Gotta Have It,* if it was so accessible to whites, was advertised as a comedy even though he had never viewed it as such, Lee said, "Anytime when there's Black people involved they put 'comedy' on it. Makes it more palatable for the white audiences. Whereas drama, they might be uneasy, might be uneven."[41] Whether or not there is truth in this statement, it indicates that African America's number one filmmaker feels the need to fight industry stereotypes even before his films are written. Films such as *Boyz N the Hood* and *Menace II Society* are condemned for catering to the Blacks-as-violent or criminal stereotypes like those dominant in the blaxploitation period. By contrast, movies featuring Blacks as neither violent nor comic, such as *Daughters of the Dust* and *To Sleep with Anger,* have been very poorly received in distribution circles.

Black films must be presented to white distributors in particular ways that are consistent with white audience stereotyping of Blacks in order to predict crossover success. Such predictions, of course, sometimes go awry, Despite the presence of Eddie Murphy, the crossover champion, for example, many observers believe that because he was in a Black business situation (similar to the Black college situation of *School Daze*), with 90 percent Black characters presented as successful professionals, white audiences found *Boomerang* inaccessible, which made it a crossover failure. Turan, for example, found that

> *the most intriguing aspect of* Boomerang *turn[ed] out to be not its story but its racial composition. . . . [T]his kind of cinematic affirmative action can be seen as*

> *very long overdue, but unlike the dramatically motivated all-black cast of* A Rage in Harlem *[a gangster film in which Blacks mutilate each other] it feels in its own way as silly and arbitrary as mainstream movies without any people of color on screen.*[42]

White audiences find Murphy accessible only when he is among 90 percent white characters in a story line aimed specifically at whites culturally. Such films' crossover revenues from a Black audience are a mere bonus since Black cultural considerations are addressed only tangentially, if at all.

Warner Bros.' 1992 release of Spike Lee's film *Malcolm X* is a case in point. When Lee demanded $35 million from Warner Bros. to produce the film he said it deserved the same budget the studio had provided for Oliver Stone's *JFK*. Warner Bros. thought otherwise on the basis that JFK as icon had a much larger potential audience than did Malcolm X. To paraphrase the famous Lloyd Bentsen quip, they were saying, "Spike, your Malcolm is no Kennedy."

That Lee thought his film could command as large an audience as *JFK* reveals how much Malcolm X's image has changed over the years, or at least the kind of image Lee was willing to fashion. Historically, JFK and Malcolm occupied entirely different political spheres. It's hard to imagine any circumstance in which Malcolm would have been invited to tea at Camelot. Nor can we visualize Kennedy, rather than Martin Luther King Jr., smiling and shaking hands with Malcolm in that famous photograph *Do the Right Thing's* Smiley lugged about. It's also doubtful that Malcolm would have issued a "chickens coming home to roost" statement had King rather than Kennedy been assassinated in 1963. Martin and Malcolm did not agree on strategies and goals, but they were not asymmetrical in the way Malcolm and JFK were. Malcolm and JFK had followings that differed radically in their racial composition, their long-range goals, and, most important, in numbers of persons. Something profound must have happened to the image of Malcolm and/or of JFK over the decades if, in the 1990s, they were considered, by the commercial film industry, capable of attracting equivalent, much less the same, moviegoing audiences. Or perhaps it is the image of Malcolm as shaped by Lee that became compatible with the image of JFK as shaped by Stone.

The major consideration for Warner Bros. regarding *Malcolm X* was whether or not it could get a crossover audience. How else could a $35 million, three-hour-plus epic bring in the nearly $90 million needed to make it a success? Malcolm had been despised by the vast majority of whites during his lifetime and disliked by a majority of Black Americans as well. JFK, in contrast, had a reasonable chance for reelection, and his death transformed him into a national martyr on the scale of President Lincoln. The conspiracy angle to *JFK* added additional dramatic dimensions that seemed lacking in the conventional version of Malcolm's assassination. Put more simply, if one assumes an average national admission price of four dollars, and if 50 percent of all thirty million African Americans bought a ticket to see *Malcolm X*, the box office return would be $60 million. If 50 percent of the two hundred million white Americans bought tickets, the return would be $400 million. This nearly seven-fold gap in returns determined Warner Bros.' consideration that a crossover audience, and not a Black audience alone, had to be the primary market for *Malcolm X*.

To meet that need, Lee dampened every controversial aspect of Malcolm's life as well as many of the period's specifically Black cultural referents. Malcolm, for instance, is the only Black person in the film to use the term "Daddy-O." This exemplifies the dilemma faced by any African American filmmaker who wants to attract mass, or crossover, market dollars. When he or she views white filmmakers and their works as the primary models, the tolerance level and cultural biases of the white audience become critical.

Unlike Warner Bros., however, KJM3 is not in the crossover business. It expects to get 100 percent of its revenues from the cultural grassroots, a segment of the Black audience numbering probably well under five million with a potential single-film revenue of $20 million maximum. Dividing this maximum revenue by the break-even ratio of 2.5 equals a maximum production cost per film of $8.8 million. Applying this same reasoning, with a budget of $50 million, projected revenues for *Boomerang* must have been $125 million. Yet, from an admittedly high ten-million-person potential Black audience, only a maximum of $40 million could be expected. Paramount must have expected the other $85 million to come from the white community. It did not. In fact, total first-year domestic receipts were $15 million short of the $85 million whites must have been projected to provide and double that expected from Blacks. At a cost of $800,000, by contrast, and revenues of $1.8 million in thirty-three rather than fifty-two weeks, with an audience that was perhaps 90 percent Black, *Daughters of the Dust* exceeded expectations.

The need to cross over in order to satisfy distribution company demands for box office return impinges on African American filmmakers' ability to depict African America's political life and culture.

Reassertion of the Majors' Dominance over Film Distribution

The majors' neglect of exhibitor needs in the 1970s allowed independent distributors and producers to gain ground. In the mid 1970s, theatrical release of films written, directed, and produced by Blacks was virtually nonexistent. The majors dominated film distribution with high-cost, culturally white blockbusters such as *Star Wars* and *Indiana Jones*. Now, in the early 1990s, by contrast, the success of tiny distribution companies, such as Kino International, has inspired the creation of still smaller, culturally focused companies such as KJM3. But this is by no means the end of the story. While only the majors can afford to experiment with the expense of making blockbusters, they are simultaneously enticing new Black filmmakers the independents have proved successful and buying existing independents and creating new, "boutique" distributors of their own.

The majors have also begun to experiment with hiring young Black filmmakers untested even in the independent arena. The best two examples of this are the Columbia Pictures financing of features by then-twenty-three-year-old John Singleton in 1990 and "twenty-something" Darnell Martin (she won't tell her age) in 1993. Singleton's film, *Boyz N the Hood,* grossed nearly $60 million on a production budget of between $6 and $8 million. Martin's *I Like It Like That,* which opened in October 1994, cost $5.5 million and grossed a very disappointing $1.2 million in its first year. It was the first feature directed by an African American woman with Hollywood financing and distribution.[43]

Spike Lee says that a small distribution company is almost doomed to failure. Of KJM3 he says, "I don't know how [they're] gonna do distribution, you gotta have tons of money. First of all anytime you start out, especially if you're Black, the majors, they're gonna try to crush you."[44] The reality of this threat is brought home by the fact that Island, which released *She's Gotta Have It* in 1986, has been forced out of domestic distribution due to severe competition from the majors. Orion, New World, and Vestron Pictures, all thought to be distribution companies with bright futures in the mid-1980s, have either filed for bankruptcy or significantly reduced their distribution activities. Samuel Goldwyn, Inc., which released Robert Townsend's *Hollywood Shuffle,* has not proved to be an aggressive player in the 1990s Black film arena. In fact, since 1990 the major players in the distribution of Black independent feature film productions have been the majors themselves. The champion of all Black independent producers, Spike Lee, is a willing participant in this reaggregation of U.S. film distribution.

Since the independent Island Pictures released his first film in 1986, Lee has gone from one major to another: first Columbia for *School Daze,* Universal for *Do the Right Thing, Mo' Better Blues,* and *Jungle Fever,* Warner Bros. for *Malcolm X,* and back to Universal for *Crooklyn* (1993) and *Clockers* (1995). Of course, it is reasonable that a talented filmmaker will outgrow a company whose financing abilities are limited, but Island is no longer sponsoring up-and-coming filmmakers. It is, rather, out of the domestic film business altogether. Lee has started to play executive producer for films by other filmmakers. He is neither writer, director, nor producer on these new projects. He merely approves a script and attaches studio production financing and distribution, as Steven Spielberg did on the *Back to the Future* series. Lee's first executive production, *The Drop Squad,* opened in October 1994. It was financed and distributed by Universal's new low-budget subsidiary, Gramercy Pictures, of which Russell Schwartz is president. Schwartz, formerly an independent distributor, is now part of the Hollywood establishment.

Like Spike Lee, the Hudlin brothers moved from independent to Hollywood distribution companies. They were with New Line for *House Party,* then a two-film deal with Columbia subsidiary Tri-Star was rumored but never realized, then they went to Paramount for *Boomerang* with Eddie Murphy and for their animated feature *Bebe's Kids*. In 1994, the Hudlin brothers moved their offices from New York City to the 20th Century Fox lot in Los Angeles. Their latest venture was *Cosmic Slop,* a ninety-minute special produced and aired on Home Box Office (HBO), which is part of the Time Warner corporation. *Cosmic Slop* was described in the *New York Times* as something "more than a multicultural 'Twilight Zone,' with a bit of 'Playhouse 90' and 'Yo! MTV Raps!' thrown in."[45]

With the success of *House Party* and *Teenage Mutant Ninja Turtles,* New Line graduated to the category of mini-major and created its own art distribution subsidiary, Fine Line. In 1994, New Line merged with Atlanta-based Turner Communications Company.

Robert Townsend went from Samuel Goldwyn for *Hollywood Shuffle* to 20th Century Fox for *The Five Heartbeats.* Charles Lane went from *Sidewalk Stories* at Goldwyn to Disney, where he was hired to direct *True Identity.*

The majors, then, are not allowing the course of feature film distribution to be taken from their hands. Rather than shun Black filmmakers, they endorse and sponsor them. In this blockbuster period, the majors may be using generally low-budget Black film productions to pad the package offered exhibitors. Traditionally "B" and genre films were used as padding. Low-budget films by African Americans, however, provide the added bonus of addressing racial inclusion complaints voiced by the NAACP and still serve the purpose of keeping the majors' competition at bay.

In a sense, Black filmmakers may be seen as pawns manipulated in white distributors' power games. While this may, in fact, be the case, the question from many African American filmmakers' point of view is really to what extent can they manipulate the distributors to continue getting their productions seen and to gain more influence in the industry. At one time, Warrington Hudlin said that Black filmmakers were the exploited cheap laborers of the industry because their productions were financed at such a low level but gained such a high relative return. But the Hudlin brothers' film *Boomerang* had a higher budget than a great number of white filmmakers have been allowed. Though it was less profitable at the box office than had been expected, this does not appear to have harmed the brothers' outlook for future production financing. In addition to the yet-to-be-realized two-picture Tri-Star deal, the Hudlins still have television offers and are in the early stages of executive producing other filmmakers' productions. Robert Townsend, whose *Five Heartbeats* also bombed despite continued good reviews from individual African American viewers, has completed his third feature, *Meteor Man.* For Gramercy, Mario Van Peebles directed *Posse,* the first Black western since the 1972 *Buck and the Preacher.* Independent distributor Miramax, now teamed with Disney, released the second feature by an African American woman, the low-budget *Just Another Girl on the IRT.* In fact, those "in the mix" generally feel that if you're Black and not getting money out of Hollywood now, something's seriously wrong with you. And, unlike the blaxploitation period of the 1970s, Black people are *behind* and *in front* of the camera now. This means that Blacks have significant decision-making authority once a studio has decided to work with a picture. True, corporate board rooms and executive suites remain largely white and male, but the Spike Lee phenomenon has allowed a few Blacks a new level of entree into the film industry.

Although there are reasons for optimism, however, it is important to remember that Hollywood's openness to African Americans is the result of a structural aberration. It is much too early to call this the norm. The majors may find new ways to make larger profits without Blacks, as happened in the beginning of the blockbuster period. The independent distributors who introduced most of the new Black filmmakers have largely joined the Hollywood establishment. The resulting structural environment, where the majors own boutique distributors and are expanding their control of cable and theatrical distribution venues, is too tight to predict success for a new crop of independents. African American filmmakers who have distribution deals are likely to support this trend because it brings a higher level of professionalism to their projects.

Notes

1. Jowett and Linton, *Communication,* p. 35
2. Donahue, *Distribution,* p. 103.
3. Jowett and Linton, *Communication,* p. 34.

4. Guerrero, *Framing*, p. 70.
5. Monaco, *Film Now*, p. 25.
6. Ibid.
7. Edgerton, *Exhibition*, p. 55.
8. Clint C. Wilson II and Felix Gutierrez, *Minorities and Media* (Beverly Hills: Sage Publications, 1985), pp. 54–55.
9. Ibid., p. 40.
10. Izod, *Box Office*, p. 181.
11. Michael Dempsey and Udayan Gupta, "Hollywood's Color Problem," *American Film* 7, no. 6 (April 1982): 68.
12. Janet Wasko, *Movies and Money* (Norwood, Conn.: Ablex Publishing, 1982), p. xix; Monaco, *Film Now*, p. 22.
13. Jowett and Linton, *Communication*, pp. 26, 30.
14. Donahue, *Distribution*, p. 83.
15. Ibid., p. 58.
16. Ibid., p. 73.
17. CNN's *Inside Business*, aired in New York on March 29, 1993, featured Home Box Office, *Variety*, and National Westminister Bank executives who spoke to this issue.
18. Spike Lee, "Class Act," *American Film* 13, no. 3 (January/February 1988): 57.
19. Monona Wali, "LA Black Filmmakers Thrive Despite Hollywood's Monopoly," *Black Film Review* 2, no. 2 (Spring 1986): 10.
20. J. Hoberman, "The Non-Hollywood Hustle," *American Film* 6, no. 1 (October 1980): 54–55.
21. Lee, "Class Act," 57.
22. Trey Ellis, "The New Black Aesthetic," *Callaloo* 12, no. 1 (Winter 1989): 237.
23. Interview with an Island Pictures executive, November 10, 1992.
24. Letter from an Island Pictures executive, March 11, 1994.
25. Dennis Greene interview, October 5, 1992.
26. Amy Dawes, "Time to 'Party' for Hudlins; Brothers Ink Film, TV Deals," *Variety*, June 27, 1990, p. 16.
27. Jacqueline Bobo, "Conference Report," *Available Visions: Improving Distribution of African American Independent Film and Video Conference*, July 24–26, 1992, San Francisco Arts Commission, December 1992, p. 11.
28. Interview with a group of KJM3 vice presidents, October 1, 1992.
29. Ibid.
30. Talmadge Anderson, *Introduction to African American Studies* (Dubuque: Kendall/Hunt, 1993), p. 252.
31. KJM3 vice presidents interview.
32. Bobo, "Conference Report," p. 15.
33. While use of the term *authentic* to delineate a cultural tradition has recently come under question, KJM3's usage reflects that of philosopher Jean-Paul Sartre. Sartre said of the European Jew within a context dominated by gentiles: "What the least favored of men ordinarily discover in their situation is a bond of concrete solidarity with other men . . . The sole tie that binds them is the hostility and disdain of the societies which surround them. Thus the authentic Jew is the one who asserts his claim in the face of the disdain shown toward him." Jean-Paul Sartre, *Anti-Semite and Jew* (New York: Schocken Books, 1976), p. 91.
34. KJM3 Entertainment Group, Inc., brochure acquired April 1995.

35. KJM3 vice presidents interview.
36. Bobo, "Conference Report," p. 14.
37. Ibid., p. 15.
38. Kenneth Turan, *"Boomerang:* Eddie Murphy's Romantic Fling," *Los Angeles Times,* July 1, 1991, p. Fl.
39. Izod, *Box Office,* p. 172.
40. Although theater attendance for *Boomerang* was less than projected, Warrington Hudlin, the film's producer, says it was the number one grosser three weeks running upon its videocassette release.
41. Spike Lee interview.
42. Turan, "Romantic Fling," p. F7.
43. Delvin Molden, *African American Film Statistics and Marketing Strategies* (Chicago: D. Molden, 1994), n.p.; Jan Hoffman, "Mom Always Said, Don't Take the First $2 Million Offer," *New York Times,* October 9, 1994, p. H28.
44. Spike Lee interview.
45. Andy Meisler, "Using Fun to Show Blacks to Whites," *New York Times,* November 7, 1994.

Spike Lee's Bed-Stuy BBQ

Marlaine Glicksman

It's the hottest day of summer in Bed-Stuy, Brooklyn, where the only thing hotter are people's tempers and a ghetto blaster not only rocks the house but burns it down. While Spike Lee's previous films looked at the under- and crosscurrents of male/female and light/dark-skinned black interactions, in his third feature, *Do the Right Thing*, Lee takes a magnifying glass-under-a-hot-sun look at black/white relations and the result—no surprise—is fire.

Do the Right Thing stars Ossie Davis, Ruby Dee, Danny Aiello, John Turturro, Richard Edson, and Lee veterans Joie Lee, Bill Nunn, Sam Jackson and Giancarlo Esposito, along with newcomer Rosie Perez. It was shot in Bed-Stuy using an almost all-black crew (a rarity in the film industry) during a recordbreaking heatwave.

To pave way for the production, Lee rejected the usual police surveillance from the Mayor's Office of Motion Pictures and instead installed members of the Fruit of Islam. With them, he also cleared the block of three crack houses. Sets were reconstructed from gutted buildings; behind the film's Korean fruit stand stood an empty shell. A pizza parlor was erected, murals painted, the street cleaned up, a block party thrown and the shoot was under way. The Antioch Baptist Church served as canteen, where lunch on some days consisted of ribs and assorted Louisiana hot sauces.

For his role as Mookie, the meandering young black man who is the film's pivotal character, and who cares less about his girlfriend and young son than getting paid, Lee donned a fade-out flat top and a gold tooth. Cinematographer Ernest Dickerson once again stood loyally behind the lens while the director's brother, David Lee, shot more of the enigmatic stills we saw in Lee's *She's Gotta Have It*.

Lee's film comes at a time when New York City is a racial tinderbox. The alleged black gang rape of a white Wall Street woman this April in Central Park angers whites, smears blacks and triggers Donald Trump to take out a full-page ad in the *New York Times* calling for reinstatement of the death penalty (yet there was no such outcry when Michael Stewart and Eleanor Bumpurs—blacks to whom Lee dedicates his film—*died* at the hands of NYC police in separate controversial incidents). The *Amsterdam News,* favored by a black readership, likened the handling of the Central Park rape to the Scottsboro boys, who were falsely convicted and nearly executed for the rape of a white woman in Alabama fifty years ago. One month later, after a twenty-five-year-old black man died in police custody, one black woman told the *New York Times,* "This is crazy. There's going to be a riot. Somebody is going to get killed and it'll probably be us."

Do the Right Thing takes up the message. Nobody wins when oppressive heat and Raheem's radio causes a meltdown in Sal's Famous Pizzeria. What bubbles up is not mozzarella but the bad feelings hidden beneath. The film, which explores the black underclass, ends with two quotes, the first by Dr. Martin Luther King in favor of non-violence, stating, "The old law of an eye for an eye leaves everybody blind," countered by Malcolm X's "I am not against violence in self-defense. I don't even call it violence when it's self-defense, I call it intelligence." It is on this quote that the film closes.

Lee is no stranger to controversy. The MPAA rated *She's Gotta Have It* with an X—later reduced to R after it was recut—because Lee included a lovemaking scene with nude black bodies. In *School Daze,* Lee broke the conspiracy of silence about prejudice between light- and dark-skinned blacks in his depiction of an all-black college campus during homecoming. *School Daze* also probes blacks' attitudes toward apartheid—income from South Africa helps keep the school running. And in one poignant scene Lee clashes Africa-identifying co-eds with their Jerri-Curled, shower-capped, local "brothers," who spout animosity like ketchup: "We're not your brothers. How come you college mother-fuckers think you run everything? You come into our town year after year and take over. We were born here, been here, will be here all of our lives, and can't find work 'cause of you."

School Daze was criticized by fellow blacks who did not want long-hidden dirty laundry on view for white eyes. But as always, Lee's films are topical. A case before the Atlanta Federal Court highlights the heretofore unmentionable: a woman is suing her former employer, alleging discrimination based on skin color. Both the woman and her employer are black; the plaintiff, however, is light-skinned.

Do the Right Thing, like Lee's other films, is a black insider's perspective on the contradictions and celebrations of African-American life. But Lee's talent lies in creating characters that transcend race and economic status and speak to us all. His Bed-Stuy comes alive with neighborhood people we know: Mother Sister (Dee), matron of the block; Da Mayor (Davis), block philosopher: Sweet Dick Willy (Robin Harris), Coconut Sid (Frankie Faison) and M.L. (Paul Benjamin), the Greek-chorus triumvirate who seek shelter from the sun in beer and beneath a beach umbrella; and even the Puerto Rican helado "icee" man carting his big block of ice and syrup bottles. It is a block where English intermingles with Spanish, where salsa meets Raheem's rap and the air is radio-active with Señor Love Daddy's We-Love show, as he does "the nasty to ya ears" with "da platters dat matter," with black music ranging from rap and juju to reggae and soul—a block where music is a main character.

Nor does this film shy from hot topics within the community. The triumvirate express anger and jealousy over the Koreans' ability to establish a successful business in their neighborhood: "Either them Korean motherfuckers are geniuses or you black asses are just plain dumb!" M.L. declares. It is also where, in a hilarious but biting scene, "You dago, wop, garlic-breath pizza slinging Vic Damone" is countered by "You gold-teeth, gold chain-wearing, fried-chicken-and-biscuit-eatin' monkey"; where "You slanty-eyed, me-no-speak-American, Korean kick-boxing, son-of-a-bitch," is met by "You Goya bean-eating, fifteen in a car, thirty in an apartment, meda-meda, Puerto Rican cocksucker" and "It's cheap, I gotta good price for you, B'nai Brith, Jew asshole!" It is where the battery-powered message carrier Radio Raheem (Nunn) blasts the word: "Fight the Power," and rules—almost to the end.

Lee's films differ not only in their black perspective—in an industry where few blacks have a voice—but also in their ability to look at both sides of the coin at once. As in real life, his characters are neither all good nor all bad.

And therein lies their—and Lee's—power: the minute he establishes our identification with a character, Lee turns him inside out to reveal the dark side in us all.

Lee's films are unmistakably Spike: direct, outspoken, no-holds-barred, tell it like it is, pointed and hard-hitting. He approaches his subject matter without hesitation, earning him a reputation as both audacious and arrogant. *Do the Right Thing* is not only an assertion of black life but, importantly, of filmmaking. It strikes you with the speed, color and style of graffiti: an urban, in-your-face declaration.

Lee's production company, 40 Acres and a Mule Filmworks, is young and black and located in the heart of Brooklyn, amidst Jamaican patty and spice parlors and other black-owned businesses. Nearby, Lee runs film workshops for minimal fees for those who can't afford the tuition and bureaucracy of film schools but still have a dream.

M G: *How did* Do the Right Thing *come about?*
S L: It started because of the whole Howard Beach incident. I wanted to do something to address that and racism. It's been reported several places that this film is the retelling of Howard Beach. This is a completely *fictional* thing. We took four things from it: the baseball bat, a black man gets killed, the pizzeria, and the conflict between blacks and Italian-Americans.

M G: *How did the ideas develop for the film, and how were they influenced by logistics? It's hot material.*
S L: I wanted it to be one twenty-four-hour period, the hottest day of the summer. I wanted the film to take place on one block in Bedford-Stuyvesant. So that's all the stuff I needed to work with, to start with. From there I could just go ahead and do what I had to do.

The script doesn't come to life till you shoot it. The finished film's always going to be different. I'm always true to what I'm saying, but the most important thing is to do what's right. If I write something, and it comes out in rehearsals that something else is better, we change it.

Every time I do a film, people ask me, 'Did you have full artistic control?' I mean, *She's Gotta Have It, School Daze* and *Do the Right Thing*—we made the films we wanted to make.

M G: *How did the character of Smiley, the Dostoyevskian "village idiot," develop?*
S L: He's not in the script at all. It came about because Roger Smith, the actor, kept hounding me. So we went for something that wouldn't seem like it was just an afterthought.

M G: *Roger Smith, who plays Smiley, doesn't have cerebral palsy in real life?*
S L: No, that was an act. We just wanted him to be a different character.

M G: *Is Smiley a symbol of the black man as handicapped. . . .*
S L: I wasn't thinking about that.

M G: *Who is Mookie, the character you play? His relationship with Tina, the mother of his child, is unresolved. We don't really know what his hopes and his dreams are, except wanting to get paid.*
S L: That's all it is. Just live to the next day. He can't see beyond the next day. Mookie is an irresponsible young black youth. He gave Tina a baby. He changes, but up to that point he doesn't really care about his son or her.

M G: *The end of the film is very powerful, and yet, somewhat ambiguous. How do you reconcile the two quotes, one from Dr. King and the other from Malcolm X?*
S L: Well, I don't think it's ambiguous. I think you really have to concentrate on what the final coda of the film is: the Malcolm X quote, not the Martin Luther King quote.

M G: *Malcolm X said, "I am not against using violence in self-defense. I don't even call it violence . . . I call it intelligence." Is the riot then, doing the right thing?*
S L: In that specific case it is, because Mookie and the people around him just get tired of blacks being killed by cops, just murdered by cops. And when the cops are brought to trial, they know nothing's going to happen. There's complete frustration and hopelessness.

They've seen it so many times: Howard Beach, Michael Stewart, Tawana Brawley, Eleanor Bumpurs. Nothing happens. The eight cops that murdered Michael Stewart—that's where we got that Radio Raheem stuff. That is the Michael Stewart chokehold. Except we didn't have his eyeballs pop out of his head like Michael Stewart's did—[the police and medical examiner] greased his eyeballs and tried to stick them back in the sockets. There's a complete loss of faith in the judicial system. And so when you're frustrated and there's no other outlet, it'll make you want to hurl the garbage can through a window.

M G: *If you read about an incident like the one in Central Park in the* Amsterdam News *and then compare it with* The New York Times *coverage there are two different perspectives. . . .*
S L: A couple days later a black woman was found raped and murdered in a park. No mention of it—you didn't see nothing—no headlines in the *Post, Newsday, Time, New York Times,* or *New York Daily News*. That's a devaluation of a black life. It's like black life doesn't mean anything, doesn't count for anything.

As long as they see, well, it's niggers killing niggers, they're animals anyway, it's no news. But if a young woman—a young *white* woman, on top of that, from Wall Street—is raped in Central Park, you might as well spit in the face of Jesus or something, because, you know, a great atrocity has happened.

This [black] woman was raped four or five days after the incident in Central Park. *Raped and murdered!* Nobody said nothing. Didn't see no outcry. I didn't see Donald Trump taking any fucking ads out behind that shit.

M G: *The fight in your film was between the most sympathetic white, Sal, and the two least sympathetic blacks. For instance, Buggin' Out, the activist, couldn't get any people on his side except Radio Raheem. John Turturro's openly racist Pino would have been his most likely counterpart.*
S L: See, that's what Hollywood would have had. But that's too easy. Pino didn't pick up that stuff out of the air. Some of it had to have been taught him by his father, Sal.

What's really troubling to some white critics is when Mookie throws the garbage can through the window. Because Mookie's one of those "nice black people." I've heard a lot of white friends tell me, "You're a nice black person, you're not like the rest." They really followed Mookie, they liked Mookie. He was a likable character. [Laughs.] They feel betrayed when he throws the garbage can through the window. Can't trust them. The Moulan yan. Telling him to get a spear. [Screams. Laughs.]

M G: *"Moulan yan" means eggplant.*
S L: Haven't you seen any Martin Scorsese movies?

M G: *Were the events leading to the riot a way to say that even the "nice" whites are willing to hide behind the colonial power structure?*
S L: Sal says, "These people love my pizza." I mean, any time you hear someone say "youse people," you know what that is.

M G: *Although he seemed proud that everyone grew up on his pizza....*
S L: Yeah, but look, as soon as the shit started to happen, all of a sudden he starts saying, "I'll break your fuckin' nigger ass." That didn't come out of thin air. It was there. It just had to be provoked. But it's still there, though.

M G: *Why provoke the fight in a seemingly safe civil arena, a gathering place, rather than on the street?*
S L: Well, that's where a fight like that would start. In the public eye. Buggin' Out's character is a direct reference to a couple days after the Howard Beach incident. Some black leaders got together and wanted all the black people in New York City to boycott pizza for a day. It was one of the most ridiculous things I ever heard in my life. It was stupid.

I mean, Buggin' Out has the right idea. But what's going to be the value of having one black photo up on Sal's wall of fame? Is that going to do anybody any good? But on the other hand, he also has a point, because let's turn it around and say, 'Look, Sal, you make all your money off black people, why don't you have enough sensitivity to have at least one photo up on the wall?' So that's the way the film is to me. Everybody has a point.

M G: *And are you advocating the riot at the end?*
S L: I'm not advocating anything. These are just characters, and this is how they act. This is how *they* acted. And if we turn that around again, I think Sal has a point, too: When you black people get together and have your own businesses, you can do what you want to do.

I don't think that blacks are going to see this film and just go out in the streets and start rioting. I mean, black people don't need this movie to riot. They've been doing it already. Just look at what happened in Miami the week before the Super Bowl, when those cops killed people. Now some people be killed in New York City in summer by the cops, and this movie's not going to help. But it's going to be tense here in New York anyway, with this whole mayoral election coming up. And it's going to be hot, you know. That was the whole premise of the film, that in 95 degrees people lose it anyway.

M G: *Do you think that the "wilding" incident in Central Park will affect the film's reception?*
S L: I never even heard of the term "wilding" before this movie came out. It's like they got this thing, they made it up, you know. I'm very sorry that the young woman got raped. It's a terrible act no matter who it happens to. But I think the whole thing was blown way out of proportion. The media just whipped white New York into a frenzy, and Donald Trump wasn't helping, taking out them ads: bring back the death penalty—they're code words. Anytime you hear Ed Koch talk about "savages" and "animals," you know he's talking about young black males. It was the whole Bernhard Goetz thing right away. And definitely this is being tied into the mayoral race. It'll

come up again: a vote for [black candidate] David Dinkins is a vote for wilding. I can see a campaign like that for sure.

M G: *White people fear that you are advocating violence.*
S L: Look, all they have to do is read the last quote of the movie. I'm not advocating violence. Self-defense is not violence. We call it intelligence. People are full of shit. Israel could go out and bomb anybody, nobody says nothing. But when black people go out and protect themselves, then we're militants, or we're advocating violence.

M G: *It seems you almost glossed over the death of Radio Raheem. When Mookie goes to see Sal at the end, he just says, "Radio Raheem is dead."*
S L: Yeah, but that's Mookie's character. What happened that night was tragic, but Mookie's whole character is not going to change overnight. And the reason why he's there that morning is because he wants to get paid. He's been saying that the whole movie, you know, get paid, get paid.

No, I don't think I glossed over it. What's the last thing that Love Daddy says? "The next record goes out for Radio Raheem. We love you, brother."

M G: *When Mookie breaks the window, it's his decision to get off the sidelines, take a stand and really explode the situation. . . . Is that you?*
S L: We've always tried to take a stand no matter what. All creative filming does. I don't think that we're going to change anything. This is just a more explosive, volatile subject matter.

M G: *Is Mookie symbolic of art taking a stand?*
S L: Of art? No. I leave that up to you journalists.

M G: *After the riot, the only people who lose out at the end of the film are the people who live in the neighborhood.*
S L: That always happens. Look at the riots in '67, '68. Anytime there's a riot, the National Guard, police—whatever—they always make sure they contain that riot to the ghetto. And so the buildings they burn down will never be built back. When there were riots in New York City, they were never on Fifth Avenue. There's never been looting in Lord & Taylor's or Saks. It was on 125th Street. So, in a way, we do lose out. But people don't *feel* they lose out, because they feel they lost already. People have nothing to lose.

M G: *Before the riot they had the pizzeria, whatever that meant. But now, the street's the same except it's filled with debris and they don't have a pizzeria anymore.*
S L: They felt better about it, though. They felt that for once in their lives, they'd taken a stand. And they felt that they had some kind of say. They felt powerful.

M G: *It's brought up several times in the film that "it's a free country." Your character brings it up at one point; Clifton, the yuppie who moves into Bed-Stuy, brings it up. It's a very ironic statement.*
S L: Well, yeah. *That* was no accident.

M G: *The street in the film—that was the cleanest street I've ever seen in New York.*
S L: I made that choice because any time you hear people say Bed-Stuy, right away they think of the rapes, murders, drugs. There's no need to show garbage piled up high and all that other stuff, because not every single block in Bed-Stuy is like that.

It would be a fallacy to say that lower-income people always live in burned-out buildings. These are hard-working people, and they take pride in their stuff just like everybody else. So there's no need for the set to look like Charlotte Street in the South Bronx.

Another thing people ask: "Where are the drugs?" Drugs is such a massive subject, it just can't be dealt with effectively as a subplot. You have to do an entire film on drugs. This film was not about that. This film was about *racism*.

M G: *The people in the film are very intelligent. The most ignorant person is Pino. Is there a difference between violence in the hands of the ignorant and violence in the hands of the intelligent?*
S L: Intelligent people will use violence to their advantage and ignorant people just use violence for violence's sake.

M G: *But if you had really ignorant people fighting back the riot would have carried a different weight.*
S L: No. I think that it is good these people were intelligent. Because then it shows this is not just a case of *random* violence. People knew *exactly* what they were doing.

M G: *And if they had jobs? Mookie says several times, "Get a job."*
S L: He gets that really from working for Sal. "Get a job"—that's really a statement on your manhood. Because everyman should be able to hold his own weight. And what's the first thing Pino says to the guys who are heckling him, when he's beating up Smiley? "Get a job!" Because a lot of these guys don't have jobs. Therefore, in Pino's eyes it means that they're not men. "All the Moulan yans are on welfare anyway."

M G: *Your screenwriting and filmmaking aren't strictly narrative. They bear a strong resemblance to a musical score. Each character is a note that you play and then bring all together for a crescendo at the end.*
S L: We just don't like to have narratives that show. They're there, but we just don't want to be out in front, because when narratives are out in front, the audience will be able to guess from watching the first ten minutes of the movie exactly where you're going to go. We like to keep them guessing, just let there be work. I think that for the most part, not enough respect is given to audiences' intelligence. They're just spoon-fed everything.

M G: *When* School Daze *was released, it was lumped together with. . . .*
S L: Shoot to Kill *and* Action Jackson. They all came out on the same day. They just think that the black audience is just one monolithic audience and has no diversity at all—which I think is very disrespectful. There's no way *Shoot to Kill* is a *black* film. Very few black people went to see that film. Sidney Poitier was the only black person in that movie.

MG: *In your book,* Do the Right Thing, *you say that blacks can't be held responsible for racism, that they're victims. It seems that one's self-perception as a victim reduces one's power—as seen in the conversation between M.L., Sweet Dick Willy, and Coconut Sid about the Korean fruit stand.*
S L: No. How is that going to be "my perception" if black people were taken from Africa as slaves? I'm not imagining that. You must acknowledge that, but not use that as a excuse.

When I was becoming a filmmaker I knew it would be harder for me to be a black filmmaker—to be a filmmaker because I was black. But I realized that you just have to be two or three—four—times better. The same thing as any black athlete. They got to be better than the white boy to make the team. You don't sit there and brood about it. This is something you just know, growing up black. It's a given. The problem starts when people say that's a given and then use that as the excuse.

M G: *I was reading an article in* Premiere *about blacks in the film industry. And one person was quoted as saying Hollywood films are based on the premise that a black man or woman can't lead you anywhere. Which is to say that whites' moral/psychological identification can't be with a black person.*
S L: I truly believe a lot of people—a lot of *executives*—believe that. There's an age-old axiom in Hollywood that black is death at the box office. Except for very few exceptions—Eddie Murphy being one. Look at *Time* the week they had *Mississippi Burning* on the cover. Alan Parker said the realities of Hollywood today demand that this film have two white leads. And I'm not going to hang Alan Parker about that statement. I think that he's just echoing what a whole lot of executives feel, the people who get pictures made.

No matter what you do—you can be as big as Michael Jackson—they still look at him as black first. So, you really can't get around it. But it doesn't bother me.

At Cannes, the jury, led by Wim Wenders, gave no award to *Do the Right Thing*. Says Spike:

"We were robbed.

"Ten films received awards and we didn't get one. I feel we entered the best of the festival.

"Most people on the jury, minus Sally Field—the biggest, most important filmmakers at the world's most important film festival—I don't think they're ready for a young black filmmaker to get the Palme d'Or. I think that it's just reality. When it comes down to between me and somebody else, they're going to give it to the white boy.

"At the party afterward, there's praise for [Soderbergh's] *sex, lies, and videotape:* 'Now we have the future of cinema.' So I guess I'm not in the future—their future at least.

"Jim Jarmusch is a really good friend of mine. I love his work. But you know that Wenders gave him that award because that's his protégé.

"I heard that Wenders said that Mookie wasn't enough of a hero. I think that they saw Spike Lee throwing that trash can through the window.

"One day Wenders is going to get off at the wrong stop on the A-train. He's supposed to get off at 59th Street and he's going to miss the stop—it's going to be express—and get off on 125th Street. And I'll be waiting for his ass. [Laughs.]

"He's going to need wings of desire. And you could say what you want, because I don't plan to be in Germany anytime soon."

LESSON FIFTEEN

Women Directors and Hollywood

Just Another Girl Outside the Neo-indie

Christina Lane

> *I'm usually reluctant to spout stuff like: 'If you're a female it's so much harder; if you're a male it's so much easier'—I hope it's a little more complicated than that. But I do think that the machine works better with boys. People are more familiar with the whole idea of a male director, especially when he's a maverick who's bucking the system.* —Christine Vachon, Shooting to Kill

In the winter of the year 2000, another 'Year of the Woman' was proclaimed in the independent film scene. Reporters had either forgotten or had never known that the Sundance Film Festival (formerly the US Film Festival) had already celebrated the Year of the Woman in 1989, 1991, and 1993. So, for trade journalists, Sundance had hit a major milestone with its notable jump in female participants: 40 percent of the candidates in the festival's dramatic competition were women, up from 20 percent in the previous eight years (Levy 2000: A1). And a woman, Karyn Kusama, won the Grand Jury Prize (as well as best direction) for her film *Girlfight*, a feminist inversion of *Rocky*, which featured a working-class teenage girl's entrance into the world of amateur boxing. Kusama, who had financed the $1 million film through her previous employer John Sayles and the Independent Film Channel, sold *Girlfight* to Sony's Screen Gems for $3 million in what was deemed the 'hottest' deal of the festival.

Around the same time, Kimberly Peirce enjoyed the success of *Boys Don't Cry* (1999). A dramatic treatment of the real-life rape and murder of Brandon Teena, a teenaged girl passing as a boy in Falls City, Iowa, this debut feature garnered critical acclaim at film festivals in Toronto, Venice, London, and New York. *Boys Don't Cry*, which Peirce had developed at Columbia University's graduate film school and the Sundance Directors' Lab, won several highly coveted Independent Spirit Awards as well as an Oscar and a Golden Globe Award for Hilary Swank's performance as Brandon. A $2 million film, *Boys Don't Cry* eventually made $11.5 million in domestic box office. It had been produced by Killer Films' maverick producers Christine Vachon and Pam Koffler and then, in a rare move, purchased by Fox Searchlight before post-production had begun.

The success of Kusama and Peirce's indie debuts had a good deal to do with casting, which is not to devalue their sophisticated sense of writing and screen direction. For *Girlfight*, a publicity campaign was developed around newcomer Michelle Rodriguez who possessed little experience in either acting or boxing when she responded to an open casting call. For *Boys Don't Cry*, Hilary Swank's status as a *Beverly Hills 90210* starlet-turned-method-actor provided immediate visibility. In addition to the attention that casting could generate, these films boasted a 'high concept,' an easily synopsized 'hook' that heightened their marketability.[1] The sensational elements of *Boys Don't Cry* aided in its packaging for an audience beyond the festival circuit as did *Girlfight*'s timely connection with the popularity of women's kickboxing.

The high visibility of Peirce and Kusama's debuts would seem to set them up for enduring careers in independent film, which is where both say they would like to stay. The experiences of women directors who came before them indicate, however, that the odds do not favor Peirce or Kusama. Perhaps this historical record is what motivated Peirce to insert her authorial control over the fifteen-second interviews she gave to television reporters as she strode down the red carpet on Oscar night 2000, when she stressed that her new two-year first-look deal with New Line included a first project commitment and granted her final cut. All that those reporters would need to do to understand Peirce's motives is rewind back to 1989 and begin to chart the filmmaking careers of independent directors such as Nancy Savoca, Julie Dash, or Allison Anders.

The problem is that women who attempt to establish careers in an independent world now dominated by 'mini-major' studios often hit a plateau after their first film. These studios have squeezed out avant-garde film and, to some extent, documentary, but what of the women who decide to direct the narrative features so valued by major film festivals and mini-major distributors?[2] Why did no woman win Sundance's Grand Jury Prize in the 1990s (with Kusama finally earning one in 2000), when four women had won the award during the 1980s (Dargis 1999: 13)? What precisely are the hurdles for women filmmakers who try to parlay their 'calling card' films into passkeys for further creative possibilities in the competitive age of the mini-majors? How and when do traditional cultural assumptions figure in the world of Sundance, Miramax, New Line, and the Independent Feature Project, even as they purport to advance the causes of (gender, racial, and sexual) diversity and 'progressive' politics? What strategies of empowerment are indie women directors crafting in the narrowly circumscribed business of mini-major cinema?

This piece examines the production–distribution context of what has become women's independent filmmaking by focusing on a number of key figures, especially Nancy Savoca, Julie Dash, Leslie Harris, Allison Anders, Rose Troche, and Lynn Hershman Leeson. It includes directors who overtly engage feminist politics as well as those who are not easily linked with feminism, for my primary interest concerns the many dilemmas confronted by women, not just feminists, given the indication of discrimination by industry statistics. This piece is not meant to be representative nor all-inclusive but rather to make broad links between the careers of fairly visible directors. Furthermore, although my major inquiry involves how these filmmakers' status as women affects their place in major independent cinema, this focus is not meant to elide the role that their ethnic, racial, or sexual identities play in their ability to navigate the system. Indeed, the decreased visibility and number of opportunities for women of color since the 1980s suggest that while African American women such as Dash and Harris, and Latina women such as Troche, have made first films, many more women of color have been denied. The numbers of women of color in independent filmmaking were higher as contemporary mini-major cinema was forming; they began to dwindle as the movement became more institutionalized.

This piece is divided according to separate historical periods. The first period, 1989–93, begins with the triumphal release of Steven Soderbergh's *sex, lies & videotape* by Miramax (after a highly publicized acquisition at the 1989 US [Subsequently Sundance] Film Festival) and ends with the 1993 purchase of Miramax by Disney, which helped solidify the mini-major's status as an economic giant with supposed autonomy. This section focuses on Savoca, Dash, Harris, all of whom initiated features sometime between 1989 and 1993. Anders is also addressed here, in relation to possibilities for women in cable and digital technology, as she serves as a bridge between the early and late 1990s. While her early films launched her career, she has managed to survive major changes in the indie industry alongside more recently emerging filmmakers. The chapter's second part, which briefly discusses Rose Troche and Lynn Hershman Leeson, focuses on further breakdowns between 1993 and 2001 in definitions of independent and studio filmmaking. By the mid-1990s, nearly all federally funded arts grants had been discontinued or drastically reduced in response to pressure from conservative and religious groups. The creative decisions made by mini-majors had also been heavily impacted by the economic phenomenon of 'independent blockbusters' such as *Pulp Fiction* (Tarantino, 1994).

At times, the piece provides a conversation with 'one-hit wonders,' films that were never made, projects that did not live up to their directors' expectations, or movies that were panned by reviewers. I would suggest, however, that it speaks volumes about the failures of contemporary independent cinema to account for those it claims to include, saying perhaps even more than the numerous success stories of certain 1990s' male directors.

Women on the Verge of an Indie Explosion, 1989–93

Directors such as Savoca, Dash, Harris, and Anders initiated their first films on the heels of a boom in women's filmmaking that had grown out of the second-wave feminist movement. They benefited from the boundless labor and energy that women had devoted to publicizing and distributing alternative cinema and documentary in the 1970s.[3] Mini-major studios such as Miramax and New Line profited from these resources as well, taking their cue from the strategies that feminist distributors had used to constitute and institutionalize a market niche within counter cinema. The debt owed to curators—for instance, the Flaherty Women's Group (who organized the early International Women's Film Festivals); start-up distributors such as New Day Films, Iris, or Women Make Movies; as well as informal networks of scores of fledgling women filmmakers in the pre-mini-major era—goes unpaid.

Two factors, in particular, placed women directors in a weak position to compete in an increasingly commercial environment. One was the way in which a number of film festivals moved from grassroots venues into mainstream publicity events and acquisition sites for independent and (eventually) major studios. Initially a state-funded festival established to promote Utah and its Film Commission, Sundance proved to be an explosive force in defining trends and the packaging of 'indie' films. The second major factor involved a shift in exhibition. Whereas a great deal of independent cinema, especially that made by women, had been shown in local sites such as traditional art theaters, museums, and schools, major independent studios found ways to show their product in mainstream theaters. As they became fixtures in multiplexes, many independent distributors channeled energy away from making a statement toward making a profit.

In 1989, the year that Sundance changed appreciably, Nancy Savoca's first feature *True Love* actually won the Grand Jury Prize. Savoca, an NYU film school graduate, had worked for seven years to make the film. Her partner and co-writer Richard Guay took on the role of producer and raised a $750,000 budget from private investors, among them John Sayles. Upon completion, *True Love* was bought by MGM–UA and went on to gross $1.3 million. The film casts a critical eye on the institution of marriage, following a working-class Italian-American bride (Annabella Sciorra) down the aisle. With this film, Savoca, who is half-Argentinian and half-Italian, established a reputation as a potent feminist voice and a purveyor of the emotional intimacies of Italian family life.[4]

Based on *True Love*'s relative box office success and its placement in several 'Top Ten' lists, Savoca was hired by Warner Bros.: to direct *Dogfight* (1991) (Maslin 1989: C10). This provocative polemic about conventions of female beauty helped cement her status with critics as a significant director. As Savoca sought to shape the $8 million production, however, Warners put pressure on her to change the film's conclusion to a more optimistic ending, revoking marketing support when she refused (Dargis 1999: 13). According to Savoca, the studio executives' attitude had been: ' "It's your movie, your name is on it but, P.S. we won't support it one iota with prints and advertising," It went straight to video. I got the movie I wanted but no one saw it' (Johnston 1993: 19).

Without promotional support from the studio *Dogfight* performed poorly, bringing in only $394,631. As a result, Savoca's third feature, *Household Saints* (1993), proved much more difficult to finance. With the support of executive producer Jonathan Demme, she reverted to earlier strategies, soliciting funds from private investors. An adaptation of Francine Prose's novel, *Household Saints* again detailed relationships and rituals of Italian-American family life. Picked up for distribution by Fine Line, the film received critical praise, but it, too, garnered little financial return ($574,152).

Savoca went from 1993 to 1999 before her next feature film, *The 24-Hour Woman*, was made. One of the major reasons for the extended delay was that *24-Hour Woman*, in which a TV producer juggles the demands of her job and new motherhood, is Latina-centered: 'Friends and potential backers suggested she change the character's ethnicity to something more "universal," meaning of course, white. . . . The character was [indeed] "whited out," and the filmmaker lapsed into an "angry, depressed period".' (Graham 1999: N7) But when she offered a minor role to Rosie Perez, the Oscar-nominated actor (for *Fearless*) asked to be considered for the lead and was cast as the protagonist soon thereafter. While this helped to restore the film to its original mission, Perez's attachment was not enough to carry the film, which was financed by Shooting Gallery and distributed by Artisan. *24-Hour Woman* gained little visibility, due in part to its perceived status as a particularized story that lacked 'universal' appeal. Reviewers were unsupportive and the $2.5 million film grossed a mere $109,000. A creative and aggressive marketing campaign could have been developed around *24-Hour Woman* for a niche audience—of Latinos—which was waiting to be targeted. Instead, the very institutions that poised Savoca for high visibility in the late 1980s positioned her for failure in the late 1990s.

In contrast, creative marketing was integral to the early 1990s' success of Julie Dash. Her *Daughters of the Dust* (1991) weaves together the stories of several generations of Gullah descendants who prepare to cross from Ibo Landing to the US mainland in the 1860s.[5] Because of *Daughters'* experimental narrative structure, Dash was continually asked to prove to Hollywood executives that an audience did indeed exist for her film. Ultimately, she financed its $800,000 budget through the National Endowment for the Arts, Women Make Movies, American Playhouse, and a number of regional grants (Dash 1992: 7). Then, with the help of New York-based distributor Kino International, publicity house KJM 3, and PBS's American Playhouse, Dash helped forge a new audience—of middle-class African American art cinema-goers—that white male executives had predicted simply was not there (Rhines 1996: 65–7). The grassroots publicity campaign 'arranged interviews on Black radio and television programs, placed stories in major Black mainstream and arts newspapers and magazines, and enlisted the support of many Black social and political organizations' (*ibid.*: 67).

Throughout the 1990s, Julie Dash has attempted to parlay the critical success of *Daughters of the Dust,* which earned back twice its budget, into an opportunity to direct more commercial films. She has been awarded many fellowships, a Sundance award for best cinematography for *Daughters,* and has several prestigious shorts to her credit. Yet Dash continues to struggle to gain the green light for a second feature. With little luck to date, Dash supports her efforts by directing music videos (Unterburger 1999: 107).

Similar biases against African American makers working on personal and political narratives have clearly affected Leslie Harris. Her status as an African American woman was a marketable 'hook' for Miramax in the early 1990s; but later her career languished. Like Dash, Harris culled funding for her $500,000 film *Just Another Girl on the I.R.T.* (1993) from grant organizations (the American Film Institute, the National Endowment for the Arts, the New York State Council for the Arts, and the Jerome Foundation). She also tapped individual supporters such as documentarian Michael Moore, cultural critic George Nelson, and novelist Terry McMillan. *Just Another Girl* tells the story of 'Chantel, a Brooklyn homegirl,' who contends with her unplanned pregnancy by ignoring it.[6] Given the atypical portrayal of an urban teen grappling with pregnancy, Harris appropriately ends her film with the tag. 'A Film Hollywood Dared Not Do.' She won the Special Jury Prize for first feature at the 1993 Sundance Film Festival and an Open Palm Independent Feature Gotham Award. Post-production of *Just Another Girl* was financed by Miramax on the basis of its newsworthy hook. Miramax's promotional strategy—which placed Harris in national and local media more than once a day during the film's opening week—netted extensive free publicity and, in fact, worked very well (Taubin 2001: 37). But, though Harris pitched several projects (including a film focusing on a female hiphop producer) to large and small studios, she has had no luck to date in securing financing for a second feature.

As the case of Allison Anders suggests, institutional support from original cable programming has provided a solution where funding has otherwise failed. Anders' 1992 debut *Gas, Food, Lodging* traced the rites-of-passage through adolescence of two sisters. It performed well at festivals and garnered a New York Critics Circle Award for best new director. But Anders faced difficulties financing her next five features, in part, she claims, because '[i]t's the boy-wonder myth. . . . The girl wonder myth doesn't exist. . . . You just end up in the girl ghetto' (quoted in Spines 2000: 45). Her second feature, *Mi Vida Loca* (1993), focused on the choices confronting four Latina teenaged gang members. It was the first project made by HBO Showcase for theatrical release. When her sixth film, *Things Behind the Sun,* proved difficult to finance, she turned again to cable, selling it to Showtime for distribution.

Anders had two reasons for negotiating with a major cable network when it came to *Things Behind the Sun.* The first was pragmatic. She said of *Grace of My Heart* (1996) and the digitally shot *Sugar Town* (1999): 'Nobody saw them. They were out for two weeks and gone. It was an awful feeling' (Weinraub 2001: El). Her second reason was the film's potential to reach a wider audience. *Things Behind the Sun* contains semi-autobiographical content related to Anders's own rape as a teenager and the resulting post-traumatic stress disorder.[7] She had already forfeited the advantage of prominent casting, losing attached star Winona Ryder and, later, Heather Graham to other projects. According to Showtime programming president Jerry Offsay, the director increased her audience tenfold by choosing the cable release over theatrical distribution *(ibid.*).[8] Although Anders' career has been celebrated for its longevity, her future remains uncertain, and in 2000 she moved to London in hope of securing European financing (Spines 2000: 47).

The most successful strategies deployed by women in their attempts to maintain the ground they gained from 1989 to 1993 have in fact occurred in cable production and a turn to digital filmmaking. Whereas in the 1980s directors such as Martha Coolidge, Donna Deitch, and Lizzie Borden were compelled to take work on existing cable series or low-budget made-for-TV movies in an effort to keep working, in the contemporary age of 'quality' cable programming women directors can, and often do, gain visibility and cultural cachet on television. HBO and Showtime, which rely on innovative counter-programming, have become major players at Sundance. They present themselves as the largest independent film companies in the contemporary indie market. According to Oscar-winning indie director Mira Nair, who made *Salaam Bombay!* (1988), 'HBO has become the independent filmmaker studio. . . . They respect your freedom, they respect your vision' (Rohan 2001: E1). This phenomenon presents both solutions and problems. Cable networks offer emerging women financing opportunities and creative freedom, but even premiere cable networks are sometimes portrayed within the industry as a 'female other' in relation to the 'masculine' sphere of theatrical indie film. This process might thus ultimately reinforce the 'girl ghetto' rather than counteract it.

Similarly, although the accessibility and low cost of digital equipment provides access to technology for disenfranchised groups, distribution remains uncertain. In general, little recognition has been given those digital features that are directed by women (while a male-dominated movement such as Dogme95 gained momentum). A promising exception occurred when Rebecca Miller won the 2002 Sundance Grand Jury Prize for *Personal Velocity* (shot by cinematographer Ellen Kuras). Of the initial ten films launched by InDiGent Films, the offshoot of Independent Film Channel (IFC) that produced Miller's film, however, only *Personal Velocity* was directed by a woman (Kaufman 2002). Furthermore, trade magazines such as *Wired,* which help set the standards and values for new technology movements such as microcinema and ifilms, have identified young, professional men as their target market. Technological developments alone clearly will not be enough to change gender power imbalances. [9]

The Comings and Goings of the Up-and-Coming, 1994–99

Two more factors had increasing influence over women's production and distribution in the mid to late 1990s: the rise of the producer–auteur and the intensification of commercial auteurism. Independent producers such as John Pierson and Christine Vachon became crucial links in the chain of acquisition.[10] During the late 1980s to mid-1990s, producers had nurtured important relationships not only with major studio executives but with festival curators and film reviewers, whose 'free' positive publicity made for invaluable promotion. They functioned as powerful gatekeepers who provided important access and mobility for filmmakers. The likelihood that independent directors would reach distributors became increasingly dependent on their ability to gain the committed interest of these producers. The second factor, a new brand of indie auteurism, grew as a result of the desire for festivals and independent studios to draw attention to their films by promoting the director as a maverick who had seized the reins of low-budget production and, in his own hip, cool way, made the system work for him. And it was nearly always a *him* because the traditional director's 'mystique' of auteurism pervaded the indie festivals and studios' marketing campaigns, excluding women from increasingly commercialized imagery. As the 1990s continued, it became less likely that films would be advertised on the basis of a 'woman director,' meaning that women filmmakers and 'female' genres became less marketable and less marketed, in a reciprocal spiral.[11] While occasional marketing campaigns would publicize films as 'made by women,' such as the promotion of both Nicole Holofcener and Tamara Jenkins as 'female Woody Allens,' mini-major marketing departments took little initiative to develop women's niche markets, thereby contributing to the homogenization of new indie cinema.

Rose Troche's *Go Fish* was one of the few films to be promoted via *difference*—on the basis of Troche's identities as woman and lesbian—and it proved successful.[12] In 1994, *Go Fish* gained notoriety as the first film to be sold to a distributor *during* the Sundance Film Festival. Troche, a Latina director, had teamed up with actor, editor, and co-writer Guinevere Turner, and they had pooled together their money (approximately $8,000) and resources to make an experimental lesbian feature. Their road to a Samuel Goldwyn $450,000 sale was a difficult one, though one made more manageable by producer Christine Vachon. Troche and Turner approached Vachon's company Killer Films when their limited financing ran out. After viewing their footage, she contributed $5,000 to keep them on track, eventually convincing Islet Films' John Pierson to bankroll a remaining $53,000 (Pierson 1995: 280–1; Vachon 1998: 137). Indie guru Pierson then initiated a 'buzz' campaign that culminated at Sundance. *Go Fish*, with its black-and-white low-budget aesthetic and loose narrative structure, was an unlikely candidate for indie success. A newly formed lesbian niche audience heightened its chances of visibility, however, and, through its charming sense of humor and innovative visual style, the film earned that audience's respect.

Without calling *Go Fish*'s quality and originality into question, the entrepreneurship and professional connections of Vachon and Pierson should not be underestimated. Pierson arranged a November 1993 private screening for Sundance programmers Geoff Gilmore and Cathy Schulman to help the film's chances of entry in the January 1994 festival. During the festival selection process, Schulman took an acquisitions job at Samuel Goldwyn and watched *Go Fish* carefully with an eye to purchasing it (Pierson 1995: 285–6). Pierson drummed up word of mouth and, by extension, a bidding war, which Goldwyn won when Miramax and New Line were slow to move *(ibid.)*. Troche's Latina identity was (problematically) written out of the marketing campaign and the film was promoted on the basis of her gender and sexuality. And the film was released during gay pride month in June 1994, which also marked the twenty-fifth anniversary of Stonewall. After word of mouth had built in New York City, Goldwyn 'counter-programmed' the film against summer Hollywood blockbusters, exhibiting it for the most part in its own Landmark Theaters chain *(ibid.: 297)*. In its opening weekend, *Go Fish* made back the purchase price ($550,000), eventually grossing $2.4 million *(ibid.)*.

Troche's immediate response to studio attention was to propose a biopic on Dorothy Arzner, the 1920s and 1930s' Hollywood director who kept her lesbian identity relatively secret.[13] A studio film on Arzner might well have capitalized on the lesbian niche market; but Troche found she was stuck in the development stage. She pitched her script to numerous studios and mini-majors with little success. After a series of disenchanting development meetings with New Line, she came to the determination that '[w]omen just get chewed up by the system' (*Filmmaker* 1996; Huisman 1999).

The director eventually made the British romantic comedy *Bedrooms and Hallways* (1999), featuring several gay male characters, one of whom comes to terms with his heterosexual identity. The film, produced and distributed by the BBC and several European finance companies, disappeared after its opening weekend, making only $16,459 in the US. Troche then returned to her previous supporter, Christine Vachon, and British financiers in order to direct *The Safety of Objects* (2002), starring Glenn Close. Initial reviews were not favorable, voicing the familiar complaint that women who have something to say lapse into tones of 'didacticism.'[14]

Though Lynn Hershman Leeson approaches style and narrative differently, she too has faced charges of didacticism for attempting to weave feminist issues into her independent features. Leeson's debut feature *Conceiving Ada* (1997) stars Tilda Swinton as Victorian-era Countess Ada Augusta Byron King of Lovelace. In real life Countess Ada was the daughter of Lord Byron and the originator of computer language. [15] A contemporary female computer scientist (Francesca Faridany) devises a virtual reality mode through which to communicate with Ada, resulting in a cyber–feminist connection that reveals the precarious status of women's bodies plagued by male-dominated industry and technology. To all intents and purposes, *Conceiving Ada* was a low-budget, high concept film, in that it re-worked the 'time machine' formula into a conceptual hook using an innovative visual style.[16] The film might have lent itself to any number of aggressive marketing campaigns, including its basis in a provocative historical figure, its topicality in relation to digitality, and its dynamic graphic design.

The Independent Feature Project saw fit to include *Conceiving Ada* in its selection of 'American Independents in the Market' showcase at the Berlin Film Festival, though with little result. At Toronto, the film received little attention from distributors and none of the major independent studios showed enthusiasm at Sundance either. But Winstar Cinema, which specializes in international art cinema and academic markets, bought domestic rights to the film there. Leeson thereby lost any chance of capturing the major indie market.

Film reviewers positioned *Conceiving Ada* for negative reception, first by comparing her virtual sets derogatively with those of big-budget male directors such as James Cameron and George Lucas, and then by belittling its female-driven content and feminist politics.[17] B. Ruby Rich, a critic known for her endorsement of feminist and queer work, was the only reviewer who apparently saw this. She proclaimed *Conceiving Ada*: 'One of the Year's Ten Best. . . . Has there ever been a film so joyous about women, knowledge, and mastery? And it's even fun' (Rich 1999).[18]

Not only was *Conceiving Ada* thus unable to find its intended market but it failed to secure Leeson any further financing. She made her second feature, a cyber–vampire movie entitled *Teknolust*, through German financiers, though she still hopes to distribute it through an outlet such as Sony Pictures Classics or Fox Searchlight. Summing up what she describes as a 'heartbreaking' experience trying to promote *Conceiving Ada*, Leeson remarked: 'Remember, it was a film about a woman by a woman' (Leeson in email correspondence with the author, 9 October 2001).

Conclusion: the Phenomenon of 'the Blair Bitch'

When these arduous career paths are analyzed collectively, and seen in conjunction with those of other indie women such as Nicole Holofcener, Maria Maggenti, Tamara Jenkins, Lisa Cholodenko, and Lisa Kreuger, they point strongly to the cultural gender biases that govern independent filmmaking.[19] From development to reception, the male-oriented gangster or thriller genres, and the quirky 'loser' film, have helped to condition major independent studios' ideas about what makes money and what makes film sense. The argument that independent women's films have not proven to be commercially viable does not suffice; such films might well have drawn indie audiences if they had been exposed to creative marketing campaigns and not been critically dismissed as didactic. No one will know what the ultimate impact of women's independent filmmaking of the 1990s might have been under other conditions.

The centralized role that Sundance has played in promotion and acquisition of indie films, and the festival's increasingly symbiotic relationship with Hollywood, have also been detrimental to women and their films. While Sundance has made some effort to serve the unique economic, institutional, and creative needs of female directors, the Institute has failed to become a potent site for fostering independent women's cinema. Its original mission was to work 'off-center' and non-commercial features 'into the public's consciousness,' and to compel mainstream audiences 'to want to see them' *(Scenario* 1995: 207). As it has grown, Sundance's mission has taken a detour (Young 1995: 22).[20]

There are concrete ways in which major independent studios might shift their marketing and distribution to enhance reception of these films. Historically, female genres, and other kinds of niche films typically made by indie women, have taken time to find their audience. In a marketplace determined by opening weekend box-office performance, many of the films mentioned here would appear unsuccessful. They are often films that, if given the chance, could develop legs, the industry term for the process of gaining steam over time.[21] However, distributors tend to presume them 'dead' before their lives have fully played out. Indeed, because distributors and marketing departments often perceive such films to be less likely to succeed in comparison to big-budget movies or male indie fare, they often fail to put the necessary resources into independent women's films before they leave the gate. Many of these features make decent comebacks at the video-rental stage; however such financial return is rarely factored in.

In the summer of 1999, just as Kimberly Peirce's *Boys Don't Cry* was picking up some publicity, 'boy wonders' appeared yet again on the scene. This time they were Eduardo Sanchez and Daniel Myrick, co-writers and directors of *The Blair Witch Project* (1999). Their film, made for a reported $30,000 and bought by Artisan for $1 million at Sundance, would go on to gross $141 million in domestic box office and another $109 million overseas. *Blair Witch,* as many trade papers pointed out, demonstrated that there were previously untapped internet resources for cultivating word of mouth around a low-budget film. Though fewer promotional articles and reviews mentioned the fact, the success of this pseudo-documentary horror movie also indicated that the support of an institutional indie such as John Pierson could go a long way in propelling word of mouth. (Six months in advance of release date, Pierson had spread the legend of the Blair Witch on his IFC program, wondering aloud whether or not this could be a true story.)

In comparison to the industry support that benefited Sanchez and Myrick, the road for independent women's films looks a lot like the menacing scenery of the low-budget horror flick. Is it any mystery that the Sanchez–Myrick project sustains its own visibility through a singular fetishized image—that of its aspiring filmmaker–female protagonist breaking down into tears as she shines an ominous flashlight on her face and apologizes profusely for ever picking up a camera in the first place? Does she really owe us, or the male members of her crew, an apology? Did we really need to see our indie woman filmmaker reduced to a sniveling, groveling victim?

It says a lot about major independent studios, structures, and audiences that such a tear-ridden, fear-driven image of the repentant *Blair Witch* woman became an industry hit. The same 'Blame the Bitch' mentality also informs industry practices of mini-majors; if a woman's film fails, executives are more likely to attribute it to her gender than if the same fate befalls a male director. Today's festival directors, mini-major executives, and film reviewers do not realize that, as taste-makers and market-shapers, they might instead raise the cultural capital of women directors and their films. As Miramax positioned itself in the independent sector in the late 1980s, Harvey Weinstein explained that the studio's strategy was to find the marketing hook in unlikely contenders. He told the *Los Angeles Times:* 'It's the distributor's responsibility to find the audience,' criticizing major studios for neglecting to create and exploit niches (1989: F1). Whereas, during their 1980s' rise, executives felt that they could define and shape the meaning of high concept, they later presumed that high concept was an objective, external value that films either had or did not have. As studios such as Miramax grew and changed through the 1990s, the 'distributor's job' shifted into a shortsighted process of catering to young, white, male audiences. Their entrepreneurial spirit stalled when it came to finding and forging niches best targeted by women directors, reinforcing Allison Anders's claim that major independents 'really don't want to know what's in a woman's head.'

Notes

I wish to thank the participants in the 2000 Society for Cinema Studies workshop 'New American Directions/New American Directors,' namely: Robert Kolker, Jon Lewis, and Devin Orgeron. Additionally, I thank Alisa Perren for the way in which her scholarship and our conversations helped shaped this piece. Finally, I thank Lynn Hershman Leeson and Nicole Holofcener for providing valuable insights.

1. See Wyatt 1994 and 1996.
2. Documentary had functioned as a stable economic force in the 1980s, and feminist distributors had carved out the genre of women's documentary as a stronghold in the independent

sector. Feminist critic B. Ruby Rich historicizes the ghettoizing of documentary by 1990s' independent institutions in gendered terms, perceiving a distinct pattern since the 1970s whereby men are associated with narrative film and women turn to documentary and the less expensive, more readily available, medium of video (Zimmerman 2000: 136).

3. In the 1970s, women, invigorated by radical consciousness-raising endeavors and feminist networking, launched film festivals, formed film co-ops, and published 'special interest' magazines: see Rosenberg 1983: 78.

4. For critical analyses of Savoca's films, see Modleski 1998 and Nardini 1991.

5. For critical analyses of Dash's films, see Alexander 1993, Bambera 1992, Guerrero 1993, hooks 1992, Jones 1993.

6. For critical analysis of Harris's film, see Phillips 1992.

7. Anders has always drawn from personal experience in the development and production of her films; but in *Things Behind the Sun,* she went so far as to film the rape scenes in the actual house (in Cape Canaveral, Florida) where the original trauma took place: see Weinraub 2001.

8. Cheryl Dunye, who made the transition from experimental art cinema to commercial narratives in the late 1990s, turned to premiere cable production as well. She made her second feature film *The Stranger Within* (2001) for HBO with the help of C-Hundred Films. Dunye explains her decision in strategic terms: 'It took me a while—making your second feature, like all the boys, you want to make it big, broad, wide, and star-studded. But I'm not one of the boys, and the key for me was that the film was going to be seen by far more people on television and that my audience would dramatically change' (Willis 2001).

9. For a discussion of digitality's gender implications, see Bolter and Grusin 1999, Leeson 1996.

10. Though Pierson and Vachon operate in similar ways, they have very different motivations and tastes. Pierson tends to promote 'quirky' and 'cool' independents geared toward a young, straight, male audience while Vachon helped usher in the 'New Queer Cinema' era, producing more experimental and 'high art' films.

11. See Perren 1998 and Corrigan 1991.

12. For critical analysis of Troche's *Go Fish,* see Henderson 1999, Hollinger 1998.

13. See Mayne 1994.

14. See, for example, Gleiberman 2001. *Safety of Objects,* which interweaves the stories of four families confronting their disillusion with suburbia, premiered at the Toronto Film Festival in 2001.

15. For critical analysis of Leeson's work, see Popper 1997: 188–90.

16. See Rich 1999.

17. Leeson was the first person to develop the technology for 'virtual sets,' a process by which she used computer software to combine photographs of Victorian bed-and-breakfasts with footage of her actors performing against a blue screen. This technology, which she patented after working for eighteen months to perfect it, was later used in James Cameron's *Titanic* (1998). It enabled her to turn a $10 million film into a $1.2 million film: see Wingfield 1998.

18. Film reviewers negatively influenced the reception of *Conceiving Ada* by playing Leeson off against the blockbuster auteur James Cameron. In a move that obscured the large power differential between Leeson and Cameron's uses of 'virtual set' technology, one reviewer asserted that *Titanic's* special effects far overpowered those of *Conceiving Ada*. Several others made unfair comparisons between Leeson's film and high-budget features such as *Phantom Menace* and *Tron*: see Sachs 1999 and Parks 1999.

19. See *Walking and Talking* (1996) and *Lovely and Amazing* (2002) by Nicole Holofcener; *Incredibly True Adventures of Two Girls in Love* (1995) by Maria Maggenti; *Slums of Beverly Hills* (1998) by Tamara Jenkins; *High Art* (1997) and *Laurel Canyon* (2002) by Lisa Cholodenko; and *Manny and Lo* (1996) and *Committed* (2000) by Lisa Kreuger. Notably, Holofcener shot *Lovely*

and Amazing on digital video when she faced resistance from top indie companies. 'They deemed it uncommercial and hard to market,' she explains. After months of struggling for financing, once she agreed to use DV she had the necessary budget (from Blow-Up Corporation) within twenty-four hours (Holofcener in a telephone interview with the author, 13 October 2001).

20. The Screenwriters and Directors' Labs at Sundance, which enable filmmakers to build alliances with festivals and distributors, accept on average one woman for every three men: see www.sundance.org
21. I thank Jon Lewis for pointing this out during the conceptualizing of this piece.

Bibliography

Alexander, K. (1993) 'Daughters of the Dust and a Black Aesthetic,' in Pam Cook and Phillip Dodd (eds.), *Women and Film: A Sight and Sound Reader,* Philadelphia: Temple University Press, 224–31.

Bambera, T.C. (1992) 'Preface,' in Julie Dash (ed.), *Daughters of the Dust: The Making of an African American Woman's Film,* New York: New Press, xi–xvi.

Bolter, J.D. and Grusin, R. (1999) *Remediation: Understanding New Media,* Cambridge, MA: MIT Press.

Corrigan, T. (1991) *A Cinema Without Walls: Movies and Culture After Vietnam,* New Brunswick, NJ: Rutgers University Press.

Dargis, M. (1999) 'Even in Independent Film, a Suit Is a Suit,' *New York Times,* 31 January, section 2: 13.

Dash, J. (1992) *Daughters of the Dust: The Making of an African American Woman's Film,* New York: New Press.

Dawtry, A. (1996) 'Revival of the Fittest,' *Variety,* 26 February–3 March: 169.

Ebert, R. (2001) 'Two More Treasures Unearthed at Telluride,' *Chicago Sun–Times,* September 4, online: www.chicagosun-times.com (accessed 11 October 2001).

Filmmaker (1996) 'Factory Outlet: Rose Troche Talks with Mary Harron' (spring), online: www.filmmakermagazine.com (accessed 9 September 2001).

Foster, G.A. (1995) *Women Film Directors: An International Bio-Critical Dictionary,* Westport, CT: Greenwood Press.

Gleiberman, O. (2001) 'Northern Views,' *Entertainment Weekly,* 25 September: 43–4, 46, 48.

Graham, R. (1999) 'A Mother's Film,' *Boston Globe,* 14 February: N7.

Guerrero, E. (1993) *Framing Blackness: The African American Image in Film,* Philadelphia: Temple University Press.

Henderson, L. (1999) 'Simple Pleasures: Lesbian Community and *Go Fish,*' *Signs,* 25, 1 (spring): 37–64.

Hollinger, K. (1998) *In the Company of Women: Contemporary Female Friendship Films,* Minneapolis: University of Minnesota Press.

hooks, b. (1992) *Black Looks: Race and Representation,* Boston, MA: South End Press.

Huisman, M. (1999) 'The Dearth of Dyke Cinema,' *City Pages,* 20, 984 (13 October), online: www.citypages.com (accessed 9 October 2001).

Jones, J. (1993) 'The Black South in Contemporary Film,' *African American Review,* 27, 1 (spring): 19–24.

Johnston, S. (1993) 'Nancy Savoca: So How Do You Follow That?' *Independent,* 24 September: 19.

Kaufman, A. (2002) 'Digital Video with Tangible Results,' *Indiewire;* 27 March, online: www.indiewire.com (accessed 1 May 2001).

Levy, E. (2000) 'Femme Force: Films Helmed by Women Span Fest Spectrum, Reach New High,' *Daily Variety,* 19 January: A1.

Leeson, L.H. (ed.) (1996) *Clicking In: Hot Links to a Digital Culture,* Seattle, WA: Bay Press.

Los Angeles Times (1989) 'Independent Miramax Mirrors the Majors,' 25 October: F1.

Maslin, J. (1989) "'True Love," As It Is in the Italian Bronx,' *New York Times,* 20 October: C10.

Mayne, J. (1994) *Directed by Dorothy Arzner,* Indianapolis: Indiana University Press.

Modleski, T. (1998) 'A Rose Is a Rose? Real Women and a Lost War,' in J. Lewis (ed.), *New American Cinema,* Durham, NC, and London: Duke University Press, 125–45.

Nardini, G. (1991) 'Is it True Love? Or Not? Patterns of Ethnicity and Gender in Nancy Savoca,' *VIA: Voices in Italian Americana,* 2,1 (spring): 9–17.

Parks, L. (1999) 'Odd "Ada" Premieres Here,' *Houston Chronicle,* 21 May: 14.

Perren, A. (1998) 'Indie, Inc.: Miramax, Independent Film, and the New Hollywood,' MA thesis, University of Texas at Austin.

Phillips, J. (1992) 'Growing Up Black and Female: Leslie Harris's Just Another Girl on the IRT,' *Cineaste,* 19, 4 (fall): 86–7.

Pierson. J. (1995) *Spike, Mike, Slackers, & Dykes: A Guided Tour Across a Decade of American Independent Cinema,* New York: Hyperion.

Popper, F. (1993) *Art of the Electronic Age,* 2nd ed. Princeton, NJ: Prentice-Hall.

——(1997) *'Conceiving Ada,'* in A. Kroker and M. Kroker (eds.), *Digital Delirium,* New York: St. Martin's Press, 188–90.

Rich, B.R. (1999) 'High Concept: *Conceiving Ada* Reinvents the Period Film,' *San Francisco Bay Guardian,* 17 February, online: www.sfbg.com (accessed 9 October 2001).

——(2000) 'Queer and Present Danger,' *Sight and Sound,* 10, 3 (March): 22–5.

Rhines, J.A. (1996) *Black Film/White Money,* New Brunswick, NJ: Rutgers University Press.

Rohan, V. (2001) 'A League of its Own,' *Record,* 7 October: E1.

Rosenberg, J. (1983) *Women's Reflections: The Feminist Film Movement,* Ann Arbor: University of Michigan Research Press.

Sachs, L. (1999) 'High-Tech Style Aside, Film Is Ill-Conceived,' *Chicago Sun–Times,* 12 March: 34.

Scenario (1995) 'Viewing Sundance: A Talk with Robert Redford,' 1, 3 (Summer): 3–5, 206–8.

Scenario (1996) 'A Talk with Nicole Holofcener,' 2, 3 (fall): 129–33, 190–4.

Spencer, L. (2001) 'Walking and Talking,' in J. Hillier (ed.), *American Independent Cinema: A Sight and Sound Reader,* London: British Film Institute, 140–2.

Spines, C. (2000) 'Behind Bars,' *Premiere* (November): 45–8.

Steinhauer, J. (1997) 'A Director Who Films What She Knows Best,' *New York Times,* 28 December, section 2: 7.

Taubin, A. (2001) 'Girl in the Hood,' in J. Hillier (ed.), *American Independent Cinema: A Sight and Sound Reader,* London: British Film Institute, 36–9.

Taylor, E. (1997) 'Girl Wonders,' *Sundance Institute Writers Fellowship Program,* online: www.sundance.org (accessed 5 September 2001).

Unterburger, A. (ed.) (1999) *St. James Encyclopedia of Women Filmmakers: Women on the Other Side of the Camera,* Seattle, WA: Visible Ink Press.

Vachon, C. with Edelson, D. (1998) *Shooting to Kill: How an Independent Producer Blasts Through the Barriers to Make Films that Matter,* New York: Avon Books.

Weinraub, B. (2001) 'Assault as Autobiography,' *New York Times,* 7 August: E1.

Willis, H. (1995) 'Christine Vachon,' *Daily Variety,* 25 July, online: www.variety.com (accessed 9 October 2001).

——(2001) 'Breaking Out,' *Independent,* June, online: www.aivf.org/independent/archives (accessed 5 September 2001).

Wingfield, N. (1998) 'Let Us Entertain You,' *Wall Street Journal,* 16 November, online: www.wsj.com (accessed 9 October 2001).

Wyatt, J. (1994) *High Concept: Movies and Marketing in Hollywood,* Austin: University of Texas Press.

——(1996) 'Economic Constraints/Economic Opportunity: Robert Altman as Auteur,' *Velvet Light Trap,* 38 (fall): 51–67.

Young, J. (1995) 'Sundown,' *New Republic,* 10 April: 22.

Zimmermann, P.R. (2000) *States of Emergency,* Minneapolis: University of Minnesota Press, 2000.

Appendix

Bibliography

Christopher Anderson, "Introduction: Hollywood in the Home," in *Hollywood TV: The Studio System in the Fifties* (Austin: University of Texas Press, 1994), 1-21.

Tino Balio, "Columbia Pictures: The Making of a Motion Picture Major, 1930-1943," in *Post-Theory: Reconstructing Film Studies*, David Bordwell and Noël Carroll, ed. (Madison: University of Wisconsin Press, 1996), 419-433.

Daniel Bernardi, "*The Birth of a Nation*: Whiteness and the Birth of the Classical Style," in *Film Analysis: A Norton Reader* (New York: W.W. Norton, 2005), 82-96.

Albert R. Broccoli, "*Goldfinger*," in *When the Snow Melts: The Autobiography of Cubby Broccoli* (Philadelphia: Trans-Atlantic Publications, 1999), 180-194.

Charlie Chaplin, "Fourteen," in *My Autobiography* (New York: Penguin, 1992), 203-211. Originally published in 1964 by Simon and Schuster.

Ian Christie and David Thompson, ed., *Scorsese on Scorsese*, rev. ed. (London: Faber & Faber, 2004), 53-67.

"Contemporary Accounts (Paul Jerrico and Herbert Biberman, Rosaura Revueltas, Jules Schwerin, Juan Chacón), from *Salt of the Earth* (New York: The Feminist Press, 1978), 169-182. Originally published in *California Quarterly*, vol. 2, no. 4 (Summer 1953).

Donald Crafton, "Pie and Chase: Gag, Spectacle, and Narrative in Comedy," in *Classical Hollywood Comedy*, Kristine Brunovska Karnick and Henry Jenkins, ed. (New York: Routledge, 1995), 106-119.

James Damico, "Ingrid from Lorraine to Stromboli: Analyzing the Public's Perception of a Film Star," in *Star Texts: Image and Performance in Film and Television*, Jeremy G. Butler, ed. (Detroit: Wayne State University Press, 1991), 240-253. Originally published in *Journal of Popular Film* 4, no. 1 (1975): 3-19.

Richard Dyer, "Introduction" to *Heavenly Bodies: Film Stars and Society*, 2nd ed. (New York: Palgrave McMillan, 1987), 1-16.

Marlaine Glicksman, "Spike Lee's Bed-Stuy BBQ," in *Spike Lee: Interviews*, Cynthia Fuchs, ed. (Jackson: University of Mississippi Press, 2002), 13-24. Originally published in *Film Comment* 25 (July-August 1989) 12-16.

D. W. Griffith, "How I Made *The Birth of a Nation*" and "The Rise and Fall of Free Speech in America," in *Focus on D. W. Griffith*, Harry M. Geduld, ed. (Englewood Cliffs, NJ: Prentice-Hall, 1971), 39-45. Originally published in Henry Stephen Gordon, "The Story of David Wark Griffith," *Photoplay* X (October 1916), 90-94 and *The Rise and Fall of Free Speech in America* (1916), pamphlet.

D. W. Griffith, "Reply to the *New York Globe*," in *The Birth of a Nation*, Robert Lang, ed. (New Brunswick, NJ: Rutgers University Press, 1994), 168-170.

Tom Gunning, "The Cinema of Attractions: Early Film, Its Spectator and the Avant-Garde" in *Early Cinema: Space, Frame, Narrative*, Thomas Elsaesser and Adam Barker, ed. (London: BFI, 1990). Originally published in *Wide Angle* 8, nos. 3-4 (1986): 66-77.

Tom Gunning, "Response to 'Pie and Chase,'" in *Classical Hollywood Comedy*, Kristine Brunovska Karnick and Henry Jenkins, ed. (New York: Routledge, 1995), 120-122.

Alfred Hitchcock, "Are Stars Necessary?" and "The Enjoyment of Fear," from *Hitchcock on Hitchcock: Selected Writings and Interviews*, Sidney Gotlieb, ed. (Berkeley: University of California Press, 1995), 76-78, 116-121. "Are Stars Necessary?" originally published in *Picturegoer*, December 16, 1933. "The Enjoyment of Fear" originally published in *Good Housekeeping* 128 (February 1949): 39, 241-243.

Lea Jacobs, "The Fallen Woman Film and the Impetus for Censorship," in *The Wages of Sin: Censorship and the Fallen Woman Film* (Madison: University of Wisconsin Press, 1991), 3-26, 163-169.

Philip Jenkinson, "John Ford Talks to Philip Jenkinson about Not Being Interested in Movies," from John Ford: Interviews, Gerald Peary, ed. (Jackson: University of Mississippi Press, 2001), 137-140. Originally published in *The Listener*, December 2, 1970.

Noel King, "'The Last Good Time We Ever Had': Remembering the New Hollywood Cinema," in *The Last Great American Picture Show: New Hollywood Cinema in the 1970s*, Thomas Elsaesser, Alexander Horwath, and Noel King, ed. (Amsterdam: Amsterdam University Press, 2004), 19-36.

Jim Kitses, "Authorship and Genre: Notes on the Western," in *The Western Reader*, Jim Kitses and Gregg Rickman, ed. (New York: Limelight, 1998), 57-68. Excerpted from *Horizons West* (Bloomington: Indiana University Press, 1969).

Christina Lane, "Just Another Girl Outside the Neo-Indie," in *Contemporary American Independent Film: From the Margins to the Mainstream*, Chris Holmlund and Justin Wyatt, ed. (London; Routledge, 2005), 193-210.

Brian Neve, "HUAC, the Blacklist, and the Decline of Social Cinema," in *The Fifties: Transforming the Screen, 1950-59*, Peter Lev, ed. (Berkeley: University of California Press, 2003), 65-86.

John E. O'Connor, "The White Man's Indian," from *Hollywood's Indian: The Portrayal of the Native American in Film* (Lexington: University of Kentucky Press, 1998), 27-38. Originally published in O'Connor's book, *The Hollywood Indian: Stereotypes of Native American in Film* (Trenton: New Jersey State Museum, 1980).

Alisa Perren, "sex, lies and marketing: Miramax and the Development of the Quality Indie Blockbuster," in *Film Quarterly* 55, no. 2 (2001): 30-39.

Jesse Algeron Rhines, "Blockbusters and Independents: 1975 to the Present," in *Black Film/White Money* (New Brunswick, NJ: Rutgers University Press, 1996), 51-78, 180-182.

Raymond Rohauer, "Interview with Marion Mack," in *Buster Keaton's The General,* Richard J. Anobile, ed. (New York: Universe Books, 1975), 11-17.

Georges Sadoul, "Founding Father: Louis Lumière in Conversation with Georges Sadoul," in *Projections 4: Film-makers on Film-making*, ed. John Boorman, Tom Luddy, David Thomson, and Walter Donahue (London: Faber & Faber, 1995), 2-13.

Mark Salisbury, ed., "*Batman,*" in *Burton on Burton*, rev. ed. (London: Faber and Faber, 2006), 70-83.

Kevin S. Sandler, "CARA and the Emergence of Responsible Entertainment," from *The Naked Truth: Why Hollywood Doesn't Make X-Rated Movies* (New Brunswick, NJ: Rutgers University Press, 2007), 42-63.

Thomas Schatz, "The New Hollywood," in *Film Theory Goes to the Movies*, Jim Collins, Hilary Radner, and Ava Preacher Collins, ed. (London: Routledge, 1993), 8-36.

Janet Staiger, "*The Birth of a Nation*: Reconsidering Its Reception," from *Interpreting Films: Studies in the Historical Reception of Cinema* (Princeton: Princeton University Press, 1992), 139-153.

Justin Wyatt, "From Roadshowing to Saturation Release: Majors, Independents, and Marketing/Distribution Innovations," in *The New American Cinema*, Jon Lewis, ed. (Durham, NC: Duke University Press, 1999), 64-86.

Jeff Young, "*A Face in the Crowd,*" in *Kazan: The Master Director Discusses His Films: Interviews with Elia Kazan* (New York: Newmarket Press, 1999), 231-254.

Supplemental Sources

Robert C. Allen and Douglas Gomery, Film *History: Theory and Practice* (New York: McGraw-Hill, 1993).

Tino T. Balio, ed., *The American Film Industry*, rev. ed (Madison: University of Wisconsin Press, 1985).

John Belton, *American Cinema/American Culture*, 2nd ed. (New York: McGraw-Hill, 2004).

David Bordwell and Kristin Thompson, *Film History: An Introduction* (New York: McGraw-Hill, 2002).

Drew Casper, *Postwar Hollywood, 1946-1962* (Malden, MA: Wiley-Blackwell, 2007).

David A. Cook, *A History of Narrative Film*, 4th ed. (New York: W.W. Norton, 2004).

Wheeler Winston Dixon and Gwendolyn Audrey Foster, *A Short History of Film* (New Brunswick, NJ: Rutgers University Press, 2008).

Louis Giannetti and Scott Eyman, *Flashback: A Brief History of Film*, 5th ed. (Upper Saddle River, NJ: Prentice-Hall, 2006).

Douglas Gomery, *The Hollywood Studio System: A History* (London: British Film Institute, 2008).

Paul Grainge, Mark Jancovich, and Sharon Montieth, ed., *Film Histories: An Introduction and Reader* (Toronto: University of Toronto Press, 2007).

Richard Jewell, *The Golden Age of Cinema, 1929-1945* (Malden, MA: Wiley-Blackwell, 2007).

Leonard J. Leff and Jerold L. Simmons, *The Dame in the Kimono: Hollywood, Censorship, and the Production Code* (Lexington: University of Kentucky Press, 2001).

Jon Lewis, *American Film: A History* (New York: W.W. Norton, 2007).

Sidney Lumet, *Making Movies* (New York: Vintage, 1996).

Geoffrey Nowell-Smith, *The Oxford History of World Cinema* (Oxford: Oxford University Press, 1997)

A Personal Journey with Martin Scorsese through American Movies (Martin Scorsese, 1995).

Andrew Sarris, *You Ain't Heard Nothin' Yet: The American Talking Film: History and Memory, 1927-1949* (Oxford: Oxford University Press, 1998).

Thomas Schatz, *The Genius of the System: Hollywood Filmmaking in the Studio Era* (New York: Holt, 1996).

Thomas Schatz, *Hollywood Genres: Formulas, Filmmaking, and the Studio System:* (New York: McGraw-Hill, 1981).

John Sedgwick, *An Economic History of Film* (New York: Routledge, 2005).

Robert Sklar, *Movie-Made America: A Cultural History of American Movies* (New York: Vintage, 2004).

Janet Wasko, *How Hollywood Works* (Thousand Oaks, CA: Sage, 2003).

Virginia Wright Wexman, *A History of Film*, 6th ed. (New York: Allyn and Bacon, 2005).

Linda Ruth Williams and Michael Hammond, *Contemporary American Cinema* (London: Open University Press, 2006).

FMS 200: Hollywood Film History
Code of Academic Integrity

You are expected to turn in original work for this course. Quotations or ideas paraphrased from other work must be properly cited. Taking credit for another's ideas or writing is plagiarism, which is a serious violation of the University's Code of Academic Integrity (http://www.asu.edu/studentaffairs/studentlife/srr/index.htm).

In the "Student Academic Integrity Manual," ASU defines "plagiarism [as] using another's words, ideas, materials, or work without properly acknowledging and documenting the source. Students are responsible for knowing the rules governing the use of another's work or materials and for acknowledging and documenting the source appropriately."

Academic dishonesty, including inappropriate collaboration, will not be tolerated. There are severe sanctions for cheating, plagiarizing, and any other form of dishonesty.

Your signature indicates your understanding of ASU's Code of Academic Integrity and definition regarding plagiarism.

_____   _____
Name   Date